GYNECOLOGIC CANCER

CONTEMPORARY ISSUES IN CLINICAL ONCOLOGY VOLUME 2

SERIES EDITOR

Peter H. Wiernik, M.D.

Gutman Professor and Chairman
Department of Oncology
Montefiore Medical Center
Chief, Division of Medical Oncology
Albert Einstein College of Medicine
Bronx, New York

Already Published

Vol. 1 Breast Cancer
Richard G. Margolese, M.D., F.R.C.P.(C), Guest Editor

Forthcoming Volumes in the Series

Vol. 3 Lung Cancer
Joseph Aisner, M.D., Guest Editor
Vol. 4 Leukemias and Lymphomas
Peter H. Wiernik, M.D., Guest Editor

GYNECOLOGIC CANCER

Edited by

Arlene A. Forastiere, M.D.

Assistant Professor
Department of Internal Medicine
Division of Hematology-Oncology
University of Michigan Medical Center
Chief, Oncology Section
Ann Arbor Veterans Administration Medical Center
Ann Arbor, Michigan

CHURCHILL LIVINGSTONE   **1984**
NEW YORK, EDINBURGH, LONDON, AND MELBOURNE

Acquisitions editor: *William Schmitt*
Copy editor: *Michael Kelley*
Production editor: *Michiko Davis*
Production supervisor: *Joe Sita*
Compositor: *The Maple-Vail Book Manufacturing Group*
Printer/Binder: *The Murray Printing Co.*

Distributed in the United Kingdom by Churchill Livingstone,
Robert Stevenson House, 1–3 Baxter's Place, Leith Walk,
Edinburgh EH1 3AF and associated companies, branches
and representatives throughout the world.

First published in 1984
Printed in U.S.A.

ISBN 0–443–08274–x
9 8 7 6 5 4 3 2 1

Library of Congress Cataloging in Publication Data
Main entry under title:

Gynecologic cancer.

 (Contemporary issues in clinical oncology ; v. 2)
 Includes bibliographies and index.
 1. Generative organs, Female—Cancer. I. Forastiere,
Arlene A. II. Series: Contemporary issues in clinical
oncology ; v. 2 [DNLM: 1. Genital Neoplasms, Female.
W1 C0769MQHD v. 2 / WP 145 G9964]
RC280.G5G87 1984   616.99'465   84-9463
ISBN 0-443-08274-X

Manufactured in the United States of America

Contributors

Hugh R.K. Barber, M.D.
Department of Obstetrics and Gynecology
Lenox Hill Hospital
Professor and Chairman
Department of Obstetrics and Gynecology
New York Medical College
Associate Dean for Cancer Programs
New York Medical College
Valhalla, New York

Kwang N. Choi, M.D.
Assistant Professor
Department of Radiation Oncology
State University of New York
Downstate Medical Center
New York, New York

Daniel L. Clarke-Pearson, M.D.
Associate Professor
Department of Obstetrics and Gynecology
Duke University Medical Center
Durham, North Carolina

William T. Creasman, M.D.
James M. Ingram Professor and Director of Gynecologic Oncology
Duke University Medical Center
Durham, North Carolina

Arlene A. Forastiere, M.D.
Chief
Oncology Section
Ann Arbor Veterans Administration Medical Center
Assistant Professor
Department of Internal Medicine
Division of Hematology-Oncology
University of Michigan Medical Center
Ann Arbor, Michigan

Henry Gerad, M.D.
Assistant Professor of Oncology
University of Maryland Cancer Center
Baltimore, Maryland

Thomas B. Hakes, M.D.
Assistant Attending Physician
Memorial Hospital
Assistant Professor of Medicine
Cornell University
School of Medicine
New York, New York

Walter Burnett Jones, M.D.
Associate Attending Surgeon
Gynecology Service
Memorial Sloan Kettering Cancer Center
New York, New York

Errol Lewis, M.D.
Assistant Professor of Radiology
Department of Diagnostic Radiology
The University of Texas System Cancer Center
M.D. Anderson Hospital
Houston, Texas

George W. Morley, M.D.
Chief
Department of Obstetrics and Gynecology
University of Michigan Medical Center
Professor of Obstetrics and Gynecology
Director, Division of Gynecologic Oncology
Ann Arbor, Michigan

Charles E. Myers, M.D.
Chief
Clinical Pharmacology Branch
Division of Cancer Treatment
National Cancer Institute
Bethesda, Maryland

Robert F. Ozols, M.D., Ph.D.
Senior Investigator
Medicine Branch
Division of Cancer Treatment
National Cancer Institute
Bethesda, Maryland

James A. Roberts, M.D.
Assistant Professor of Obstetrics and Gynecology
Associate Director
Department of Obstetrics and Gynecology
Division of Gynecologic Oncology
University of Michigan Medical Center
Ann Arbor, Michigan

Marvin Rotman, M.D.
Professor and Chairman
Department of Radiation Oncology
State University of New York
Downstate Medical Center
New York, New York

Gary A. Schnur, M.D.
Department of Internal Medicine
Division of Hematology-Oncology
University of Michigan Medical Center
Ann Arbor, Michigan

James Tate Thigpen, M.D.
Associate Professor of Medicine
Department of Medicine
Assistant Professor of Obstetrics and Gynecology
Department of Obstetrics and Gynecology
The University of Mississippi
School of Medicine
Jackson, Mississippi

David B. Thomas, M.D., Dr.P.H.
Head
Program in Epidemiology
Fred Hutchinson Cancer Research Center
Professor of Epidemiology
University of Washington
Seattle, Washington

Sidney Wallace, M.D.
Professor of Radiology
Department of Diagnostic Radiology
The University of Texas System Cancer Center
M.D. Anderson Hospital
Houston, Texas

Noel S. Weiss, M.D., Ph.D.
Department of Epidemiology
University of Washington
Program in Public Health Sciences
Fred Hutchinson Cancer Research Center
Seattle, Washington

Robert C. Young, M.D.
Chief
Medicine Branch
Division of Cancer Treatment
National Cancer Institute
Bethesda, Maryland

Jesus Zornoza, M.D.
Radiologist
Department of Diagnostic Radiology
Danbury Hospital
Danbury, Connecticut

Preface

Invasive gynecologic malignancies represent approximately 18 percent of newly diagnosed malignancies in women in the United States each year. These cancers rank second in incidence only to breast cancer. As a cause of cancer mortality in women, cancer of the ovary and cancers of the uterus (corpus and cervix) rank fourth and fifth, respectively. This represents a 57 percent decrease in the death rate from uterine cancers over the past 30 years while the death rate from ovarian cancer has remained essentially unchanged. The mortality rate has been reduced for those sites of gynecologic malignancies for which we have an effective means of early diagnosis (such as the Papanicolaou cytologic screening test for cancer of the uterine cervix) and for those in which a sensitive tumor marker and effective chemotherapy have been identified, such as gestational trophoblastic disease and ovarian germ cell malignancies. However, for other sites, such as epithelial ovarian cancer, in which the majority of patients are diagnosed at an advanced stage, an understanding of the role of each therapeutic modality and the exploration of investigational approaches are critical to improving survival.

Achievements in the specialty of gynecologic oncology today are a reflection of advances in multiple areas: epidemiology, diagnostic techniques, radiation therapeutics, surgical expertise, chemotherapeutics, and investigative approaches. The purpose in writing this book was *not* to compile a reference of standard treatment practices but to provide a comprehensive discussion of current knowledge in each of these areas by experts in the field.

Each contributor has attempted to present a readable and easily comprehensible discussion of the indications for and limitations of conventional diagnostic and therapeutic strategies, areas of controversy, and new directions in clinical management. The subjects selected were those felt to be most important to the practicing community physician, residents in training, and other health care professionals who are involved with the care of the patient with a gynecologic malignancy. Major epidemiologic issues, the role of each diagnostic and therapeutic modality, and investigative approaches are discussed with recommendations for clinical management summarized and amply referenced. A risk for the development of a second malignancy following "curative" therapy has been recognized, and a chapter is devoted to a comprehensive discussion of this important area.

I would like to acknowledge the effort of all the contributors to make this book a comprehensive and up-to-date reference. We all hope that this endeavor will have a beneficial impact on the survival and care of the patient with gynecologic cancer.

Arlene A. Forastiere

Contents

1. Radiologic Techniques in the Diagnosis and Therapeutic
   Management of Gynecologic Malignancies 1
   Jesus Zornoza, Errol Lewis, and Sidney Wallace
2. Epidemiology of Cervical Cancer: The Herpes
   Virus Question 33
   David B. Thomas
3. The Staging and Surgical Therapy of Cervical Carcinoma 47
   James A. Roberts and George W. Morley
4. Radiation Therapy in the Management of Invasive
   Cervical Carcinoma 67
   Kwang N. Choi and Marvin Rotman
5. Cervical Cancer: Role of Chemotherapy........................... 93
   Arlene A. Forastiere and Gary A. Schnur
6. Ovarian Cancer: Diagnosis and Surgical Management 119
   Hugh R. K. Barber
7. Ovarian Cancer: Postoperative Management 139
   William T. Creasman and Daniel L. Clarke-Pearson
8. Chemotherapy of Advanced Ovarian Carcinoma 155
   Thomas B. Hakes
9. New Investigational Techniques in Ovarian Cancer................... 177
   Robert F. Ozols, Charles E. Myers, and Robert C. Young
10. Epidemiology of Endometrial Cancer: A Review of
    Hormonal and Non-Hormonal Risk Factors 199
    Noel S. Weiss
11. Approaches to the Evaluation and Management of
    Endometrial Carcinoma 215
    James Tate Thigpen
12. Gestational Trophoblastic Disease: Prognostic Factors
    and Management 249
    Walter Burnett Jones
13. Second Malignancies After Alkylating Agent Therapy or
    Radiation Therapy 275
    Henry Gerad
Index.. 301

1 | Radiologic Techniques in the Diagnosis and Therapeutic Management of Gynecologic Malignancies

Jesus Zornoza
Errol Lewis
Sidney Wallace

In the U.S., gynecologic malignancies comprise 28 percent of all cancers in women (endometrium 13 percent, ovary 6 percent, uterine cancer 6 percent, and others 3 percent). The radiologic armamentarium available to define the site, nature, and extent of these gynecologic neoplasms includes conventional radiography, intravenous urography, gastrointestinal barium studies, radionuclide scintigraphy, ultrasonography, computed tomography (CT), lymphangiography, angiography, and percutaneous biopsy. Pelvic pneumography and hysterosalpingography are rarely used today and only to define specific problems. The roles of digital subtraction angiography (DSA) and nuclear magnetic resonance (NMR) are yet to be determined.

Because of the relatively late stage in which these patients often present, the diagnostic effort is directed primarily to establish the extent of the disease. More recently, the radiologist has become increasingly involved in the management of patients with gynecologic malignances by transcatheter intraarterial infusion and occlu-

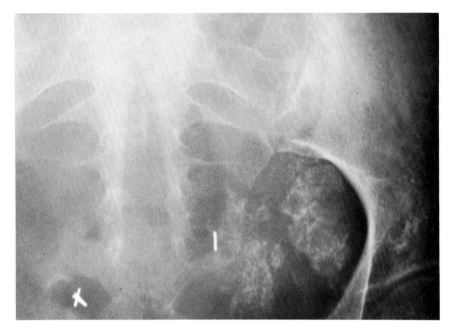

Fig. 1-1. Radiograph of the pelvis demonstrates psammomatous calcification within a cystadenocarcinoma of the ovary.

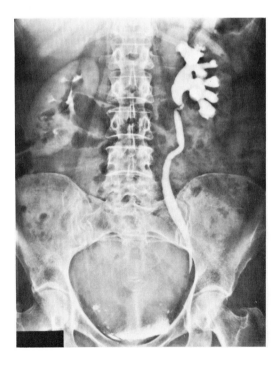

Fig. 1-2. Soft tissue mass in the pelvis causing left sided hydronephrosis and lateral displacement of the left ureter. Pelvic mass was related to a sarcoma of the uterus.

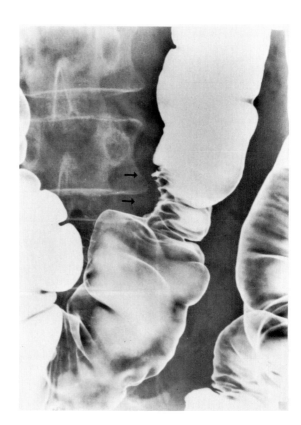

Fig. 1-3. Submucosal and serosal metastasis from ovarian carcinoma. Double contrast barium enema demonstrates areas of spiculation and tethering. (arrows)

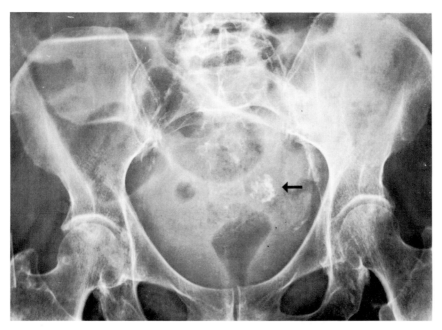

Fig. 1-4. Plain radiograph of the pelvis demonstrates coarse calcification (arrow) within uterine fibroid.

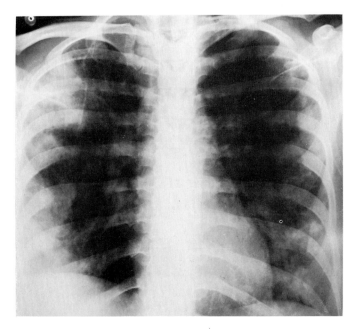

Fig. 1-5. Radiograph of the chest shows bilateral parenchymal masses simulating an inflammatory process; however, these were due to hemorrhagic metastasis from choriocarcinoma. (Courtesy of Herman I. Libshitz)

sion, percutaneous aspiration and injection of cystic or necrotic neoplasms, and nephrostomy.

The diagnostic sequence utilized is individualized depending upon the clinical presentation and is intended to minimize superfluous studies that result in financial burden, inconvenience, radiation exposure, morbidity, and mortality. To warrant the risks and cost, the information so gathered should influence management. The availability of the equipment and personnel and the expertise in performance and interpretation of the various procedures must also be considered.

CONVENTIONAL RADIOGRAPHY

Ovary

Plain radiography of the abdomen may reveal a soft tissue mass within the pelvis that displaces gas-filled loops of bowel. The presence of calcification, dental structures, or fat within the mass may indicate a benign dermoid. Approximately 12 percent of patients with serous cystadenoma or cystadenocarcinoma develop psammomatous calcification in the primary tumor or the metastases (Fig. 1-1). The malignant nature of this tumor may be suggested by the presence of distorted bowel, ascites, or, rarely, skeletal metastases.[1]

Chest radiography is useful for detecting pulmonary metastases and pleural effusions and for monitoring their response to chemotherapy. Routine chest tomography is not recommended because lung metastasis represents advanced disease usually preceded by other findings such as peritoneal carcinomatosis and ascites.

Intravenous urography is frequently performed to detect the presence of a pelvic mass distorting the bladder or obstructing the ureters (Fig. 1-2). Barium enema has been used routinely to define extension from the pelvic neoplasms or its metastases. Displacement of the hollow viscera and fixation and tethering are indicative of metastasis (Fig. 1-3). Meyers described the spread of abdominal malignancy as related to the dynamics and distribution of ascites.[2] Four sites of ovarian metastases are common: the pouch of Douglas, the right lower quadrant, the sigmoid colon, and the right paracolic gutter. In Meyers' series of 35 cases with ascites and abdominal carcinomatosis, 15 were of ovarian origin.[2-5] Following therapy, barium studies can also indicate the degree and extent of radiation effect on the bowel.

Metastases to the ovaries most frequently originate from neoplasms of the gastrointestinal tract, breast, lung, and reticuloendothelial system. Metastases are usually bilateral. Krukenberg tumor, originally described as bilateral solid ovarian tumors metastatic from a gastric carcinoma, now encompasses all ovarian metastases arising from carcinoma of the gastrointestinal tract.[1,6,7]

Uterine Corpus

In mesodermal tumors, conventional radiography of the abdomen and pelvis will demonstrate a nonspecific mass indenting the adjacent colon and bladder. When large, the tumor may obstruct the urinary tract. The presence of calcifications, which may be irregular, coarse, and scattered or in aggregates, indicate a uterine fibroid (Fig. 1-4). Rapid growth and invasion of pelvic viscera suggest malignant degeneration.

Aside from a usually obvious uterine mass, trophoblastic tumors may be associated with an adnexal mass in the pelvis due to theca lutein cyst. Direct injection of water-based iodinated contrast material through the wall into the uterine cavity will outline the vesicles of the hydatidiform mole.

Pulmonary metastases from choriocarcinoma are usually rounded nodular densities, but, on occasion, are less well-defined, without sharp margins, and simulate an inflammatory process, i.e., an alveolar pattern (Fig. 1-5). This appearance is caused by metastases with a surrounding halo of hemorrhage. Rarely, it may result from embolic occlusion of pulmonary arteries, without evidence of masses in the lung. Persistent nodules in the lungs of a patient with a normal HCG titer, with choriocarcinoma after adequate treatment, may represent necrosis or fibrosis without viable tumor.[8]

Uterine Cervix

Pulmonary and skeletal metastases seldom appear until the local disease is advanced. Excretory urography demonstrates deviation of the ureters or hydronephrosis in 20 percent. Barium studies occasionally detect invasion of the bowel.

Complications of therapy include a small, elevated bladder with thickened wall,

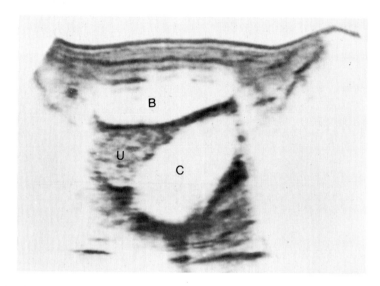

Fig. 1-6. Ovarian cyst. Transverse sonogram of the pelvis demonstrates a cystic mass (C) to the left of the uterus (U) B = bladder.

a narrow rigid rectum, and increased pelvic fat with a widened presacral space.[9] Rectovaginal and vesicovaginal fistulas occur in 1.2 percent of patients, more frequently when hysterectomy is combined with radiation therapy.[10] Development of ureteral obstruction after treatment is almost invariably due to recurrent tumor (9 percent) rather than radiation fibrosis (5 percent) and is frequently associated with lower extremity edema secondary to compression of an iliac vein. Radionecrosis of the bony pelvis and aseptic necrosis of the femoral heads may complicate therapy.[11]

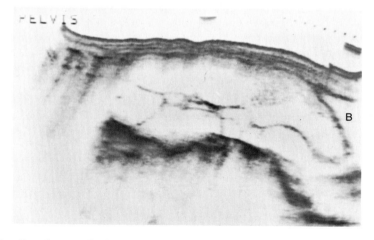

Fig. 1-7. Cystadenoma. Sagittal sonogram through the pelvis demonstrates a large predominantly cystic mass with thin septation arising from the pelvis. B = bladder

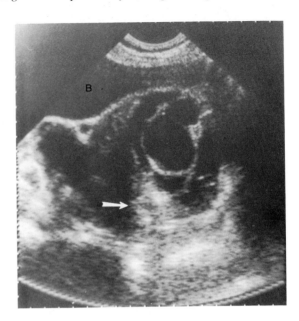

Fig. 1-8. Cystadenocarcinoma. Transverse sonogram through the pelvis demonstrates a multiseptated mass with solid nodules (arrow). B = bladder

ULTRASONOGRAPHY

Ovary

Ultrasound is the most revealing method for the detection of ovarian masses, although it is the most technically dependent. Bladder distention is a prerequisite for a good examination, because it displaces loops of intestine out of the pelvis. Fluid-filled loops of bowel create pseudolesions difficult to distinguish from pelvic masses. Both static and real-time examinations are frequently necessary to demonstrate the change in configuration from peristalsis. A water enema may help to distinguish the colon from a mass. A technically adequate study may disclose a cystic mass smaller than 2 cm in diamter because of its echo-free nature and sharply defined margins; however, a solid mass less than 2 to 3 cm may escape recognition.

The accuracy of ultrasound in the detection of a pelvic mass and in determining its size, location, and consistency is as high as 91 percent.[12] However, the appearance is nonspecific, except for a few conditions with specific features that suggest the histologic diagnosis. These include simple ovarian cyst (Fig. 1-6), cystadenoma with fine septation (Fig. 1-7), and cystadenocarcinoma with solid nodules (Fig. 1-8).[12–17] Ovarian teratomas exhibit attenuation of the sound beam with distal shadowing, the "tip of the iceberg sign" (Fig. 1-9), a fluid level, and solid mural components.[12,13]

Ultrasonic findings that suggest malignancy include: a multiloculated cystic mass over 5 cm in diamter; thick septation, especially with coexistent solid nodules; a complex mass inseparable from the uterus; ascites; "omental cake" (mesenteric metastases) (Fig. 1-10); paraaortic lymph node enlargement; and hepatic metastases. In two re-

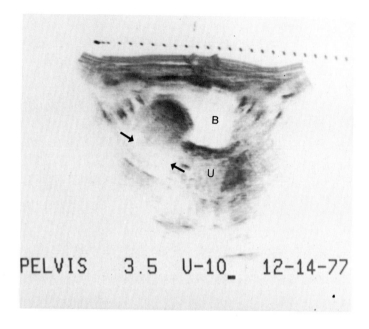

Fig. 1-9. Ovarian teratoma. Transverse sonogram through the pelvis shows an echogenic mass with distal shadowing. (arrows) B = bladder U = uterus

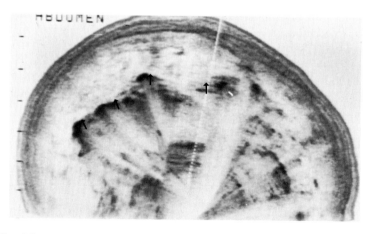

Fig. 1-10. ''Omental cake'' Transverse sonogram through the midabdomen reveals a solid mass (arrows) posterior to the anterior abdominal wall.

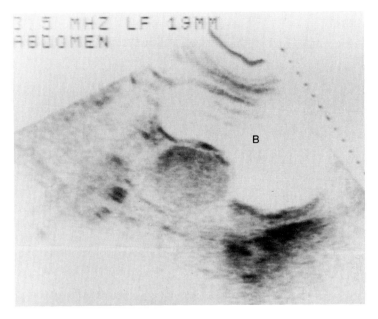

Fig. 1-11.   Uterine fibroid. Longitudinal sonogram through the pelvis demonstrates an echogenic mass in the body of the uterus indenting the bladder (B).

cent studies of ovarian carcinoma,[16,17] ultrasonography disclosed ascites in 37 to 41 percent, extrapelvic disease in 40 percent, and hydronephrosis in 14 percent. Omental or peritoneal involvement was discovered in 20 percent with a high false negative rate probably related to the presence of small implants that are impossible to differentiate from omental fat and bowel gas. Ascites also hinders the recognition of omental and mesenteric metastases.

Sonography may predict uterine involvement by showing that the mass is inseparable from the uterus, but it is insensitive in defining bladder or bowel invasion.[18] Once a suspected malignant mass is detected, full abdominal sonography should be performed to determine the presence of ascites, hydronephrosis, retroperitoneal disease, and liver metastases. Because of the absence of ionizing radiation, sonography is useful in defining an ovarian mass in the pregnant patient.

Uterine Corpus

The diagnostic accuracy of identifying leiomyoma by ultrasonography is 90 percent.[12] Sonographic features include nodular enlargement of the uterus and sonolucent to echogenic masses (Fig. 1-11), which in the presence of calcifications exhibit acoustical shadowing. Fibroids become more sonolucent during pregnancy. A pedunculated fibroid may be confused with an adnexal mass. The echo-free fundus of the retroverted uterus may simulate a fibroid.[7,13,15,19]

The distinction by ultrasonography between benign and malignant disease in an

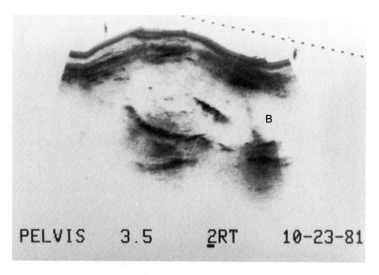

Fig. 1-12. Endometrial carcinoma. Longitudinal sonogram through the pelvis shows an enlarged uterus with mixed echogenicity due to tumor and debris. B = bladder

enlarged uterus is not particularly accurate. In 21 patients with adenocarcinoma of the uterus, Requard et al.[20] demonstrated a normal or bulbous uterus with a normal echo pattern in 94 percent of patients in Stages I and II; 80 percent of Stage III or IV cases had a lobular uterus with mixed echo pattern. Features suggestive of malignant tumor are absent of the normal central echoes of the endometrial cavity and sonolucency with irregular echoes in the endometrial cavity (Fig. 1-12), probably due to hematometra or pyometra. Causes of hematometra are cervical or endometrial ex-

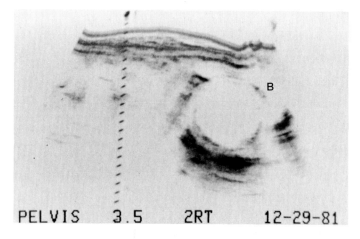

Fig. 1-13. Hematometra. Longitudinal sonogram reveals sonolucency within a distended endometrial cavity. B = bladder

tension of the carcinoma, radiation fibrosis, or postsurgical scarring (Fig. 1-13).

Ultrasonography is the method of choice in establishing the presence and recurrence of a hydatidiform mole.[21] A homogenous vesicular intrauterine mass is the most common finding (Fig. 1-14).[22] Invasive trophoblastic disease is recognized by clusters of high amplitude echoes within the myometrium. Theca lutein cysts of the ovary can be identified in 44 percent of patients with persistent trophoblastic disease. Sonography is the most effective approach for detecting these cysts (Fig. 1-14).[23]

Uterine Cervix

In the early stages of carcinoma of the uterine cervix, ultrasound offers little, except in patients in whom clinical examination is difficult and in those with a large exophytic or fungating mass (Fig. 1-15). A mass involving the cervix and parametrium with enlargement of the pelvic lymph nodes, Stages III or IV carcinoma, can be demonstrated by ultrasound. Involvement of the pelvic wall, bladder, and rectum may be difficult to define by ultrasonography. The kidneys should be examined routinely for hydronephrosis, which indicates Stage III disease.[7,20]

COMPUTED TOMOGRAPHY

Ovary

With the ability of CT to demonstrate subtle differences in density, the nature of the primary neoplasm can often be defined by detecting fat (dermoid), calcifications (psammomatous or dental), a cystic or solid mass, or septations (Fig. 1-16).[24] Local and extrapelvic extension of disease is recognized by the invasion of the adjacent viscera or the pelvis or by retroperitoneal lymph nodes. Involved paraaortic nodes are more readily identified than pelvic nodes because of the surrounding retroperitoneal fat. Large matted, nodular masses are almost invariably due to nodal metastasis (Fig. 1-17). Enlargement of isolated nodes (1.5 cm or greater in diameter) must be verified by biopsy or lymphangiography. Metastatic peritoneal and omental nodules (Fig. 1-18) greater than 2.0 cm, as well as ascites, can be demonstrated by CT.[25,26] With the use of intraperitoneal water-soluble contrast material, smaller peritoneal metastases may be detected.[27] In addition to staging by determining the extent of disease, CT is effective in defining radiation therapy fields,[28] monitoring response to treatment, and detecting recurrent tumor (with an accuracy of 87.5 percent).[24]

The differential diagnostic considerations include nonneoplastic mass, such as functional ovarian cyst (Fig. 1-19), ovarian hyperstimulation syndrome,[29] endometriosis, and pelvic inflammatory disease, as well as nongynecologic masses such as metastasis, lymphoma, presacral tumor, fluid-filled loops of bowel fixed by adhesions, lymphocele, hematoma, and pelvic kidney.

Liver metastasis from ovarian neoplasm is relatively uncommon (10 percent). Of the imaging techniques, CT is the best single examination for determining the presence and extent of an hepatic mass.[30] A practical and accurate screening plan consists of scintigraphy, followed only as clinically indicated by CT. Angiography is the last resort to solve a clinical problem or in preparation for transcatheter management.

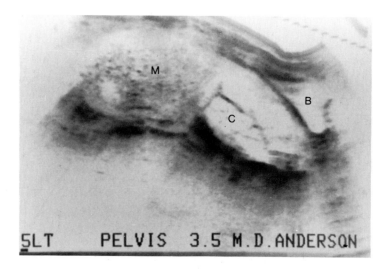

Fig. 1-14. Hydatidiform mole. Longitudinal sonogram demonstrates a solid mass (M) with sonolucent areas in the uterus. A multiseptated cyst (C) consistent with a theca lutein cyst is present. B = bladder

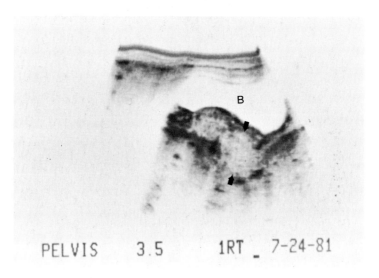

Fig. 1-15. Cervical carcinoma. Longitudinal scan through the pelvis demonstrates a mass (arrows) in the cervix. B = bladder

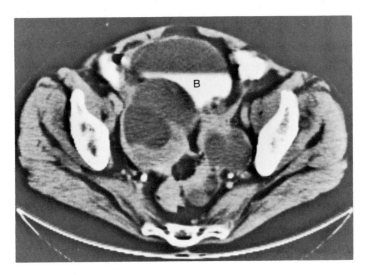

Fig. 1-16.   Bilateral ovarian cystadenocarcinoma. CT of the pelvis demonstrates bilateral partially cystic masses with intramural nodules. B = bladder

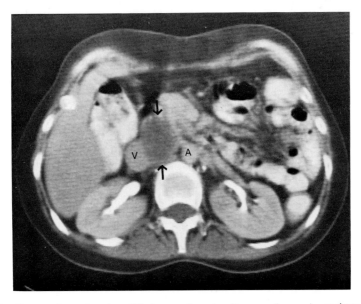

Fig. 1-17.   Retroperitoneal nodes. CT shows a low density mass (arrows) consistent with adenopathy between the aorta (A) and inferior vena cava (V).

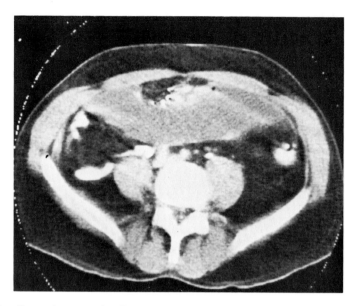

Fig. 1-18. Omental metastasis. CT demonstrates a solid mass posterior to the anterior abdominal wall.

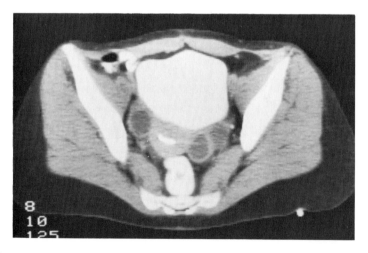

Fig. 1-19. Bilateral ovarian cyst. CT of the pelvis with bilateral cystic masses lateral to the uterus. Incidentally noted is an IUD within the endometrial cavity.

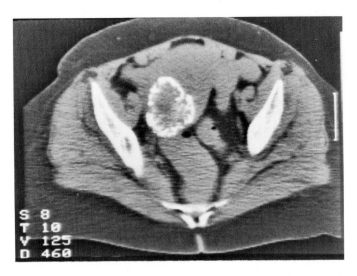

Fig. 1-20.   Uterine fibroid. CT reveals irregular coarse calcification within an enlarged uterus.

Uterine Corpus

CT findings in leiomyoma were described by Tada et al.[31] and include a lobulated enlarged uterus, a soft tissue mass distorting or obliterating the uterine cavity, and calcifications or an area of decreased attenuation within the mass (Fig. 1-20). In their study, the sensitivity of CT was 76 percent in 83 cases. Most false positive diagnoses were the result of adenomyosis of the uterus. Malignant change is difficult or impossible to detect unless there is invasion of adjacent structures with a loss of the fat planes.

Because the majority of patients with endometrial carcinoma present with the tumor confined to the uterus, the value of CT is minimal in Stages I and II. With contrast enhancement, Hamlin et al.[32] detected hypodense carcinomas confined to the uterus. CT is helpful in determining local pelvic and extrapelvic extension. Staging and the setting of planning radiation therapy portals are thus assisted by CT. The diagnostic considerations for enlarged uterus are pregnancy, benign and malignant neoplasm, fluid-filled uterus (pyo-, hemato-, or hydrometra), and congenital bicornuate uterus.

In patients with choriocarcinoma, CT could identify an enlarged uterus and theca lutein cysts. CT is the best screening technique for the detection of liver metastases, which occur in 10 percent of cases of choriocarcinoma.[33] In general, gynecologic malignant neoplasms seldom spread to the liver.

Brain metastases, which occur in 10 percent of choriocarcinoma, are clearly defined by cranial CT. Because of the associated hemorrhage, these metastases are frequently seen on the precontrast scans as areas of increased attenuation that usually enhance with the infusion of contrast material (Fig. 1-21). Subarachnoid hemorrhage and occlusion of vessels may also occur in metastatic choriocarcinoma.

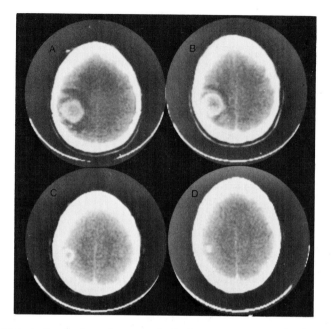

Fig. 1-21. Metastastic choriocarcinoma to the brain. A. Increased attenuation of the metastasis. B. Enhancement after the infusion of contrast material. C&D. Improvement in the metastases following methotrexate chemotherapy.

Uterine Cervix

The main role of CT in cervical carcinoma is to determine the extent of disease, i.e., tumor size, endometrial invasion, parametrial and pelvic side wall extension, and pelvic lymphadenopathy. Extrapelvic metastases to the liver, skeleton, and paraaortic lymph nodes, as well as hydronephrosis, are readily detected.

Primary neoplasms of the cervix are frequently the same density as water and are best seen at the level of the femoral heads (Fig. 1-22). Recurrent neoplasm usually occurs as an irregular soft tissue mass in the center of the pelvis between the bladder and rectum. Parametrial invasion is determined by extension to the obturator internus or pyriformis muscles. Bladder invasion with fistula formation and rectal involvement (Fig. 1-23) are difficult to assess but may be manifested by irregular thickening of the adjacent walls with obliteration of the posterior perivesical and anterior rectal fat planes. Differentiation between fibrosis and tumor recurrence can be established by CT-directed percutaneous biopsy. The obturator, hypogastric, external, and common iliac lymph nodes (Fig. 1-24) are the most frequent sites of metastasis and are considered abnormal if they are 1.5 cm or greater in diameter. Because of the frequency of secondary infection in patients with carcinoma of the cervix, the presence of lymph node metastases producing isolated enlargement of lymph nodes must be established histologically. Metastases to nodes of normal size and microscopic spread will escape detection.[34–38]

Only a few references regarding CT in the diagnosis of lymph node metastases from carcinoma of the uterine cervix have appeared in the radiological literature. Whitley

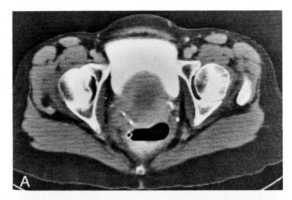

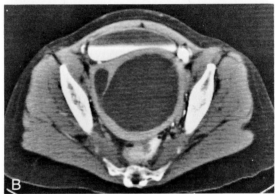

Fig. 1-22. Cervical carcinoma. A. CT scan demonstrates a large mass with central low density area in the region of the cervix. B. Hematometra of the uterine cavity with central low density due to the obstruction caused by the cervical tumor.

et al.[37] reported 17 patients with carcinoma of the cervix studied preoperatively by CT. In their study, the sensitivity of CT was 80 percent (4/5), the specificity 83 percent (10/12), and the accuracy 83 percent (14/17). The false positive rate was 11.7 percent (2/17), caused by lymphoid hyperplasia, while the false negative rate was 5.8 percent (1/17) due to microscopic metastases in nodes less than 1.5 cm in diameter. In 75 selected patients with primary untreated cervical carcinoma evaluated for staging by CT, Walsh and Goplerud[35] found 19 patients with pelvic and inguinal node metastases with pathological correlation. CT was correct in 14 of the 19 patients (accuracy 74 percent).

CT has been used to map the portals for radiation therapy. The detection of pelvic wall and retroperitoneal disease allows the radiotherapist to adapt the treatment to the tumor bulk and to alter the portals in response to changes in tumor size.

LYMPHANGIOGRAPHY

Ovary

The importance of lymphatic metastases from carcinoma of the ovary has been underestimated. The extent of local and peritoneal spread is usually the dominant factor in determining treatment.

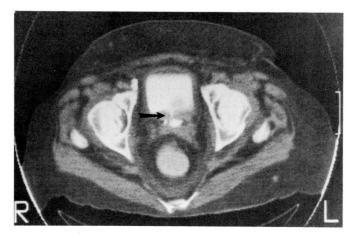

Fig. 1-23.   Vesico-vaginal fistula. Fistulous tract (arrow) between bladder and vagina.

Ovarian lymphatic drainage is to the paraaortic lymph nodes (Fig. 1-25) from the aortic bifurcation to the renal pelvis and occasionally to the nodes of the middle chain of the external iliac lymph node group. Once there is neoplastic involvement of the ovarian capsule or fallopian tubes, metastases are more likely to occur in the iliac and inguinal nodes. Anastomoses exist between the ovarian lymph vessels and those of the uterus and fallopain tubes, so that other pathways may be involved.

Fuks[39] found a positive lymphangiogram in 21 percent of 289 patients with Stage I or II epithelial carcinoma of the ovary. Aortic node dissections confirmed lymph node involvement in all 20 patients with a positive lymphangiogram and in 8 or 48 patients with negative studies (17 percent false negative rate). Athey et al.,[40] in a retrospective study of 72 lymphangiograms performed on 66 patients, described the distribution of metastases from ovarian neoplasms. The paraaortic nodes were involved in 70 percent, the iliac nodes in 58 percent, and the inguinal nodes in 27 percent. In germ cell tumor, there was a 90 percent incidence of paraaortic and 30 percent of iliac node metastases. Epithelial carcinoma metastasized to iliac lymph nodes in 73 percent, to aortic lymph nodes in 60 percent, and to inguinal nodes in 41 percent. Metastases to the paraaortic nodes were found by lymphangiography in 8 (18 percent) of 44 patients by Douglas et al.,[41] in 44 (38 percent) of 117 patients by Musumeci et al.,[43] and in 19 (48 percent) of 39 patients by Fuchs.[43]

Uterine Corpus

The yield of lymphangiography in the detection of metastases in carcinoma of the endometrium is small unless reserved for the more advanced bulky cancer or those extending into the cervix. Douglas et al.[44] reported an overall incidence of lymph node metastases of 19 percent in 76 patients prior to treatment of carcinoma of the uterine corpus. About half of the patients had paraaortic lymph node metastases. Kademian et al.[45] performed lymphangiography on 108 patients with adenocarcinoma of the endometrium and found lymph node metastasis in 32 patients (29.6 percent);

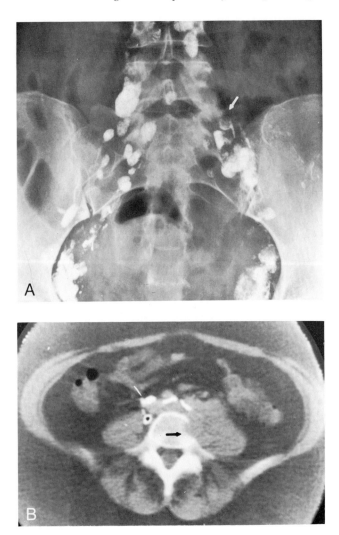

Fig. 1-24. Nodal metastasis from carcinoma of the uterine cervix. A. Nodal phase of the lymphangiogram demonstrates defect in left common iliac node (arrow). B. CT shows left common iliac nodal metastasis with associated destruction of the vertebrae (arrow) not appreciated on the lymphangiogram.

paraaortic node involvement was present in 8 (7.4 percent). Histologic confirmation was seldom obtained, but short term follow-up indicated that a positive interpretation was associated with an extremely poor prognosis.

Uterine Cervix

The lymphatics of the uterine cervix form a rich plexus. The collecting trunks drain to the lymph nodes of the external iliac and hypogastric chains as well as to the

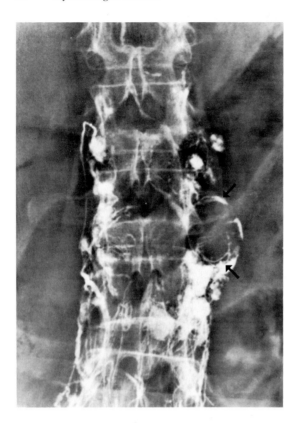

Fig. 1-25. Nodal metastasis from carcinoma of the ovary in the paraaortic region. The lymphatics do not traverse the area replaced by the tumor (arrows).

presacral area.

The yield of lymphangiography in the detection of metastases in patients with Stage I carcinoma of the cervix is small. The metastases in this group are usually in the pelvis and are most likely included within the usual radiation portals.

At M.D. Anderson Hospital, of 103 patients with advanced cancer of the cervix including bulky Stage I lesions and postirradiation recurrences, 42 were diagnosed by lymphangiography as having metastases (Fig. 1-24A).[46] Exploratory laparotomy confirmed the presence of metastases in 41 of these patients (sensitivity 77 percent). Of the 61 patients considered negative by lymphangiography, 49 were true negative (specificity 98 percent) and 12 were found to have lymph node metastases. The overall accuracy was 87 percent. The high percentage of false negatives (12 percent) supports our contention that only a diagnosis of definitely positive disease is of any clinical use.[47,48] Microscopic neoplastic foci are not detected by lymphangiography, nor are all the pelvic and paraaortic lymph nodes opacified.

In our institution, 48 patients with carcinoma of the uterine cervix examined by lymphangiography and followed within 2 to 3 weeks by CT were reviewed to assess the findings and their impact on management.[49] Lymphangiography was negative in 33 and positive for lymph node metastases in the remaining 15. CT was negative in 32 patients and positive in 16. Pathologic correlation by biopsy or surgery was ob-

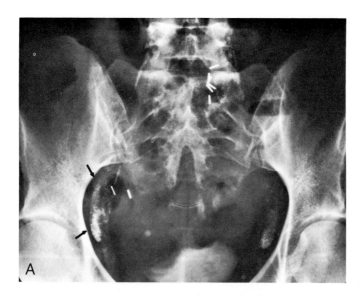

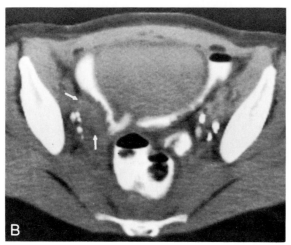

Fig. 1-26. Post radiation fibrosis in a patient with carcinoma of the uterine cervix.
A. Lymphangiogram demonstrates poorly opacified nodes in the right external iliac region (arrows).
B. CT scan shows enlarged node greater than 1.5 cm in diameter in the right internal iliac region considered abnormal (arrows).

tained in 20 patients. Lymphangiography showed evidence of nodal metastasis in 7 and an overall accuracy of 95 percent. Six patients had nodal metastases by CT and the overall accuracy was 75 percent. There were 2 false negatives (10 percent) with CT. Three cases (15 percent) showed false positive findings on CT resulting from lymphoid hyperplasia and postirradiation fibrosis (Fig. 1-26).

In advanced lesions and postirradiated or postsurgical patients, when lymphangiography showed lymphatic obstruction in the pelvic region with nonopacification of the nodes above the interruption, CT demonstrated either normal nodes with no evidence of metastases or nonopacified nodal metastases in the paraaortic area. In addition, CT revealed local extension of the cervical lesion and extranodal metastases, such as to the urinary tract, liver, and skeleton (Fig. 1-24B).

ANGIOGRAPHY

Ovary

Angiography is seldom used in the diagnosis of ovarian tumors except in selected cases. The arterial supply to the ovary originates from two sources: the ovarian arteries usually arising from the aorta and the adnexal branches of the uterine arteries from the interal iliac arteries. Fernstrom[50] described the use of arteriography in the diagnosis of gynecologic neoplasms. With the advent of ultrasound and CT, arteriography is rarely utilized to demonostrate an ovarian mass.

Arteriography is still valuable in the delineation of hepatic metastases. Hepatic angiography, especially with superselective catheterization technique, is now reserved for staging and in preparation for interventional management.

Most ovarian malignancies and their metastases are relatively hypovascular.[50] The angiographic evaluation of the left lobe of the liver remains difficult, but selective catheterization of the left hepatic artery adds immeasurably to the diagnostic capabilities.[51] Angiography and CT make a most exquisite combination for specific situations.[52]

Ovarian venography, i.e., the retrograde injection of the catheterized gonadal vein, is seldom done. However, when there is a need to determine the site of origin of a pelvic mass, ovarian venography may be helpful. An enlarged ovary separates the adnexal venous plexus (usually three major vessels) that surrounds the ovary. A mass adjacent to the ovary, usually of uterine origin, will displace these draining veins in the same direction. As the ovarian neoplasm progresses, it invades adjacent pelvic veins, especially the external and common iliacs.

Uterine Corpus

A leiomyoma will usually opacify as a hypervascular mass on uterine arteriography. The vessels are frequently bizarre, especially when the tumor is small. As the neoplasm enlarges, there is often a central area of decreased vascularity (from degeneration) while the periphery remains hypervascular.[50] It is possible to suggest the presence of sarcoma only if the vascularity is obviously neoplastic with arteriovenous shunting.

Trophoblastic neoplasms are usually hypervascular (Fig. 1-27), so arteriography may detect lesions as small as 5 mm in diameter. This is most important in the search for metastasis or residual uterine tumor in patients with a rising HCG and no obvious focus of disease on the usual screening techniques of scintigraphy, ultrasonography, and CT. Small metastases in the vagina, pelvis, liver, and brain can be opacified by arteriography. Occasionally, cerebral angiography is necessary to define the meta-

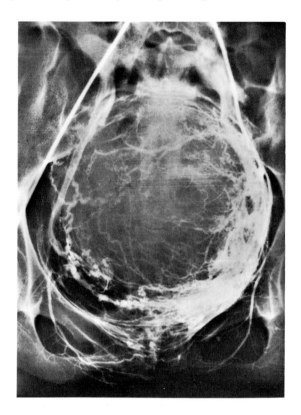

Fig. 1-27. Choriocarcinoma. Arteriography demonstrates a markedly hypervascular mass with irregular vessels in the pelvis.

static tumor thrombus or pseudo-aneurysm as a cause of subdural or subarachnoid hemorrhage or cerebral infarction.

Following therapy for choriocarcinoma, arteriovenous shunts may persist in the absence of residual tumor as defined by a normal HCG titer and no change on follow-up examination. Arteriovenous shunts may be seen with any trophoblastic metastasis or at a site of previously treated metastasis.[53]

HYSTEROGRAPHY

Hysterography, the opacification of the uterine cavity, may help define the size, location, shape, and microscopic appearance of a neoplasm. A small lesion may be detected, especially in the cornua, where it may be out of the reach of currettage. A neoplasm originating in the endometrium and extending into the cervix (corpus et collum) may be delineated with greater accuracy. Hysterography may also be useful to guide the accurate placement of radium capsules or tandem and to follow tumor regression or recurrence after irradiation. In a series reported by Schwartz et al.[54] in 1975, unexpected findings were present in 42 of 105 patients (40 percent) examined by hysterography for unexplained bleeding, discharge, or known endometrial carcinoma. In spite of these advantages, hysterography has little popularity.[55]

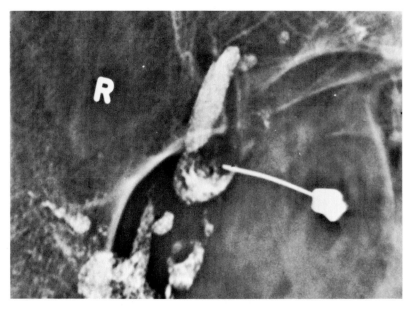

Fig. 1-28. Percutaneous lymph node biopsy of metastastic cervical carcinoma. The biopsy of the right external iliac node was performed under fluoroscopic guidance.

PNEUMOGRAPHY

Pelvic pneumography has been available to outline the uterus and ovaries since its introduction by Goetze in 1918.[56] Its value in the assessment of uterine size in carcinoma of the uterus was restated by Stevens[57] and Brascho.[58] Pelvic pneumography was made safer by the intraperitoneal injection of nitrous oxide or carbon dioxide rather than air or oxygen and is especially helpful in the obese patient in whom palpation is futile. By outlining the size and shape of the uterus, a more accurate estimation of the extent of disease was accomplished. Extension beyond the uterus could be suspected, but neoplastic involvement could not be differentiated from inflammatory change. At times, the combination of hysterography and pelvic pneumography demonstrated the uterine cavity, the thickness of the myometrium, and the size of the uterus. This information was useful when radium capsules were utilized. Ultrasonography has almost completely replaced pneumography and hysterography.

PERCUTANEOUS BIOPSY

Historically, the radiologist has employed the least invasive technique available to diagnose abnormality. Recently, radiologic techniques such as computed axial tomography, ultrasonography, selective angiography, and interventional procedures have changed diagnostic radiology. With percutaneous needle biopsy, an accurate

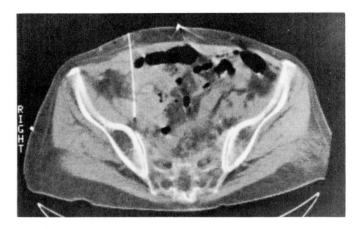

Fig. 1-29. Percutaneous lymph node biopsy of metastastic cervical carcinoma. CT of the pelvis demonstrates a needle in the mass in the right external iliac region.

pathologic diagnosis can be made without surgery in patients with probable metastatic disease. Consequently, the patient is spared the risk and expense of surgery. Percutaneous needle biopsy has been successfully employed to establish the diagnosis of lesions of the lymph nodes, abdominal viscera, and other organs.[59,60] Although cytologic methods will never eliminate the need for histologic diagnosis, clinical experience over the past decade has shown that percutaneous needle aspiration biopsy has a definite place in the management of patients with metastatic neoplastic disorders.

The percutaneous approach to the paraaortic and pelvic lymph nodes represents a simple technique to confirm the presence of neoplasm and thereby to determine the extent of disease and to facilitate treatment planning (Fig. 1-28). Because the contrast medium for a lymphangiogram remains in the lymph nodes for a prolonged period of time, approximately 15 months, changes in the lymph nodes in response to treatment can be evaluated at varying intervals. When possible recurrent disease is noted, percutaneous biopsy offers the possibility of a tissue diagnosis, and a more appropriate treatment can be started (Fig. 1-29).

Percutaneous retroperitoneal lymph node biopsy was performed on 129 patients with carcinoma of the cervix in whom a lymphangiogram had been reported as positive or suspicious for metastatic disease at M. D. Anderson Hospital.[61] Of the 159 biopsies, 114 were done on external iliac lymph nodes and 45 on paraaortic nodes. An overall accuracy of 68 percent was obtained without significant complications. The sensitivity of the test was 58 percent and the specificity 100 percent. This reiterates the fact that only a positive biopsy is of significance.

Percutaneous needle biopsy is a safe technique that can be performed on an outpatient. Potential complications, such as intra-abdominal bleeding, bowel perforation, peritonitis, or tumor dissemination along the biopsy tract, were not encountered during either clinical follow-up or surgical exploration.

PERCUTANEOUS NEPHROSTOMY

In the female with gynecologic malignancy, the most common reason for performing a nephrostomy is ureteral obstruction secondary to pelvic or retroperitoneal disease. Urinary tract diversion by percutaneous nephrostomy has been used for postoperative or postradiotherapy fistula. Prior to arterial chemotherapy with cis-diammine dichloroplatinum (CDDP), a renal toxic agent, a nephrostomy to relieve ureteral obstruction is necessary and is performed under fluoroscopic or ultrasonic guidance.[62]

TRANSCATHETER MANAGEMENT

Renewed interest in transcatheter management of malignant gynecologic tumors has been stimulated by the development of techniques of percutaneous transcatheter infusion and occlusion. These methods allow ready access to the vascular supply of the neoplasms for intraarterial treatment with decreased morbidity and mortality compared to a surgical approach.

Ovary

Pelvic recurrence of ovarian neoplasm has been managed by bilateral internal iliac arterial infusion of chemotherapy. A combination of CDDP, adriamycin, and alkeran or thiotepa has considerable potential. Control of hemorrhage has been accomplished by embolization.

Metastatic ovarian carcinoma in the liver is relatively uncommon and difficult to treat. Hepatic arterial infusion or embolization has been successful. Sensitivty of the neoplasm for the chemotherapeutic agents is usually apparent after a single course. The treatment is repeated at monthly intervals as long as the response continues. With stable or progressive disease, sequential embolization of the hepatic arteries with Ivalon is undertaken. One lobe is embolized each month, and then the entire liver is reembolized with Ivalon.[63] A combination of infusion and embolization may also be effective.

Uterine Corpus

Transcatheter arterial infusion and embolization have been valuable adjuncts in the management of trophoblastic disease in the pelvis or metastatic to the liver (Fig. 1-30A,B). In view of the propensity of this tumor to bleed, embolization has been effective in controlling bleeding.

Uterine Cervix

The rationale for arterial infusion is to expose the neoplasm to a high local concentration of chemotherapeutic agent (as compared to the intravenous administration) without an increase in toxicity. Bilateral internal iliac artery infusion of bleomycin alone or in combination with mitomycin C and vincristine has been used for the treat-

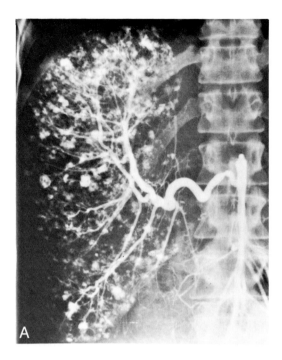

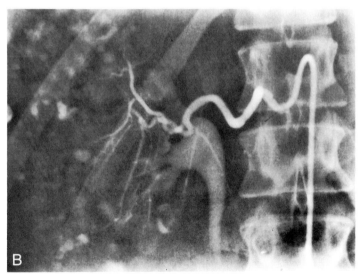

Fig. 1-30. Hepatic artery embolization for metastastic choriocarcinoma of the uterus to the liver. A. Hepatic arteriography demonstrates multiple hypervascular metastasis. B. Re-examination following embolization reveals marked reduction in the hepatic metastasis.

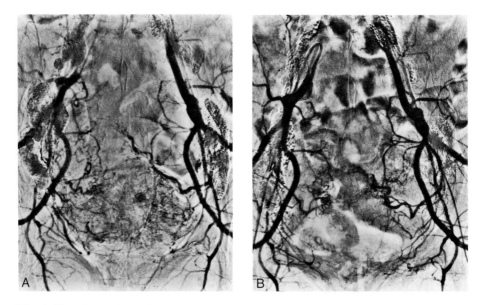

Fig. 1-31. Transcatheter intraarterial chemotherapy for advanced carcinoma of the cervic. A. The carcinoma is hypervascular. B. Following three courses of intraarterial cisplatinum and bleomycin, and intravenous vincristine and mitomycin C, there is marked improvement. The patient was subsequently treated by radiation therapy.

ment of recurrent cervical carcinoma. Morrow et al.[64] observed 2 of 16 objective remissions, while Swenerton et al. reported 3 of 20.[65] Ohta and other Japanese investigators suggested employing arterial infusion prior to definitive radiation therapy.[66]

At M. D. Anderson Hospital, 9 patients with squamous cell carcinoma of the uterine cervix were treated by bilateral internal iliac artery infusion of CDDP.[67] Of these, 6 had an unresectable pelvic recurrence following radiation therapy and 3 had a previously untreated, large volume primary tumor. Three patients (33 percent) experienced a partial response.

More recently, CDDP has been combined with bleomycin intraarterially while vincristine and mitomycin C were delivered intravenously. All 7 patients treated thus far have had a partial response (50 percent or more reduction in size of the pelvic mass) with 2 qualifying for curative local radiation therapy (Fig. 1-31).

The control of hemorrhage in patients with carcinoma of the cervix is, at times, life saving and may allow more specific therapy by surgery, irradiation, or chemotherapy. We prefer Ivalon particles (250–500 μm) and Gelfoam cubes (3mm) or peripheral embolization and Gelfoam segments and stainless steel coils for central vascular occlusion. Embolization of the arterior branches of both internal iliac arteries has been helpful in controlling vaginal hemorrhage from carcinoma of the cervix.[68] Bleeding from the cervix, bladder, and rectum following radiation therapy has been successfully treated in approximately 50 percent of patients by embolization of the internal iliac or inferior mesenteric arteries.

REFERENCES

1. Stevens GM: The Female Reproductive System. An Atlas of Tumor Radiology. Chicago, Year Book Medical Publisher, 1971.
2. Meyers MA: Distribution of intra-abdominal malignant seeding: Dependency on dynamics of flow of ascitic fluid. AJR 119:198, 1973.
3. Meyers MA, McSweeney J: Secondary neoplasms of the bowel. Radiology 105:1, 1972.
4. Meyers MA: Metastatic seeding along the small bowel mesentery. AJR 123:67, 1975.
5. Khilnani MT, Marshak RH, Eliasoph J, et al: Roentgen features of metastases to the colon. AJR 96:302, 1966.
6. Novak ER, Woodruff JD: Gynecological and Obstetric Pathology with Clinical and Endocrine Relations, ed 2. Philadelphia, WB Saunders, 1979.
7. Sanders RC, James AE: The Principles and Practice of Ultrasonography in Obstetrics and Gynecology, ed 2. New York, Appleton-Century Croft, 1980.
8. Brewer JI, Rinehart JJ, Dunbar RW: Choriocarcinoma. Am J Obstet Gynecol 81:574, 1961.
9. Green B, Libshitz HI: Bladder and uterer. In Libshitz HI (ed): Diagnostic Roentgenology of Radiotherapy Change. Baltimore, Williams & Wilkins, 1979, pp 123–136.
10. Strockbine MF, Hancock JE, Fletcher GH: Complications in 831 patients with squamous cell carcinoma of the intact uterine cervix treated with 3,000 rads or more whole pelvis radiation. AJR 108:293, 1970.
11. Cunningham JJ, Fuks ZY, Castellino RA: Radiographic manifestations of carcinoma of the cervix and complications of its treatment. Rad Clin North AM 12:93, 1974.
12. Lawson TL, Albarelli JN: Diagnosis of gynecologic pelvic masses by gray scale ultrasonography: Analysis of specificity and accuracy. AJR 128:1003, 1977.
13. Fleischer AC, James AE, Millis JB, et al: Differential diagnosis of pelvic masses by gray scale sonography. AJR 131:469, 1978.
14. Berland LM, Lawson TL, Albarelli JN, et al: Ultrasonic diagnosis of ovarian and adnexal disease. Semin Ultrasound 1:17, 1980.
15. Walsh JW, Taylor KJW, Wasson JF, et al: Gray-scale ultrasound in 204 proved gynecologic masses: Accuracy and specific diagnosis criteria. Radiology 130:391, 1979.
16. Requard CK, Mettler FA Jr, Wicks JD: Preoperative sonography of malignant ovarian neoplasms. AJR 137:79, 1981.
17. Paling MR, Shawker TH: Abdominal ultrasound in advanced ovarian carcinoma. J Clin Ultrasound 9:435, 1981.
18. Bowie JD: Ultrasound of gynecologic pelvic masses: The indefinite uterus and other patterns associated with diagnostic error. J Clin Ultrasound 5:323, 1977.
19. Callen PW, DeMartini WJ, Filly RA: The central uterine cavity echo: A useful anatomic sign in the ultrasonographic evaluation of the female pelvis. Radiology 131:187, 1979.
20. Requard CK, Wicks JD, Mettler FA: Ultrasonography in the staging of endometrial adenocarcinoma. Radiology 140:781, 1981.
21. Fleischer AC, James AE Jr, Krause DA, et al: Sonographic patterns in trophoblastic diseases. Radiology 126:215, 1978.
22. Sauerbrei EE, Salem S, Fayle B: Coexistent hydatifidiform mole and live fetus in the second trimester. Radiology 135:415, 1980.
23. Requard CK, Mettler FA: The use of ultrasound in the evaluation of trophoblastic disease and its response to therapy. Radiology 135:419, 1980.
24. Amendola MA, Walsh JW, Amendola BE, et al: Computed tomography in the evaluation of carcinoma of the ovary. J Comput Assist Tomogr 5:179, 1981.
25. Lee JKT, Stanley RJ, Sagel SS, et al: Accuracy of CT in detecting intraabdominal and pelvic lymph node metastases from pelvic cancers. AJR 131:675, 1978.

26. Walsh JW, Amendola MA, Konerding KF, et al: Computed tomographic detection of pelvic and inguinal lymph-node metastases from primary and recurrent pelvic malignant disease. Radiology 137:157, 1980.

27. Dunnick NR, Jones RB, Doppman JL, et al: Intraperitoneal contrast infusion for assessment of intraperitoneal fluid dynamics. AJR 133:221, 1979.

28. Brizel HE, Livingston PA, Grayson EV: Radiotherapeutic applications of pelvic computed tomography. J Comput Assist Tomogr 3:453, 1979.

29. Rankin RN, Hutton LC: Ultrasound in the ovarian hyperstimulation system. J Clin Ultrasound 9:473, 1981.

30. Snow JH, Goldstein HM, Wallace S: Comparison of scintigraphy, sonography, and computed tomography in the evaluation of hepatic neoplasms. AJR 132:915, 1979.

31. Tada S, Tsukioka M, Ishii C, et al: Computed tomographic features of uterine myoma. J Comput Assist Tomogr 5:866, 1981.

32. Hamlin DJ, Burgener FA, Beecham JB: CT of intramural endometrial carcinoma: Contrast enhancement is essential. AJR 137:551, 1981.

33. Goldstein DP, Berkowitz RS: The management of gestational trophoblastic neoplasms. Curr Prob Obstet Gynecol 4:1, 1980.

34. Kilcheski TS, Arger PH, Mulhern CB, et al: Role of computed tomography in the presurgical evaluation of carcinoma of the cervix. J Compute Assist Tomogr 5:378, 1981.

35. Walsh JW, Goplerud DR: Prospective comparison between clinical and CT staging in primary cervical carcinoma. AJR 137:997, 1981.

36. Ginaldi S, Wallace S, Jing BS, et al: Carcinoma of the cervix: Lymphangiography and computed tomography. AJR 136:1087, 1981.

37. Whitley NO, Brenner DE, Francis A, et al: Computed tomographic evaluation of carcinoma of the cervix. Radiology 142:439, 1982.

38. Walsh JW, Amendola MA, Hall DJ, et al: Recurrent carcinoma of the cervix: CT diagnosis. AJR 136:117, 1981.

39. Fuks Z: External radiotherapy of ovarian cancer: Standard approaches and new frontiers. Semin Oncol 2:253, 1975.

40. Athey PA, Wallace S, Jing BS, et al: Lymphangiography in the ovarian cancer. AJR 123:106, 1975.

41. Douglas B, MacDonald JS, Baker JW: Lymphography in carcinoma of the ovary. Proc R Soc Med 54:400, 1971.

42. Musumeci F, Banfi A, Bolis G: Lymphangiography in patients with ovarian epithelial cancer: An evaluation of 289 consecutive cases. Cancer 40:1444, 1977.

43. Fuchs WA: Malignant tumors of the ovary. In Fuchs WA, Davidson JW, Fischer HW (eds): Recent Results in Cancer Research-Lymphography in Cancer. New York, Springer-Verlag, 1969, pp 119–123.

44. Douglas B, MacDonald JS, Baker JW: Lymphography in carcinoma of the uterus. Clin Radiol 23:286, 1972.

45. Kademian MT, Buchler DA, Wirtanen GW: Bipedal lymphangiography in malignancies of the uterine corpus. AJR 129:903, 1977.

46. Piver S, Wallace S, Castro J: The accuracy of lymphangiography in carcinoma of the uterine cervix. AJR 111:278, 1971.

47. Wallace S, Jing BS: Carcinoma. Lymphangiography in carcinoma. In: Clouse ME (ed): Clinical Lymphography. Baltimore, Wilkins & Williams, 1977, pp 185–273.

48. Wallace S, Jing BS, Zornoza J, et al: Is lymphangiography worthwhile? Current concepts in cancer: Updated cervix cancer II. Stages IB and II. Int J Radiat Oncol Biol Phys 5:1873, 1979.

49. Jing BS, Wallace S, Zornoza J: Metastases to Retroperitoneal and Pelvic Lymph Nodes: Computed Tomography and Lymphangiography. Radiol Clin N Am 20:511, 1982.
50. Fernstrom I: Arteriography of the uterine artery. Acta Radiol Suppl No. 122, 1955.
51. Wallace S, Chuang VP: The radiologic diagnosis and management of hepatic metastases. Der Radiologe 22:56, 1982.
52. Prando A, Wallace S, Bernardino ME, et al: Computed tomographic arteriography of the liver. Radiology 130:697, 1979.
53. Cockshott WP, Hendrickse JP, de V: Persistent arteriovenous fistulae following chemotherapy of malignant trophoblastic disease. Radiology 88:329, 1967.
54. Schwartz PE, Kohorn EI, Knowlton AH, et al: Routine use of hysterography in endometrial carcinoma and postmenopausal bleeding. Obstet Gynel 45:378, 1975.
55. Wallace S, Jing BS, Medelin H: Endometrial carcinoma: Radiologic assistance in the diagnosis, staging, and management. Gynecol Obstet 2:287, 1974.
56. Goetze O: Die Rontgendiagnostik bei gasgefüllter bauchhohle, eine neue methode. Med Wochenschr 65:1275, 1981.
57. Stevens MG: Pelvic pneumography. Semin Roentgenol 4:252, 1969.
58. Brascho DJ: Use of pelvic pneumography in planning radiotherapy of endometrial carcinoma. Radiology 97:113, 1970.
59. Zornoza J: Percutaneous Needle Biopsy. Baltimore, Williams & Wilkins, 1981.
60. Zornoza J, Lukeman JM, Jing BS, et al: Percutaneous retroperitoneal lymph node biopsy in carcinoma of the cervix. Gynecol Oncol 5:43, 1977.
61. Edeiken-Monroe ES, Zornoza J: Carcinoma of the cervix: Percutaneous lymph node aspiration biopsy. AJR 138:655, 1982.
62. Pfister RC, Yoder JC, Newhouse JH: Percutaneous uroradiologic procedures. Semin Roentgenol 16:135, 1981.
63. Chuang VP, Wallace S, Soo CS, et al: Therapeutic Ivalon embolization of hepatic tumors. AJR 138:289, 1982.
64. Morrow CP, DiSaia PJ, Mangan CF, et al: Continuous pelvic arterial infusion with bleomycin for squamous carcinoma of the cervix recurrent after irradiation therapy. Cancer Treat Rep 61:1403, 1977.
65. Swenerton KD, Evers JA, White GW, et al: Intermittent pelvic infusion with vincristine, bleomycin, and mitomycin C for advanced recurrent carcinoma of the cervix. Cancer Treat Rep 63:1379, 1979.
66. Ohta A: Basic and clinical studies on the simultaneous combination treatment of cervical cancer with a carcinostatic agent and radiation. J Tokyo Med Coll 36:529, 1978.
67. Oku T, Iwasaki M, Tojo S: Study on surgical chemotherapy for advanced carcinoma of the uterine cervix-particularly on the problem of clinical effect and drug concentration. Acta Obstet Gynecol Jpn 31:1833, 1979.
68. Schwartz PE, Goldstein HM, Wallace S, et al: Control of arterial hemorrhage using percutaneous arterial catheter techniques in patients with gynecologic malignancies. Gynecol Obstet 3:276, 1975.

2 | Epidemiology of Cervical Cancer: The Herpes Virus Question

David B. Thomas

HISTOLOGY AND PATHOGENESIS

The pathogenesis of cervical cancer has recently been reviewed by Cramer.[1] The columnar epithelium of the endocervical canal meets the stratified squamous epithelium of the ectocervix at the squamocolumnar junction. The location of this transitional zone varies. In the prepubertal female, the columnar epithelium often extends onto the ectocervix. At puberty, the ectocervical columnar epithelium undergoes squamous metaplasia, and the squamocolumnar junction becomes located within the endocervical canal. During pregnancy the cervix may undergo eversion, and columnar epithelium may again be exposed to the vagina until it too undergoes squamous metaplasia. The squamous epithelial cells resulting from the metaplastic process probably arise from reserve cells in the lower layer of the epithelium in the transition zone. They may develop in part in response to the low ph of the vaginal secretions. The roles of sexual intercourse and microorganisms in the normal metaplastic process are unknown.

Cervical neoplasms develop in the transitional zone, and probably also arise from the totipotential basal reserve cells. Neoplasms that do not penetrate the basement membrane of the epithelium are called cervical intraepithelial neoplasia (CIN), and include carcinoma in-situ and squamous dysplasia (hereafter referred to as dysplasia). The former is characterized by proliferation of round stem cells with no evidence of differentiation (squamatization or keratinization). Dysplastic lesions consist of lesser disorders of epithelial differentiation, with, for example, some evidence of squamatization or preservation of underlying glandular structures. Dysplastic lesions may be graded according to their degree of anaplasia, and pathologists may disagree as to the criteria for distinguishing the more severe ones from carcinoma in-situ.

Approximately 85 percent of all invasive carcinomas are of the squamous cell type, and the most probable sequence leading to their development is that the epithelium of the squamocolumnar junction undergoes continuous change from mild to severe dysplasia, to carcinoma in-situ, to invasive disease. This is a process, requiring years, or even decades before invasion occurs. The steps leading to severe dysplasia are reversible, and that from dysplasia to carcinoma in-situ may also be so. Screening programs in some areas have detected numbers of carcinomas in-situ in excess of those expected from prior incidence rates of invasive cancer, suggesting that not all in-situ carcinomas eventually lead to invasive disease.

In addition to the histologic appearance of the individual lesions, there is other evidence for the hypothesized sequence of events leading to invasive squamous carcinoma. The simultaneous occurrence of dysplasia and carcinoma in-situ, and of carcinoma in-situ and invasive carcinoma, have been observed in the same lesions; women with dysplasia tend to be younger than those with carcinoma in-situ, and the latter in turn tend to be younger than those with invasive disease; and follow-up studies have shown women with dysplasia to be at high risk of developing carcinoma in-situ.

Adeno and adenosquamous carcinomas of the uterine cervix each constitute from 5 to 8 percent of invasive cervical neoplasms. With the exception of clear cell adenocarcinomas resulting from prenatal exposure to diethylstilbesterol, their origin is unclear. Also with the exception of the clear cell tumors, epidemiologic studies have generally not distinguished the individual histologic types of cervical carcinoma. Because most are of the squamous cell type, unless otherwise stated it may be assumed that the information summarized in the remaining portions of this chapter pertains to squamous carcinomas.

DESCRIPTIVE EPIDEMIOLOGY

An initial step in utilizing epidemiologic methods to elucidate the etiology of a disease is to determine how incidence or mortality rates vary geographically, over time, and with respect to certain personal characteristics. Particular caution must be exercised in interpreting variations in rates of cervical cancer for the following reasons:

1. The practice of classifying cervical cancer as simply uterine cancer can influence rates. Until about 1950, mortality rates of cancers of the uterine cervix and corpus were combined in the United States; and even today the proportion of uterine cancers classified as "not otherwise specified" varies among countries.

2. Pathologists may differ over time and from place to place (as well as among themselves within the same area) as to which lesions are considered dysplasia, carcinoma in-situ, and invasive carcinoma.

3. The amount of cytologic screening will influence the incidence rates of both in-situ and invasive disease, as well as the mortality rates. Initially, the incidence rates of invasive and in-situ disease increase following initiation of screening in a

population, as prevalent cases are detected. If there is no actual change in the rate of occurrence of the initial neoplastic process, with continued screening the observed incidence and mortality rates subsequently decline and then reach a steady state at levels dependent not only on the rates of occurrence of new disease, but also on the proportion of the population being screened.

4. Only women with a cervix are at risk of cervical cancer, and observed rates of cervical cancers in a population will underestimate the rate of occurrence of new disease in women at risk if the proportion of women in the population that have had hysterectomies for benign conditions is not taken into account.

Although differences in classification, diagnosis, and rates of screening and hysterectomy present special problems, variations in rates of cervical cancer, if considered with appropriate caution, do provide information of etiologic relevance.

Cervical cancer has a high frequency rate in certain Latin American nations and probably also in some less developed countries in Africa and Asia; intermediate rates are reported in Europe, Canada, and the United States; and Israel has the lowest rates in the world.[2] With some exceptions, migrants from lower to higher rate countries tend to develop cervical cancer at the higher rates,[3] strongly suggesting that the international differences in rates are due to environmental, rather than genetic factors.

Variations in rates within countries also suggest that environmental factors are of etiologic importance. Rates of cervical cancer are inversely related to social class in Britain[4] and socioeconomic status as measured by income and education in the United States.[5] In the latter country, rates are highest for blacks and American Indians, intermediate for whites, and lowest for Japanese and Chinese; but a recent study[4] showed that two-thirds of the excess risk in non-whites compared to whites could be explained by differences in socioeconomic status.

A woman's sexual behavior plays a role in her exposure to the environmental factors of etiologic importance. The disease does not occur before puberty, and rates are lower in single women than in women who have ever been married.[3]

Sexual behavior of men may also affect women's exposures to the environmental causes of cervical cancer. It has been suggested[6] that the high rates in Latin America, where virginity prior to marriage and female fidelity afterwards are encouraged, are due to frequent use of prostitutes by men. Also, in Britain, women in each social class whose husbands engaged in occupations requiring travel or frequent contact with travelers were found to be at increased risk;[5] and rates of cervical cancer in women in various social class and occupational categories were strongly correlated with rates of syphilis in men in these same categories.[5]

Finally, there is evidence from descriptive epidemiology that sexual exposure early in adult life is of particular etiologic importance. Starting at about age 15, rates of carcinoma in-situ increase with age until about age 30, and then decline; and rates of invasive disease increase with age after about age 25, reach a peak in the 50's, and then decrease.[1] This is the pattern one would expect if carcinoma in-situ is a precursor of invasive cancer, and if exposure at onset of sexual maturity is followed by a latent period before clinically apparent disease develops. Studies of time trends provide additional evidence for the etiologic role of early sexual exposure. Age-adjusted mortality rates of cervical cancer in succeeding birth cohorts in both England

and Wales, and in Scotland, have been shown to be correlated with the incidence of gonorrhea in the cohort when its members were in their twenties.[5] In addition, following the liberalization of sexual practices in the late 1950's to early 1960's, mortality rates of cervical cancer in Britain,[7] the United States,[8] New Zealand,[9] and Australia[10] have increased during the 1970's in young women (below about age 35), but not in older women; and in China, where prostitution and sexual promiscuity were markedly reduced following the revolution of 1949, rates of cervical cancer have declined, and the disease now occurs primarily in women who had reached sexual maturity before the revolution.[11]

RISK FACTORS

We have been able to infer from variations in incidence and mortality rates of cervical cancer that this disease is probably caused by one or more environmental factors that are most likely transmitted as a result of sexually promiscuous behavior by women or their male partners, and that exposures early in life may be of particular etiologic importance. Some prospective studies in groups of women with known sexual practices, and large numbers of case-control studies, have provided additional support for the hypothesis that cervical cancer is a veneral disease. These have been previously reviewed.[1,12] Rates are low in nuns, virgins, and generally monogamous religious groups such as the Seventh Day Adventists and Mormons; and rates are high in prison inmates and prostitutes. Other factors that distinguish women at high risk include a history of illegitimate children, induced abortion, marital separation or divorce, pre- and extra-marital relations, multiple partners, and such venereal diseases as syphilis, gonorrhea, trichomoniasis, and genital herpes. In addition, use of occlusive contraceptives may be associated with a reduced risk.

Evidence that males can transmit the causative agent is supported by several pieces of evidence. In one study, the risk of cervical cancer was found to be increased in the second wives of men whose first wife had had cervical cancer.[13] This finding, however, was based on small numbers, and the possibility that the second wives were similar to the first wives with respect to other risk factors for cervical cancer was not adequately considered. Several studies have shown increased risks of cervical cancer in women who were married to men with cancer of the penis.[14,15,16] This finding might suggest a common etiology for cancers of the cervix and penis, although rates of the two diseases in various populations are weakly correlated at best,[14] and the epidemiologic features of cancer of the penis do not suggest a veneral etiology. More convincingly, compared to husbands of normal women, those of women with cervical cancer have more frequently had a history of multiple sexual partners and extra-marital relations; and in one study of women with only one admitted partner, risk was found to increase with the number of partners that the husband was known to have had.[17]

It is uncertain whether the young cervix is particularly vulnerable to the carcinogenic effects of the venerally transmitted agent for cervical cancer. Most studies have shown that cases tend to have their first pregnancy, marriage, or intercourse at an earlier age than unaffected controls. However, early age at onset of sexual activitiy is related to number of partners in many cultures, and this relationship has not been considered in many investigations. In one recent study,[18] relative risk of dysplasia or carcinoma in-situ was found to be highly related to number of sexual partners, but after controlling for the confounding effect of this variable, relative risk was not related to age at first intercourse. It may be, therefore, that sexual exposure early in adult life is a determinant of risk simply because that is the period of maximal sexual activity and consequently maximal risk of contracting venerally transmitted pathogens.

The low rates of cervical cancer in Jewish women have lead to the suggestion that circumcision of the male partner reduces risk, but results of careful case-control studies have not supported this hypothesis. However, the increased risk of cervical cancer in wives of men with penile cancer, and the probable relationship of penile hygiene to cancer of the penis, suggest that penile cleanliness could also play a role in the genesis of cervical cancer.

After controlling for sexual factors, parity and other variables related to child-bearing have not been shown to be related to cervical cancer. Menstrual factors such as age at menarche, frequency or duration of menstrual periods, or history of irregular menses, have also not been associated with cervical neoplasia.

The apparent venereal nature of cervical cancer has lead to a search for specific sexually transmitted agents that might be of etiologic importance. A number of studies have shown more cases than normal controls to have had syphilis, gonorrhea, trichomoniasis and chlamydial infection, but none of these pathogens have been shown to have oncogenic potential in experimental systems, and many cases have not had prior exposure to these organisms. It is likely that their associations with cervical cancer, like their associations with each other, are due simply to their common mode of transmission.

A number of sexually transmitted viruses have come under consideration as possible etiologic agents for cervical cancer. To date, the most work has been done on herpes simplex virus Type-2 (HSV-2), and there is more evidence to implicate this virus than any other as a causal agent.

HERPES SIMPLEX VIRUS TYPE-2

Experimental Studies

There are two known types of herpes simplex virus (HSV). Type-1 (HSV-1) is generally responsible for oral lesions (cold sores, fever blisters) and Type-2 (HSV-2) most frequently causes genital herpetic lesions, although oral infections by HSV-2 and genital infections by HSV-1 have been demonstrated. Age-specific prevalence rates of antibodies against HSV-1 and HSV-2 suggest that HSV-2 is usually transmitted sexually, and that HSV-1 is usually not: in most countries the prevalence of HSV-1 antibodies rises rapidly with age from birth, whereas the prevalence of HSV-2 antibodies increases with age only after the usual age of puberty.[19] Also, individuals with evidence of HSV-2 infection tend to have multiple sexual partners.[19]

The herpes simplex viruses are large DNA viruses. In infected cells, their genetic material is produced and organized in the nucleus, the virions acquire an envelope by budding through the nuclear membrane, and the complete virus particles are released by cell lysis. HSV-2 often infects the epithelial cells of the cervix; and it may remain in a latent state in the sacral dorsal root ganglion, and be periodically reactivated, resulting in repeated epithelial insults. Theoretically, therefore, this virus is in a position to affect changes in the genetic material of the same cells from which cervical neoplasms probably arise.

Attempts to induce cervical neoplasia in experimental animals by infection of the cervix with whole HSV-2 virus have met with only limited success. Dysplasia and invasive carcinomas developed in mice in whose vaginas were inserted cotton tampons saturated with HSV-2 that had been inactivated by formalin or ultraviolet light (to reduce mortality due to acute infection).[20] However, none of the 129 monkeys that had received repeated inoculations of live HSV-2 into the epithelium of their cervices developed carcinomas, although 13 developed cellular atypia.[21]

Other experimental studies, however, have clearly shown HSV-2 to have oncogenic potential. These studies have recently been reviewed by Rapp and Jenkins.[22] Hamster embryo fibroblasts have been transformed morphologically by HSV-2 viruses that have been inactivated photo-dynamically or by ultraviolet light, the transformed cells have resulted in the development of tumors when injected into newborn hamsters, and antibodies against HSV-2 have been detected in serum from these affected animals. Human embryonic lung cells, chicken embryo fibroblasts, and cell lines derived from rats, hamsters and humans, have also been transformed by growth with HSV-2 at high temperatures (to reduce the cytopathic effect of the virus).

Studies of transformed hamster cell lines have shown the transformed cells to contain fragments of HSV-2 DNA, but not the entire viral genome, suggesting that only a portion of the viral DNA is needed for maintenance of the transformed cells. Also, it has been shown that only certain DNA fragments are necessary to induce transformation of rodent cells, and that cells so transformed can produce tumors when injected into nude and newborn mice. Thus, if HSV-2 does produce cervical neoplasms in humans, production of incomplete virions that do not cause acute lesions and cell lysis could be involved.

Seroepidemiologic Studies

A large number of case-control studies have been conducted in which serologic tests have been used to attempt to distinguish women with and without a prior HSV-2 infection. A variety of neutralization tests to measure HSV-2 antibodies have been developed and utilized in these studies. Unfortunately, HSV-1 and HSV-2 share some common antigens and exhibit a degree of cross-reactivity in all assays. Therefore, none of the tests that have been used in these studies distinguish women who have previously been infected with HSV-2 from those who have not with 100 percent sensitivity or specificity. Such women with prior HSV-2 infections have been misclassified as not having been infected and some uninfected women have erroneously been considered previously infected.

Because the magnitude of this misclassification undoubtedly varies according to the tests used, and because the actual prevalence rates of HSV-1 and HSV-2 antibodies vary among normal population, comparisons of prevalence rates of HSV-2 antibodies observed in different case-control studies are of little value.

Prevalence rates of HSV-2 antibodies in cases and controls are used to estimate relative risks of cervical neoplasia (risks in women with HSV-2 antibodies relative to rates in women without such antibodies). If the degree of misclassification as to prior exposure to HSV-2 is the same for cases and controls, then, if there is really no association between cervical neoplasia and HSV-2, spuriously elevated relative risks will *not* be observed. If there is a real association, misclassification of those previously infected will result in underestimation of the true relative risks. However, the magnitude of this error is sufficiently small that comparisons of relative risks from different studies can be meaningful.

The results of serologic case-control studies, when compared in this way, are remarkably consistent. These have been summarized in several different reviews.[1,23,24,25] Nearly all studies show relative risks of cervical neoplasia to be elevated in women with HSV-2 antibodies. These include investigations conducted in countries and racial groups with markedly varying risks of cervical cancer.

The magnitude of the relative risks have consistently been found to vary with the severity of the cervical lesion.[25] Relative risks of invasive cervical cancer are the highest, those of carcinoma in-situ somewhat smaller, those of severe dysplasia smaller yet, and those of mild dysplasia or atypia the least elevated.

One possible interpretation of the results of these serologic studies is that women with cervical neoplasia suffer either primary or recurrent infections with HSV-2 more frequently than other women. Three lines of evidence argue against this hypothesis. One is that women with cervical cancer do not have increased rates of clinical genital herpes. Another is that one case-control study[25] showed the relative risk of both carcinoma in-situ and dysplasia in women with HSV-2 antibodies to be greater for women with an early than late first pregnancy. Since age at first pregnancy was probably related to age at first intercourse in the population in which that study was conducted, this observation suggests that exposure to HSV-2 probably occurred prior to the onset of cervical neoplasia (and also that the young cervix may be particularly vulnerable to the carcinogenic effects of HSV-2). Finally, two prospective studies have shown subsequent rates of dysplasia[26,27] and carcinoma in-situ[26] to be higher in women with than without virological[27] or serological[26,27] evidence of infection with HSV-2. Although based on small numbers, these results strongly suggest that HSV-2 infection preceded the neoplasia.

Another interpretation of the results of serologic investigations (which is applicable to the prospective as well as the case-control studies) is that HSV-2 and cervical neoplasia are not causally related, and that they are statistically associated only because of their common mode of venereal transmission. If this is true, then controlling for differences in sexual behavior between cases and controls would result in estimates of relative risks in relation to HSV-2 antibodies close to one. This was not found in three case-control studies,[23,25,28] in which reasonable attempts were made to control for a number of sexual variables. Melnick et al.[23] reported values for relative risks of cervical carcinoma (largely in-situ) in whites of 2.3 and 1.8, and in blacks of 2.7 and 2.6 after controlling for age at first intercourse and number of sex partners, respectively; Thomas and Rawls[25] found relative risks of 1.9 and 2.0 for carcinoma in-situ and dysplasia, respectively, after controlling simultaneously for 12 different variables, including premarital conception of first child, marital dissolution, and husband with previous marriages; and Graham et al.[28] found relative risks of carcinoma in-situ of 2.5 and 1.6, and relative risks of invasive disease of 3.3 and 3.6, in women with one and more than one sexual partner, respectively. In addition, after controlling for the possible confounding influence of HSV-2 antibodies, Graham et al.[28] found multiple sexual partners *not* to be a risk factor; and Thomas and Rawls[25] found HSV-2 antibodies to be the only one of 13 variables considered that was associated with carcinoma in-situ after simultaneously adjusting relative risks associated with each of the 13 factors for the possible confounding effects of all the others using a linear regression model. These findings provide strong evidence that the association between HSV-2 and cervical cancer is not a spurious one due to the confounding effect of sexual variables.

A third interpretation of the results of seroepidemiological studies is that the association between HSV-2 and cervical neoplasia is causal. This is supported by virologic studies which have successfully demonstrated viral components and products in human cervical cancer cells, and antibodies against these products in serum from cervical cancer patients.

Virologic Studies

The results of these types of studies have been summarized in recent reviews.[22,29] A number of early viral antigens have been identified. Aurelian et al.[30] detected an HSV-2-induced antigen in cervical cancer tissue, which they called AG-4, and which was found to be antigenically identical to IPC-10, an early viral antigen detected in infected hamster embryo cells grown in tissue culture. Melnick et al.[31] isolated a non-structural protein from HSV-2 infected cells, which they called VP-134. Others[32,33] have reported what was termed an HSV-tumor-associated antigen (HSV-TAA). Studies have consistently shown a high proportion of women with cervical neoplasia to have antibodies against these antigens, and both tumor-free women and women with non-cervical neoplasms to infrequently have such antibodies.

Another antigen, called AG-e, and consisting of two viral proteins (ICP-12 and ICP-13) has been described[34] that stimulated cell mediated immunity and is reactive with lymphocytes from a high proportion of cervical cancer patients, but only a low percentage of controls.

In cells infected with HSV-2, the ICP-10 protein appears in the cytoplasm and perinuclear region before the whole virus is assembled. It may be a surface protein for the complete virion. ICP-10 antibodies can only be detected early in persons acutely infected with HSV-2, presumably because they are IgM antibodies produced in response to stimulation by the viral surface protein. After about four days, when the complete virion is formed, antibodies against the complete HSV-2 virion appear, and those against ICP-10 are no longer present.[29] Since AG-4 and ICP-10 are closely related, or identical, and since AG-4 is present in women with cervical neoplasia, it appears that cervical neoplasia may be related to infection characterized by the production of incomplete virions, and in particular with production of viral surface protein. If incomplete virion production is indicative of the presence in the infected cell of incomplete viral DNA, then these findings are consistent with the observations in tissue culture systems that only certain fragments of DNA are necessary for cell transformation and their maintenance in a transformed state.

Furthermore, AG-4 appears to be associated with tumor progression in humans. The prevalence of antibodies against AG-4 are lowest in women with mild dysplasia, higher in women with more severe dysplasia, higher yet in women with carcinoma in-situ, and highest in women with Stage I invasive carcinomas.[29] In addition, AG-4 antibodies disappear in cases following surgical removal of their tumor, and reappear in conjunction with tumor recurrences. Also, AG-4 antibodies increase following radiation therapy, perhaps in response to the presence of incomplete virions that are released from cells damaged by the treatment. The prevalence of AG-4 antibodies is, however, lower in women with Stage II or III than Stage I disease. The reason for this is conjectural, but a compromised immune response due to advanced disease could explain this inconsistent finding.

One group of investigators[35] showed more cases of cervical cancer than normal controls to have antibodies against two different proteins derived from HSV-2. This group also reported that the production of one of these proteins is governed by the same fragment of HSV-2 DNA that can induce conversion of rodent cells in tissue culture.

Using indirect immunofluorescence techniques, several investigators have demonstrated the presence of HSV-2 antigens in exfoliated cervical cancer cells[36,37] and tissue slices from cervical dysplasia and carcinoma.[38] Royston and Aurelian[36] found antigens only in exfoliated neoplastic cervical cells, and not in normal cells from the same patients, or in cells from tumor-free women or women with other neoplasms. The percentage of women in whose cervical cells HSV-2 antigens were demonstrated was found by Pasca et al.[37] to be 94 percent, 65 percent and 9 percent for women with invasive cancer, dysplasia, and normal cervices, respectively; and Dreesman et al.[38] found these percentages in women with carcinoma (in-situ or invasive), severe dysplasia, moderate dysplasia, mild dysplasia, metaplasia, and normal cervices to be 40 percent, 36 percent, 10 percent, 3 percent, 4 percent and 0 percent, respectively.

Using in-situ nucleic acid hybridization techniques, several groups of investigators[39,40,41,42] have demonstrated HSV-2 RNA sequences in cervical cells from patients with carcinoma or dysplasia.

Finally, using molecular hybridization, one group of investigators[43] detected DNA fragments that were homologous to HSV-2 DNA in one cervical cancer specimen. Others[44,45] have failed to confirm these findings, but, as noted by Rapp and Jenkins,[22] this could be due to the low sensitivity of the hybridization techniques used, which would be a particular problem if (as expected) only a small portion of the HSV-2 genome is present in the neoplastic cells.

Summary

In summary, the evidence that HSV-2 is a cause of cervical cancer is strong. The virus has oncogenic potential in experimental systems; its venereal mode of transmission is compatible with the epidemiologic features of cervical carcinoma; it produces latent infection; it can infect the tissues from which cervical neoplasms arise;

and individuals with serologic and virologic evidence of HSV-2 infection are at increased risk of cervical neoplasia.

It is likely that the development of cervical cancer is related to the incomplete production of HSV-2 virions in cervical cells. This hypothesis is supported by a number of independent observations. Only fragments of HSV-2 DNA are needed to transform cells in tissue culture and maintain them in a transformed state; various early viral antigens (but not whole viruses) have been demonstrated in cervical cancer cells (but not in normal cells from cases or controls); antibodies against these antigens have been demonstrated in a high proportion of cervical cancer cases but less frequently in normal women and women with other neoplasms; the production of one antigenic viral protein was reported by one group to be governed by the same portion of HSV-2 DNA that can induce conversion of rodent cells in tissue culture; and both DNA and RNA fragments homologous to portions of the HSV-2 genome have been demonstrated in cervical cancer cells. The production of only incomplete virions in women with cervical cancer could (along with the insensitivity of the available serologic tests) also explain why HSV-2 neutralizing antibodies are not present in all women with cervical cancer.

Additional work needs to be done to confirm some of these observations, and to characterize more specifically the portion(s) of the HSV-2 genome that are responsible for these findings. Evidence that HSV-2 is a cause of cervical cancer would be particularly strong if the HSV-2 DNA and RNA fragments that have been identified in cervical cancer cells by hybridization techniques, those that induce one or more of the early viral antigens that have been identified in women with cervical cancer, and those that transform cells in tissue culture, are confirmed to be the same or closely related.

OTHER INFECTIOUS AGENTS

There are causes of dysplasia other than HSV-2, and it is reasonable to ask whether dysplastic lesions of non-herpetic etiology are also precursors of carcinoma. A number of differing features of women with dysplasia and carcinoma suggest that they are not.

The seroepidemiologic features of dysplasia and carcinoma differ. A case-control study by Thomas and Rawls[25] showed evidence of *Trichomonas vaginalis* on histologic slides, and antibodies against adenoviruses and *Mycoplasma pneumoniae* (as well as a history of vaginal discharge) to be most strongly related to mild dysplasia, less strongly related to severe dysplasia, and most weakly related to carcinoma in-situ. They also found risk of dysplasia, but not carcinoma in-situ to be related to antibodies against cytomegalovirus; and the relative risk of dysplasia increased more strongly than that of carcinoma in-situ with the number of different organisms by which a woman had previously been infected (including HSV-2, cytomegalovirus, *M. pneumoniae*, trichomonads, and adenovirus). Others have also reported associations between cervical atypia and CMV antibodies,[46] and between atypia[47] or dysplasia[48] and *Chlamydia trachomatis* antibodies. A recent case-control study[48] also showed the latter antibodies to be more prevalent in a mixed group of patients with varying degrees of dysplasia, carcinoma in-situ, and microinvasive carcinoma, than in a control group.

The human papillomavirus, that causes condyloma acuminata, can infect the cervix, where it causes flat lesions that have the histologic appearance of dysplasia. Intracellular viral particles have been identified in electron micrographs of these lesions, and intracellular viral antigens have been demonstrated using immunofluorescent techniques. However, the percentage of lesions that stain positive decreases with the severity of the lesion, and carcinomas only rarely have evidence of papillomavirus.[49]

It thus appears that dysplasia is a non-specific response of the cervical epithelium to infection by a variety of organisms, probably including, in addition to HSV-2, cytomegalovirus, trichomonads, *Chlamydia trachomatis,* and papillomavirus. That prior infections with these agents are less strongly related or unrelated to carcinoma, suggest that dysplasias caused by them are not precursors of cervical cancer. On the other hand, the prevalence of HSV-2 and AG-4 antibodies, and of AG-4 antigens in cervical cells, all increase with the severity of the lesion, suggesting that those dysplastic lesions of HSV-2 origin are the ones that progress. Although epidemiologic studies based on data obtained from interviews[18,50,51] have shown women with cervical dysplasia and carcinoma to be similarly characterized by early ages at first marriage and intercourse, multiple sexual partners, parity and non-use of barrier methods of contraception, these observations are likely due to the common sexual mode of transmission of HSV-2 and the various other causes of dysplasia.

PROSPECTUS

The most likely sequence of events in the genesis of cervical cancer is that exposure to HSV-2 is followed by an infection involving the stem cells in the transition zone of the cervix. Incomplete viral genomes, rather than complete virions, are produced, which are replicated along with the infected cells. The viral DNA in the cells in some way prevents them from undergoing normal differentiation, and as they proliferate they develop first into mildly dysplastic lesions. With the passage of time, less differentiation occurs, the dysplasia becomes more severe, and eventually carcinoma in-situ results. After a number of years, the proliferating carcinomatous cells eventually penetrate the basement membrane of the cervical epithelium, resulting in invasive cervical carcinoma.

If HSV-2 is a cause of cervical cancer, it may or may not be a necessary cause. In some studies, close to 100 percent of the cases have some evidence of HSV-2 infection, and if those cases that are not classified as having been infected are erroneously so designated due to the insensitivity of the tests that were employed, then HSV-2 could be a necessary causal agent. Studies based on better methods to identify individuals with prior evidence of HSV-2 infection will hopefully eventually clarify whether all cases of cervical cancer have been infected by HSV-2.

HSV-2 is certainly not a sufficient cause. Most women who are infected with HSV-2 do not develop cervical cancer. Other factors undoubtedly play a role. One mechanism by which these could operate is to somehow cause the production of incomplete HSV-2 virions in infected cells. Factors that would do this are unknown.

They might be related to age, which could explain the possible vulnerability of the young cervix to cervical carcinogenesis. Nutritional factors might play a role, which could explain the relationship of cervical cancer to Vitamin A intake that has been postulated;[52] and recent studies linking smoking to cervical cancer[18,50,53,54] suggest that chemicals could be involved.

Additional studies are needed to clarify the role of HSV-2 in the genesis of cervical cancer. In addition to those already mentioned, these include follow-up studies to measure lesion progression in women with dysplasias of varying etiologies (including HSV-2), and studies to determine the conditions under which infection by HSV-2 leads to incomplete production of the viral genome.

Although one cannot state with certainty that HSV-2 causes cervical cancer, the evidence that it does is strong, and other organisms that have so far been considered are much less likely to play a causal role.

REFERENCES

1. Cramer DW: Uterine Cervix. In Schottenfeld D, Fraumeni JF (eds): Cancer Epidemiology and Prevention. Philadelphia, WB Saunders Co., 1982.
2. Waterhouse J, Muir C, Shanmugaratnam K, et al: Cancer Incidence in Five Continents, Volume IV. Lyon, IARC Scientific Publication No. 42, 1982.
3. Lilienfeld AM, Levin ML, Kessler II: Cancer in the United States. Cambridge, Harvard University Press, 1972.
4. Devesa SS, Diamond EL: Association of breast cancer and cervical cancer incidences with income and education among whites and blacks. JNCI 65:515, 1980.
5. Beral V: Cancer of the cervix: a sexually transmitted infection? Lancet 2:1037, 1974.
6. Skegg DCG, Corwin PA, Paul C: Importance of the male factor in cancer of the cervix. Lancet 2:581, 1982.
7. Yule R: Mortality from carcinoma of the cervix. Lancet 1:1031, 1978.
8. Anello C, Lao C: U.S. trends in mortality from carcinoma of the cervix. Lancet 1:1038, 1979.
9. Chang AR, Hudson DG: Trends in the incidence and age at diagnosis of carcinoma of the cervix over a twenty-year period. Proceedings of the University of Otago Medical School, Dunedin, N.Z., Volume 59, No. 1, 12–13, 1980.
10. Armstrong B, Holman D: Increasing mortality from cancer of the cervix in young Australian women. Med J Aust 1:460, 1981.
11. Gao YT, Tu JT, Jin F et al: Cancer mortality in Shanghai during the period 1963–77. Br J Cancer 43:183, 1981.
12. Thomas DB: An epidemiologic study of carcinoma in situ and squamous dysplasia of the uterine cervix. Am J Epidemiol 98:10, 1973.
13. Kessler II: Venereal factors in human cervical cancer. Cancer 39:1912, 1977.
14. Smith PG, Kinlen LJ, White GC, et al: Mortality of wives of men dying with cancer of the penis. Br J Cancer 41:422, 1980.
15. Graham S, Priore R, Graham M, et al: Genital cancer in wives of penile cancer patients. Cancer 44:1870, 1979.
16. Martinez I: Relationship of squamous cell carcinoma of the cervix to squamous cell carcinoma of the penis. Cancer 24:777, 1969.
17. Buckley JD, Harris RWC, Doll R, et al: Case-control study of the husbands of women with dysplasia or carcinoma of the cervix uteri. Lancet 2:1010, 1981.

18. Harris RWC, Brinton LA, Cowdell RH, et al: Characteristics of women with dysplasia or carcinoma in situ of the cervix uteri. Br J Cancer 42:359, 1980.

19. Rawls WE, Campione-Piccardo J: Epidemiology of herpes simples virus type-1 and type-2 infections. Department of Pathology, McMaster University, Hamilton, Ontario, Canada, 1981.

20. Wentz WB, Reagan JW, Heggie AD, et al: Induction of uterine cancer with activated herpes simples virus, types 1 and 2. Cancer: 48:1783, 1981.

21. Palmer AE, London WT, Nahmias AJ, et al: A preliminary report on investigation of oncogenic potential of herpes simples virus type-2 in cebus monkeys. Cancer Research 36:807, 1976.

22. Rapp F, Jenkins FJ: Genital cancer and viruses. Gyn Oncology 12:S25, 1981.

23. Melnick JL, Adam E, Rawls WE: The causative role of herpesvirus type-2 in cervical cancer. Cancer 34:1375, 1974.

24. Melnick JL, Adam E: Epidemiological approaches to determining whether herpesvirus is the etiological agent of cervical cancer. Prog Exp Tumor Res 21:49, 1978.

25. Thomas DB, Rawls WE: Relationship of herpes simplex virus type-2 antibodies and squamous dysplasia to cervical carcinoma in situ. Cancer 42:2716, 1978.

26. Catalano LW, Johnson LD: Herpesvirus antibody and carcinoma in situ of the cervix. J Am Med Assoc 217:447, 1971.

27. Nahmias AJ, Naib ZM, Josey WE, et al: Prospective studies of the association of genital herpes simplex infection and cervical anaplasia. Cancer Research 33:1491, 1973.

28. Graham S, Rawls W, Swanson M et al: Sex partners and herpes simplex virus type-2 in the epidemiology of cancer of the cervix. Am J Epidemiol 115:729, 1982.

29. Aurelian L, Kessler II, Rosenshein NB et al: Viruses and gynecologic cancers: herpesvirus protein (ICP10/AG-4), a cervical tumor antigen that fulfills the criteria for a marker of carcinogenicity. Cancer 48:455, 1981.

30. Aurelian L, Schumann B, Marcus RL, et al: Antibodies to HSV-2 induced tumor specific antigens in serums from patients with cervical carcinomas. Science 181:161, 1973.

31. Melnick JL, Courtney RJ, Powell KL, et al: Studies on herpes simplex virus and cancer. Cancer Research 36:845, 1976.

32. Notter MFD, Docherty JJ: Comparative diagnostic aspects of herpes simplex virus tumor-associated antigens. J Natl Cancer Inst 57:438, 1976.

33. Hollingshead AC, Chretien PB, Lee O, et al: In vivo and in vitro measurements of the relationship of human squamous carcinomas to herpes simplex virus tumor-associated antigens. Cancer Research 36:821, 1976.

34. Bell RB, Aurelian L, Cohen GH: Proteins of herpesvirus type-2. IV. Leukocyte inhibition responses to type common antigen(s) in cervix cancer and recurrent herpetic infections. Cell Immunol 41:86, 1978.

35. Gilman SC, Docherty JJ, Clark A, et al: Reaction patterns of herpes simplex virus type-1 and type-2 proteins with sera of patients with uterine cervical carcinoma and matched controls. Cancer Research 40:4640, 1980.

36. Royston I, Aurelian L: Immunofluorescent detection of herpes simplex virus antigens in exfoliated cells from human cervical carcinoma. Proc Natl Acad Sci, USA 67:204, 1970.

37. Pasca AS, Kummerländer L, Pejtsik B, et al: Herpes simplex virus-specific antigens in exfoliated cervical cells from women with and without cervical anaplasia. Cancer Research 36:2130, 1976.

38. Dreesman GR, Burek J, Adam E, et al: Expression of herpesvirus-induced antigens in human cervical cancer. Nature 283:591, 1980.

39. Jones KW, Fenoglio CM, Shevchuk-Chaban M, et al: Detection of herpes simplex virus type-2 m RNA in human cervical biopsies by in-situ cytological hybridization. In de Thé

G, Henle W, Rapp F (eds): Oncogenesis and Herpesviruses, III. Lyon, IARC, 1978.

40. MacDougall JK, Galloway DA, Fenoglio CM: Cervical carcinoma: detection of herpes simplex virus RNA in cells undergoing neoplastic change. Int J Cancer 25:1, 1980.

41. Eglin RP, Sharp F, MacLean AB, et al: Detection of RNA complementary to herpes simplex virus DNA in human cervical squamous cell neoplasms. Cancer Research 41:3597, 1981.

42. Maitland NJ, Kinross JH, Busuttil A, et al: The detection of DNA tumour virus-specific RNA sequences in abnormal human cervical biopsies by in-situ hybridization. J Gen Virol 55:123, 1981.

43. Frenkel M, Roizman B, Cassai E, et al: A DNA fragment of herpes simplex 2 and its transcription in human cervical cancer tissue. Proc Natl Acad Sci, USA 69:3784, 1972.

44. Cassai E, Rotola A, Meneguzzi G, et al: Herpes simples virus and human cancer. I. Relationship between human cervical tumours and herpes simplex type-2. Europ J Cancer 17:68, 1981.

45. ZurHausen H, Schulte-Holthausen H, Wolf H, et al: Attempts to detect virus-specific DNA in human tumors. II. Nucleic acid hybridization with complementary RNA of human herpes group viruses. Natl J Cancer 13:657, 1974.

46. Pasca AS, Kummerländer L, Pejtsik B, et al: Herpesvirus antibodies and antigens in patients with cervical anaplasia and in controls. J Natl Cancer Inst 55:775, 1975.

47. Paavonen J, Vesterinen E, Meyer B: Genital Chlamydia trachomatis infections in patients with cervical atypia. Obstet Gynecol 54:289, 1979.

48. Schachter J, Hill EC, King EB, et al: Chlamydia trachomatis and cervical neoplasia. J Am Med Assoc 248:2134, 1982.

49. ZurHausen H: Human papillomaviruses and their possible role in squamous cell carcinoma. Curr Top Microbiol Immunol 78:1, 1977.

50. Wright NH, Vessey MP, Kenward B, et al: Neoplasia and dysplasia of the cervix uteri and contraception: A possible protective effect of the diaphragm. Br J Cancer 38:273, 1978.

51. Ory H, Naib Z, Conger SB, et al: Contraceptive choice and prevalence of cervical dysplasia and carcinoma in situ. Am J Obstet Gynecol 124:573, 1976.

52. Wynder EL: Epidemiology of carcinoma in situ of the cervix. Obstet Gynecol Surv 24:697, 1969.

53. Stellman SD, Austin H, Wynder EL: Cervix cancer and cigarette smoking: A case-control study. Am J Epidemiol 111:383, 1980.

54. Clarke EA, Morgan RW, Newman AM: Smoking as a risk factor in cancer of the cervix: Additional evidence from a case-control study. Am J Epidemiol 115:59, 1982.

3 The Staging and Surgical Therapy of Cervical Carcinoma

James A. Roberts
George W. Morley

In 1983, it is estimated that 16,000 women will be diagnosed as having invasive cervical cancer, thus making it the sixth most common cancer afflicting women and accounting for 3.7 percent of all cancers seen in women.[1] At the same time, it is estimated that 44 percent or 7000 of these women will die of this disease, making it the fifth most common cause of cancer related deaths in women. However, improvement in therapeutic modalities and detection in earlier stages has resulted in a decline in both of these rates over the past five decades. Thus it would appear that the war against this disease has been successful until one considers that routine cervical cytology should eliminate this disease completely.

CERVICAL CYTOLOGY

In 1941 Papanicolaou and Traut[2] reported on the success they had in detecting cervical cancer by evaluating the exfoliated cells present in vaginal smears. Their technique called for the evaluation of cells present in the vaginal pool. It was soon realized that this technique resulted in an unacceptably high false negative rate. Ayre later devised a wooden spatula that would allow one to obtain cells directly from the

Supported in part by Junior Clinical Faculty Fellowship from the American Cancer Society cervix itself. This device provided a more readable and representative sample of the neoplastic activity present in the cervix. However, false negative rates continued to be reported in the range of 30–50 percent.[3,4] Rylander[5] reviewed the negative cervical smears of 56 women found to have invasive cervical cancer. She identified two sources of error to explain these false negative smears: (1) cytological interpretation and (2) sampling. Kern and Zivolich[6] evaluated the reproducibility of histologic classification of cytologic smears and found that the overall concurrence rate between cytology and histology was 78 percent. When the slides were reread by the same cytologist, the cytologic classification was reproduced in over 90 percent of cases. Thus it would appear that the false negative rate due to cytologic interpretation should be quite low. A feature not reviewed in their work was that of fatigue. Sandmire et al.[7] reviewed 40,000 consecutive smears and found a significant neoplasia rate of only one lesion per 400 cytologic specimens. Under such circumstances one would expect the dulling of diagnostic accuracy. Therefore they stress the need for establishing strict quality control programs to minimize the occurrence of these errors.

The problem of sampling errors has been reviewed by several groups. Many adaptations of the Ayre spatula have been introduced to overcome this problem. Since the majority of neoplastic lesions arising in the cervix occur at the squamocolumnar junction, these designs are intended to collect cells from this area. In the young patient where this junction is on the ectocervix, there is little problem in obtaining a satisfactory specimen. However, in women where this junction has receded into the endocervical canal, either as a result of the natural cervical aging or artificial changes induced by surgery, cryotherapy, cautery, or laser therapy, the endocervix must be sampled. The modified spatulae which are available do not always provide such a specimen. Shingleton et al.[8] and Johansen et al.[9] evaluated the contribution of endocervical smears to the accuracy of cervical cytology. They reported an increase in accuracy when the traditional ectocervical sample and an endocervical swab sample are combined. It was found that a high rate of unsatisfactory swab specimens were obtained when a dry swab was used. Therefore, when this technique is employed, the swab should be premoistened with saline. It has been suggested that cells obtained with a swab will become entangled in the cotton fibers and not be released to the slide. This can be overcome by obtaining the specimen employing a clockwise rotation of the swab and applying it to the slide using a counterclockwise rotation.

Several manufacturers have developed spatulae which will function as endocervical aspirators to provide an endocervical specimen. While these cost more than a cotton swab, Shingleton et al.[8] suggest that they provide little or no improvement over the moistened swab.

In order to provide the cytologists with the best possible specimen and thus decrease the chance of a false negative smear, one must: (1) sample the squamocolumnar junction, (2) apply the ectocervical and swab specimen to two different slides, and (3) be certain that the smearing and fixation are done promptly.[10] As a check for the completeness of sampling, the cytologists should observe and report on the presence of endocervical cells.

Another disturbing fact is the relatively high rate of false negative cytologic smears in women with frankly invasive cancer. This can be a result of a number of factors, i.e., massive infection, bleeding, etc. Therefore, if a cervix is found to have a visible lesion on it, a biopsy of that lesion *must* be done regardless of what the cytological screening demonstrates.

A great deal of debate has been generated by the recently released American Cancer Society guidelines on cervical cytology.[11] This has centered around the frequency that such specimens should be collected. Before considering this, it is important to point out that while it seems that this screening test should decrease the incidence of cervical cancer, there is no randomized prospective study which proves this. Data reported in the Walton Report[12] show that a decrease in the incidence of cervical cancer has been seen in Canada but that this was occurring before cytological screening began. Fruchter et al.[13] reported that "between 1960 and 1975, the number of new cases of invasive cervical cancer did not decrease significantly despite a fourfold increase in preinvasive cancer." Further, a study of the population in San Diego by Martin[14] concludes "that while many individual invasive cervical cancers appear to be preventable, in general this disease cannot be considered completely preventable." Therefore, while it seems obvious that this test should play a large role in the early detection and diagnosis of cervical cancer, this has not been scientifically proven.

Since the introduction of cytological screening, most sources have recommended that a smear be obtained annually. This remained unchallenged until the publication of the most recent American Cancer Society cancer screening guidelines.[11] Their recommendation is that once a woman has had two consecutive negative annual smears, it is unnecessary to repeat a cytologic smear more often than every three years unless she were considered to be at high risk for developing cervical cancer. This recommendation is based on the Walton Report[12] and the Society's own medicoeconomic evaluation of cervical cytology.

One of the benefits of cervical cytology was that it allowed one to detect asymptomatic preinvasive cervical neoplasia. With large screening programs, one could detail the natural history of this disease from its earliest form to advanced cancer. Using this data the Walton Report concluded that it took an average of 35 years for an in situ lesion to become invasive. This length is in sharp contrast to the 10 year period which many, such as Fidler et al.,[15] suggest when using the same methods to determine natural history. Earlier works reported prospective evaluations of women progressing from carcinoma in situ to invasive cancer, and they seem to support the 10 year natural history rather than the much longer 35 years. While it would seem that this large variation in the length of the natural history of cervical cancer would have a strong influence on the outcome of a medicoeconomic evaluation for the ideal frequency for obtaining cervical cytology, this is not the case. Such diverse sources as Schneider and Twiggs[16] at the University of Michigan and the British National Health Service have used this shorter duration and found it to be cost efficient to repeat cytological smears every three years. This entire debate on frequency becomes a moot point when one considers how infrequently the average woman obtains a pap smear.[17]

When making recommendations about the frequency in which cervical cytology should be obtained, it is always stated that those who are at high risk should be screened more frequently. There are several conditions which are said to place a woman in this group, the most important of which are sexual exposure at a young age (generally before age 18) and exposure to genital herpes. Low socioeconomic status has been said also to be a high risk factor; however, Nealon and Christopherson[18] reported a study of 96,600 women of low socioeconomic status under the age of 21, and they found no cases of carcinoma in situ or invasive cancer. This report would tend to downplay the importance of the socioeconomic factor. It has also been suggested that circumcision status of marital partners is of importance, but work by Terris, Wilson and Nelson[19] found no difference in cervical cancer rates when this factor was evaluated. Finally, oral contraceptives have possibly allowed changes in sexual habits which could result in an increased incidence of cervical cancer, but when looked at as an independent factor, there is no difference in the rates of cervical cancer between those on oral contraceptives and a control group.[20,21]

Once it is found that a woman has abnormal cytology, it must be remembered that this is merely a screening test and not a diagnostic procedure even though the cytology report may give a histological diagnosis. Thus, under no circumstances should a woman ever be treated on the basis of a cytological specimen alone. Once such a cytologic report is obtained there are two diagnostic procedures available: (1) colposcopy and directed biopsies or (2) cervical conization.

Colposcopy

Colposcopy was introduced in 1925 by Hinselman to study the morphological features of various cervical diseases. This technique quickly gained wide acceptance in Europe. At first it was used as a method for screening patients for cervical disease. While the cost and training required to do colposcopy have resulted in cervical cytology replacing it as a screening technique, colposcopy is still used as such in some areas. Acceptance of this procedure was much slower in North America. There was great concern that serious disease would be misdiagnosed. However, several groups showed a very high correlation between colposcopically directed biopsies obtained from women found to be satisfactory for this exam, i.e., the entire squamocolumnar junction is seen, when compared to cervical cone biopsy or hysterectomy diagnoses (Table 3-1).[22-27] When invasive cancer was present the correlation rate reported was generally greater than 99 percent. Thus the fears surrounding this procedure were resolved and colposcopy has become an invaluable tool for evaluating patients with abnormal cervical cytology.

At the present time women presenting to the University of Michigan with abnormal ctology are managed as shown in Figure 3-1. Prior to the use of colposcopy, all women with abnormal cytology were required to undergo cervical conization in order to diagnose the cause of this abnoramlity. With colposcopy, less than 10 per-

Table 3-1. The Percent of Patients Having a Colposcopically Directed Biopsy Diagnosis Confirmed by Cervical Cone or Hysterectomy

Author	Number of Patients	% Correlation
Benedet et al.[22]	620	87
Kirkup and Hill[23]	201	98
Savage[24]	50	96
Cecchini et al.[25]	107	83
Knutzen and Sherwood[26]	150	93
Hovadhanakuletal et al.[27]	100	94

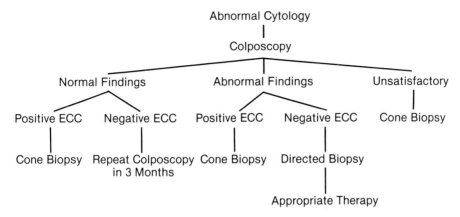

Fig. 3-1.   The approach taken at the University of Michigan to evaluate a woman with abnormal cervical cytology (ECC = endocervical curettage)

cent of those now seen require cervical conization. This has resulted in a large reduction in cost and morbidity borne by those so treated. As noted in the scheme, it is imperative that an endocervical curettage be performed on all patients undergoing colposcopic evaluation.[28] In several cases where this procedure was deleted and therapy administered, serious and fatal recurrences have been encountered.[29,30]

Since colposcopy allows one to identify the most severely affected area of the normal appearing cervix, those women with a grossly obvious lesion are not candidates for colposcopy. Rather, they should simply undergo a punch biopsy of the cervix to diagnosis their condition.

Directed biopsies are an important part of the colposcopic evaluation but the pregnant patient presents a special situation where biopsies may result in excessive bleeding and possible abortion. Thus rather than subjecting the woman to this risk, a biopsy is often not performed but rather frequent reevaluations with the colposcope are indicated with a standard evaluation being performed postpartum.[31]

Cervical Cone Biopsy

Prior to the introduction of colposcopy, the only way to evaluate an abnormal cervical cytology was with cervical cone biopsy. Thus the frequency with which this procedure has been performed has greatly decreased. The major diagnostic use of cone biopsy is in those with unsatisfactory colposcopy or those with a lesion in the endocervical canal. The diagnostic accuracy of this procedure has been documented by numerous reports. Van Nagell et al.[32] reported the results of 756 women subjected to cone biopsy. They found a correlation between cytology and cone biopsy in 86 percent of women with cervical intraepithelial neoplasia grade 3 (CIN III) while this correlation was 75 percent in those with invasive cancer. When random biopsies were done the correlations were 77 and 29 percent, respectively.

The major drawback besides the high cost of cone biopsy over colposcopy is the complication rate. While colposcopy is nearly free of complications, van Nagell et al.[32] report major postconization complications requiring hospitalization in 3.4 percent of nonpregnant women and in 7.5 percent of pregnant women. These included heavy bleeding, uterine perforation, pelvic infection and pregnancy loss.

At the University of Michigan, cervical cone biopsy has been used mainly as a therapeutic tool. In those patients with extensive CIN III lesions which would be poorly treated by cryotherapy or laser ablation, a cone biopsy, whose limits have been tailored by the colposcopic findings, is used as treatment. Such an approach allows one to obtain adequate surgical margins while sparing the maximum amount of normal tissue. This results in a minimum of postcone complications. The initial experience with this approach seems to confirm the data from New Zealand and Norway,[33-35] i.e., in selected cases the cure rate and recurrence rate are equal to that obtained with hysterectomy.

STAGING

The diagnostic procedures outlined above are needed to evaluate those women who present with subtle asymptomatic lesions. Unfortunately all too often a woman will present with the classic symptoms of bright red, painless, and irregular vaginal bleeding. Upon examining such a patient one will often find a large ulcerative mass replacing the cervix. In these cases, a punch biopsy of the lesion should provide the diagnosis.

Once the diagnosis has been made, the extent of disease is determined and a clinical stage must be assigned (Table 3-2). In order to better understand the strengths and weaknesses of this staging system, one must look at the route of spread of this disease. After a lesion becomes invasive it will generally spread in a lateral direction along the paracervical tissues and cardinal ligaments. In some cases it will spread downward and involve the vagina. In both of these situations different lymphatic drainage becomes involved and thus will affect the stage. However, in four to 17 percent of women the endometrial cavity will become involved.[36,37] This factor is not

Table 3-2. FIGO International Classification of Cervical Carcinoma

Stage 0	Carcinoma in situ, intraepithelial carcinoma
Stage I	Carcinoma strictly confined to the cervix (extension to the corpus should be disregarded)
Stage Ia	Microinvasive carcinoma (early stromal invasion)
Stage Ib	All other cases of stage I. Occult cancer should be marked occ.
Stage II	Carcinoma extends beyond the cervix but has not extended onto the pelvic wall. Carcinoma involves the vagina, but not the lower third
Stage IIa	No obvious parametrial involvement
Stage IIb	Obvious parametrial involvement
Stage III	Carcinoma has extended onto the pelvic wall. On rectal examination there is no cancer-free space between the tumor and the pelvic wall. Tumor involves the lower third of the vagina. All cases with hydronephrosis, or nonfunctioning kidney.
Stage IIIa	No extension onto the pelvic wall
Stage IIIb	Extension to the pelvic wall or hydronephrosis, or nonfunctioning kidney, or both
Stage IV	Carcinoma has extended beyond the true pelvis or has clinically involved the mucosa of the bladder or rectum. Bullous edema as such does not permit a case to be allotted to stage IV.
Stage IVa	Spread of the growth to adjacent organs
Stage IVb	Spread to distant organs

addressed in the staging system in spite of the fact that Perez et al.[38] have shown that this involvement of a different lymphatic drainage does seem to worsen the prognosis. Also not included in the staging system are such factors as tumor size, depth of invasion, and vascular infiltration. All of these variables have been found to affect the outcome of treatment.[39]

Due to its location close to the cervix, the ureter will often become involved. Bosch et al.[40] found this to be the case in 14 percent of untreated cases of cervical cancer. This involvement is found to be at the ureterovesical junction in most cases.[41] Such involvement generally results from external pressure rather than true invasion of the ureter by tumor.[42]

Most distant spread is via the lymphatic spaces which are found within 0.51 mm of the basement membrane.[43] Nodal involvement occurs in an orderly fashion with the external iliac and obturator nodes most commonly involved.[44,45] Following involvement of these nodes the common iliac, paraaortic and finally supraclavicular nodes become involved.

In those cases where the differentiation is particularly poor or the tumor is advanced, blood borne metastases develop. These involve the lung in over 25 percent of cases with liver and bone the next most common sites.[42]

With these factors in mind, it can be seen that bone scans, liver scans, barium enemas, and upper gastrointestinal studies need not be done except in far advanced or poorly differentiated diseases.[46,47] The studies which are most informative and thus should be done are IVP, cystoscopy, sigmoidoscopy, chest x-ray and a careful pelvic examination. The single most important of these is the pelvic exam which van Nagell et al.[48] report is best done with the aid of anesthesia. In spite of the most careful efforts at clinical staging, some 35 percent of patients are found to be incorrectly staged when surgical staging is employed.[49,50]

Since the errors in staging most commonly occur because lymph node spread is not detected, it has been suggested that lymphangiogram be included in the staging procedure. This test is not universally available so it has not been included. In addition, while Piver and Barlow[51] report a high degree of correlation between lymphangiogram and surgical findings, others, including Averette et al.,[52] find that in some stages the correlation between these evaluations is no better than the 50 percent obtained by chance.

STAGING LAPAROTOMY

In an effort to identify these high risk women, several authors have reported the results of pretherapy exploratory laparotomy and lymphadenectomy.[52–63] Initially both pelvic and paraaortic nodes were removed but as experience was gained it became apparent that the nodes of major importance were those located outside the radiated field. It is felt that involvement of these nodes can be equated with systemic disease. This concept seems to be borne out by the work of Welander et al.,[63] who found that in those with paraaortic involvement 54.8 percent developed distant metastases while only 25 percent in the control group did likewise. Due to the anatomical variability of the aortic bifurcation, Berman et al.[61] have suggested that the high common iliac nodes carry a similarly poor prognosis. When the results of these reports are reviewed, it is surprising to find that, regardless of stage, about 25 to 35 percent of women staged surgically had involvement of the paraaortic nodes (in the case of stage IB, only high risk patients were surgically staged). An additional finding was that about 15 percent of women had intraabdominal disease, a route of spread not appreciated in the past. Both of these high risk groups require some alteration in the standard form of therapy in order to afford them a chance for cure.

In those women who were surgically staged, it was found that a very high price was paid in terms of serious complications during treatment with radiation therapy. Berman et al.[61] found that in the 31 women they staged with the transperitoneal approach used by others, 30 percent experienced severe small bowel damage and 7 percent died as a result of this complication. These high morbidity and mortality rates caused most surgeons to abandon this method. The retroperitoneal approach described by Berman et al.[61] has resulted in a morbidity rate of 2.5 percent and a zero mortality rate. Thus, if surgical staging is to be done this approach should be used.

The initial reason to perform surgical staging was to outline the high risk paraaortic node positive group and provide them with therapeutic alterations which would effect a cure. Most authors have found that extending the field of radiation has not significantly increased survival in this group.[64-76] Since paraaortic nodal involvement most likely indicates systemic spread, some form of effective chemotherapy should be given in addition to the radiation therapy. At the present time there is no proven effective chemotherapy for cervical cancer; thus staging laparotomy should be considered a research tool unless one plans to use it to identify this high risk presently incurable group and deliver smaller palliative courses of radiation therapy.

An additional step to the surgical staging has been the addition of a scalene node biopsy. Delgado et al.[68] found that this group of nodes was rarely involved and suggested that sampling this area in all women with cervical cancer was not indicated. However, Lee et al.[69] and Buchsbaum and Lifshitz[76] found that when this area is sampled in those women with proven paraaortic involvement, 30–35 percent were found to be involved with metastatic tumor. Most of these women had no clinical findings to suggest the presence of this involvement. Thus in a selected population, this procedure will provide valuable information about the extent of disease.

RADICAL HYSTERECTOMY

The technique of radical surgical excision of a cancerous cervix has generally been attributed to Wertheim because of his report of its use in 500 cases in 1912.[71] However, reports of this technique by Rumpf, Clark, Kelly, and Reis predate Wertheim's paper by several years. At first this procedure was used for nearly all cases of cervical cancer because no other effective form of therapy existed. Under these circumstances these authors reported operative mortality rates of 15 to 20 percent. This remained the case until radium became available for treating advanced lesions. As technology in radiation therapy improved, it became apparent that this was a far superior way to treat cervical cancer and radical surgery became the treatment for early disease (stage IB and IIA) only.

Over the years even the treatment of early disease with radical surgery was challenged by radiotherapists who felt that radiation provided the best route for cure. This question was settled when Morley and Seski[72] reported the results of a 30-year prospective series comparing these modalities. They found that there was no difference in the rate of survival between these groups. Further, they found that the therapeutic morbidity and mortality were comparable. These findings confirmed the results reported by Newton[73] in a smaller series.

When the group treated with radical surgery is reviewed it is found that the corrected five-year survival rate is 91.3 percent (136/146). When the status of the pelvic lymph nodes is analyzed, it is found that 12.6 percent of those undergoing surgery had nodal involvement. This group had a corrected five-year survival rate of 55.6 percent (10/18) while the node negative group rate was 96 percent (120/125) (p<0.001). The addition of radiation to this group with nodal involvement seems to be of little benefit. These results have been confirmed by several other authors.[74–83]

The presence of the less common adenocarcinoma has generally been associated with a poorer survival rate when compared to squamous cell carcinoma. This has prompted radiotherapists to suggest a surgical treatment and surgeons to consider radiation to be the more favorable approach. In stage IB disease, Morley and Seski[72] found a corrected five-year survival for the squamous lesion of 91.2 percent while the rate for adenocarcinomas was 61.9 percent (p=0.0006). Two other factors which the authors point out as affecting survival are: (1) differentiation and (2) lymphatic or vascular involvement. The well-differentiated group had a 96.3 percent five-year survival (103/107) while the poorly differentiated group had a survival of 87.5 percent (56/64) (p=0.03). With lymphovascular involvement the survival was 72.7 percent versus 97.4 percent (p<0.01).

As noted above, the complication rate with this procedure was quite high. However, with the introduction of better anesthesia, blood banking, and antibiotics, postoperative mortalities became very rare. The most common severe complications are related to urinary dysfunction with fistulas forming in about 5 percent of patients.[72] Cystometric and electromyographic evaluation of the bladder reveals a hypertonic phase resulting from increased myogenic tonicity of the detrusor muscle.[84] This coupled with the partial detrusor denervation which results from the dissection leads to the inability to urinate effectively with the resulting increase in bladder pressure and, in the case of reflux, ureteral pressure. Such pressure increases can compromise effective blood flow to these structures with fistula formation resulting. This problem can be overcome by employing catheter drainage until the bladder recovers. Van Nagell et al.[85] suggest that suprapubic drainage may be the route of choice.

The largest reduction in ureteral fistulas occurred with the induction of suction catheter drainage applied to the retroperitoneal spaces around the lymphadenectomy and existing either through the vagina[86] or the abdominal wall.[87] Use of this technique has resulted in a fistula rate of 1 or 2 percent.

Thus with the present day technology and operative techniques, survival and complication rates for women with early stage cervical cancer are equal when either surgery or radiation therapy are used. It has been suggested that the ability to maintain ovarian function makes the surgical approach more desirable particularly in the younger women.[88–90] Parente et al.[88] reviewed 105 radical hysterectomy specimens and were unable to find a case with ovarian involvement. In this same series there was a 16 percent incidence of nodal involvement. Therefore, it is unnecessary to perform an oophorectomy in these women. In addition, there seems to be less alteration in vaginal anatomy and sexual function in those women undergoing surgical therapy when compared to those treated with radiation therapy. With these factors in mind, radical hysterectomy would seem to be the treatment of choice for women with early staged cervical cancer.

In an effort to improve survival further, some authors[91–93] have suggested combining radical hysterectomy and preoperative radium implants. In all three cases the survival rates were not improved over the 92 percent reported by Morley and Seski.[72]

MICROINVASIVE CERVICAL CANCER

The definition of microinvasive cervical cancer has been put forth and debated by many.[94–100] Its importance lies in the belief that a group of women with early invasion can be defined such that no nodal involvement will be present and thus more conservative surgery is possible. To date the best definition has been proposed by the Society of Gynecologic Oncologists (SGO). It states that for a lesion to be considered as microinvasion it must be limited to a depth of less than three mm of the stroma and be without evidence of lymph-vascular invasion by tumor.[99] The Gynecologic Oncology Group Study[97] suggested that confluence of invasion and lateral spread of tumor less than four mm be added to the definition. Boronow,[96] using the SGO definition, reviewed 35 cases that fit the definition and found no case of lymph node involvement while his control group had involved nodes in 21 percent of the cases. Thus it would seem that women who fit this definition, and it can be determined only after cone biopsy, can be treated by a standard hysterectomy. The abdominal approach is favored since it allows for evaluation of the parametrium and pelvic lymph nodes. This conservative approach has been taken one step further by Rubio et al.[100] who suggest that in selected women treatment with conization only is adequate. This approach requires much more evaluation and patient follow-up before it can be considered as a therapeutic alternative.

STANDARD HYSTERECTOMY FOR INVASIVE DISEASE

For many years it was felt that microinvasive cervical cancer should be treated with a radical hysterectomy plus pelvic lymphadenectomy or a modified radical hysterectomy (type II radical hysterectomy as per Piver et al.[101]). As is noted above, in selected cases the lymphatic involvement appears to be zero. Thus it would appear that pelvic lymphadenectomy is unnecessary. The concept of an extended or modified radical hysterectomy for treatment of microinvasive cancer has been compared to the use of a standard extrafascial hysterectomy. When this is done, most report that a standard hysterectomy is as successful at providing a cure as a more radical dissection.[102–104] Since the most common site for these women to have recurrences is the vaginal apex, annual exams and vaginal cytology are required as part of their follow-up.

In the case of frankly invasive cervical cancer the use of standard hysterectomy is strictly contraindicated. Women treated by this approach have a very high recurrence rate and poor overall survival.[105] In most cases the use of this procedure in the face of cancer can be eliminated by a careful preoperative visual and cytological evaluation of the cervix. In those cases where cancer is an unexpected finding, some additional therapy is necessary. Green and Morse[106] suggest that these women should undergo immediate reoperation with "radical surgical removal of the residual tumor-bearing area by means of the Wertheim, Schauta, or pelvic-exenteration procedure. . . ." They found, as did Barber et al.,[107] that this affords the best cure for these women. With the development of new high energy radiation units, Andras et al.[108] and Davy et al.[109] have found that immediate treatment with radiation therapy can result in a prognosis as good as in those treated more conventionally.

The use of bilateral salpingo-oophorectomy in women with cervical cancer is unnecessary and should be condemned except in those women to be treated with cesium application who have known salpingo-oophoritis. Another practice which is contraindicated in this disease is surgical debulking of tumor prior to radiation therapy. In most cases such an approach results in the formation of adhesions which will result in a greater complication rate while interfering with the blood supply to the tumor which will decrease its response to radiotherapy.

POSTRADIATION THERAPY HYSTERECTOMY

Women with bulky stage I or II cervical cancer have generally been treated with radiation therapy. Most of the women have extensive endocervical and often myometrial involvement which would not be adequately treated with standard radiotherapy. Thus one would predict a high rate of residual disease after radiation with treatment failures resulting. In an effort to test this theory, Crawford et al.[110] looked at 137 women with stage I or II cervical cancer who underwent hysterectomy after radiation therapy and found that 20 percent had residual disease in the surgical specimen. This problem was first noted by Fletcher and Rutledge and prompted them to suggest the addition of extrafascial hysterectomy to the treatment course of women with early staged bulky disease.[111] In the scheme they developed, such a patient would receive 4,000 rads of external therapy and a single cesium implant of 4,000 to 5,000 mg-hr. Six weeks later an extrafascial hysterectomy would be performed. The initial reports of this approach showed no improvement in survival in spite of a marked reduction in the rate of central recurrences. It was found that their survival was affected by the systemic disease which developed. At the same time these women suffered a high complication rate. The addition of pelvic lymphadenectomy served only to further increase complications.[112–114] A later review indicated that if careful sharp dissection was used in these women and if those women with a history of diagnosed or suspected pelvic inflammatory disease were excluded from the surgical group, there was a great reduction in morbidity and mortality in the operative group.[115] Unfortunately, no significant improvement in survival was noted. At the present time efforts are underway in the Gynecologic Oncology Group to study this approach in women with stage I cervical cancers measuring greater than five cm.

Stevenson[116] has suggested that radical hysterectomy and pelvic lymphadenectomy be used to complete treatment of cervical cancer after standard pelvic radio-therapy. His data seems to suggest some improvement in results but this is at the cost of a significant rate of complications. Many other reports have been published using variations of the above treatment protocols. In most cases there was little improvement in survival while morbidity and mortality rates were adversely affected.[117–122]

SURGICAL MANAGEMENT OF RECURRENT CERVICAL CANCER

Most women who present for surgical treatment of recurrent cervical cancer have in the past undergone pelvic radiation therapy and as a result will have changes in the pelvic tissues that will make evaluation of both physical findings and cytologic specimens very difficult. Serial pelvic exams will allow the detection of changes which often can be evaluated with cytology or directed needle biopsies. However, with this approach there is a 10 percent false-negative rate.[123] Follow-up intravenous pyelogram may demonstrate the development of ureteral obstruction which in all but 3 percent of these will be the result of tumor recurrence.[124]

Once a recurrence is documented histologically one is faced with treating a woman who has received the limit of radiation which the normal pelvic tissues can tolerate and thus is no longer eligible for additional radiotherapy. As a result of its tendency to remain localized in the pelvis, many of these women remain candidates for some form of regional therapy. In the case of small recurrences limited to the cervix, radical hysterectomy with or without pelvic lymphadenectomy can be used.[99] In special cases where isolated extension to the bladder or rectum has been encountered, Symmonds et al.[83] have used radical hysterectomy with segmental resection of involved organs. While this proves effective in resecting the neoplasm, the unacceptably high fistula rate makes this approach too morbid for general use.

In 1948 Brunschwig[125] reported the treatment of 22 women with what he termed a "one-stage abdominoperineal operation with end colostomy and bilateral ureteral implantation into the colon above the colostomy." In spite of an operative mortality rate of 23 percent, he reported general acceptance of this procedure by all women presented with the prospect of undergoing it. It is of interest that he states that the complete deperitonealization of the pelvis can be done without subsequent development of intestinal obstruction. The literature is replete with data indicating the error of this observation as well as methods of correcting it.[126,127]

With this initial success in treating these terminal patients, Brunschwig and Daniel[128] reported on the use of pelvic exenteration in 441 women. They suggested that the extent of the disease present and not previous treatment was the basis for indicating the need for this procedure. As a result of this they performed this procedure in 93 women who had not had previous treatment. When they reviewed survival it was found that the procedure was not effective in women with distant metastases or indurated, painful and swollen legs. In addition, when the operation was for palliation, i.e., macroscopic disease was left behind, the survival was 3 percent. Thus, before this procedure is started, a careful exploration is needed to illustrate that all of the disease can be removed.

In spite of their better patient selection, the surgical mortality was 16 percent. In most cases, the cause was surgical shock in those who died within 30 days of surgery and small bowel fistula in those dying more than a month after surgery. In spite of this mortality rate, they report an 18 percent five-year survival rate.

In 1956 Bricker et al.[129] reported the results of pelvic exenteration in 118 women. They experienced long operative times and extensive blood loss at the beginning of their series but with additional experience they were able to complete the procedure in 4 hours with a need for only five to six units of blood. Operative deaths continued to be a problem with 16 women (13.5 percent) not surviving. On the other hand, 23 percent of women operated upon 3 or more years before the report were alive and well.

A major advance for which Bricker is credited is the isolated ileal loop for use as a bladder substitute.[130] In his report only two women (2 percent) developed fatal urinary complications. This success has resulted in the universal adoption of the technique or a variant of it in pelvic exenterative surgery.

As was noted by Brunschwig, Bricker found this procedure to be of no use for palliation or in women who had nodal involvement. He also pointed out the ominous nature of ureteral obstruction, leg edema, and leg pain of sciatic distribution and its association with inoperatibility.

More modern experience has been reported by several major centers.[131–134] In general, improved blood banking, antibiotics, intensive care units, and experience have resulted in lower operative mortality and morbidity, as well as increased survival (Table 3-3). Most report that of those presenting for consideration for pelvic exenterative surgery, only 50 to 75 percent are found to be operative candidates, with only about 50 percent of this group being found to be resectable at the time of exploratory laparotomy. If one assumes a five-year survival of 50 percent, under the best of situations only 18.5 percent of those presenting with recurrent disease will undergo pelvic exenteration and survive to 5 years. This is a low figure until one considers that this represents a cancer cure in the face of failure of at least first line and in some cases second line therapy.

Early in his experience Bricker found that often there was a profound effect of this procedure on the stability of the woman's marriage as well as her feeling of self worth. Because of the overwhelming concern about cure and the high morbidity and mortality rates associated with this procedure, attention to this problem was limited. In recent years with the drop in morbidity and mortality rates, quality of life after

Table 3-3. Changes in Survival and Operative Mortality Reported with Pelvic Exenteration

Author	Number of Patients	Mortality Rate	5 Year Survival
Brunschwig (1948)[124]	22	23	—
Brunschwig & Daniel (1956)[125]	441	16	18
Bricker et al. (1956)[128]	118	13.5	40
Symmonds et al. (1968)[130]	118	12.0	25.9
Symmonds et al. (1975)[131]	198	8.1	33
Morley & Lindenauer (1977)[133]	70	1.4	61.8
Rutledge et al. (1977)[132]	296	13.3	48.3

these procedures has been addressed. This has resulted in the development of several reconstructive procedures.[135,136] Using those procedures, women may have vaginal and sexual function restored as well as restoration of normal bowel function. In addition to these reconstructive procedures, women considered for pelvic exenterative surgery at the University of Michigan are seen, with their husband, by a social worker-sexual counselor to address the potential problems they both may encounter as a result of this surgery. To date this has seemed to provide the couple with a more solid basis with which to tackle the problems and setbacks they all encounter during and after the surgery.

REFERENCES

1. Silverberg E, Lubera JA: A review of American Cancer Society estimates of cancer cases and deaths. Ca—A Cancer Journal for Clinicians 33:2, 1983.
2. Papanicolaou GN, Traut HF: Diagnostic value of vaginal smears in carcinoma of uterus. Am J Obstet Gynecol 42:193, 1941.
3. Sedlis A, Walter AT, Balin H, et al: Evaluation of two simultaneously obtained cervical cytological smears. Acta Cytol 18:291, 1974.
4. Richart RM, Barron BA: Screening strategies for cervical cancer and cervical intraepithelial neoplasia. Presented at the American Cancer Society National Conference on Cancer Prevention and Detection, Chicago, April 17–19, 1980.
5. Rylander E: Negative smears in women developing invasive cervical cancer. Acta Obstet Gynecol Scand 56:115, 1977.
6. Kern WH, Zivolich MR: The accuracy and consistency of the cytologic classification of squamous lesions of the uterine cervix. Acta Cytol 21:519, 1977.
7. Sandmire HF, Austin SD, Bechtel RD: Experience with 40,000 Papanicolaou smears. Obstet Gynecol 48:56, 1976.
8. Shingleton HM, Gore H, Straughn JM, et al: The contribution of endocervical smears to cervical cancer detection. Acta Cytol 19:261, 1975.
9. Johansen P, Arffmann E, Pallesen G: Evaluation of smears obtained by cervical scraping and an endocervical swab in the diagnosis of neoplastic disease of the uterine cerix. Acta Obstet Gynecol Scand 58:265, 1979.
10. Love RR: How you can make the Pap test more sensitive and reliable. Your Patient and Cancer 2:76, 1982.
11. Eddy D: ACS report on the cancer-related health checkup. Ca—Cancer J Clinicians 30:215, 1980.
12. Cervical cancer screening programs. I. Epidemiology and natural history of carcinoma of the cervix. CMA Journal 114:1003, 1976.
13. Fruchter RG, Boyce J, Hunt M, et al: Invasive cancer of cervix: failures in prevention. II. Delays in diagnosis. NY State J Med 80:913, 1980.
14. Martin PL: How preventable is invasive cervical cancer? A community study of preventable factors. Am J Obstet Gynecol 113:541, 1972.
15. Fidler HK, Boyes DA, Lock DR, et al: The cytology program in British Columbia. II. The operation of the cytology laboratory. Can Med Assn J 86:823, 1962.
16. Schneider J, Twiggs LB: The costs of carcinoma of the cervix. Obstet Gynecol 40:851, 972.
17. LaFerla JJ, Zuniga M, Naylor B, et al: Relative frequency of cervical cytology screening by age groups in the United States, 1981. (Manuscript in preparation.)

18. Nealon NA, Christopherson WM: Cervix cancer precursors in young offspring of low-income families. Obstet Gynecol 54:135, 1979.
19. Terris M, Wilson F, Nelson JH Jr: Relation of circumcision to cancer of the cervix. Am J Obstet Gynecol 117:1056, 1973.
20. Boyce JG, Lu T, Nelson JH Jr, et al: Cervical carcinoma and oral contraception. Obstet Gynecol 40:139, 1972.
21. Boyce JG, Lu T, Nelson JH Jr, et al: Oral contraceptives and cervical carcinoma. Am J Obstet Gynecol 129:761, 1977.
22. Benedet JL, Boyes DA, Nichols TM, et al: Colposcopic evaluation of patients with abnormal cervical cytology. Br J Obstet Gynaecol 83:177, 1976.
23. Kirkup W, Hills AS: The accuracy of colposcopically directed biopsy in patients with suspected intraepithelial neoplasia of the cervix. Br J Obstet Gynaecol 87:1, 1980.
24. Savage EW: Correlation of colposcopically directed biopsy and conization with histologic diagnosis of cervical lesions. J Reprod Med 15:211, 1975.
25. Cecchina S, Bonardi L, Cipparrone G, et al: Contribution of cytology, colposcopy, target biopsy and conization to the early diagnosis of precancerous and cancerous lesions of the cervix uteri. Tumori 64:389, 1978.
26. Knutzen VK, Sherwood AGB: Colposcopy and selective biopsy in patients with abnormal cervical cytology. S Afr Med J 52:478, 1977.
27. Hovadhanakul P, Mehra U, Terragno A, et al: Comparison of colposcopy directed biopsies and cold knife conization in patients with abnormal cytology. Surg, Gynecol and Obstet 142:333, 1976.
28. Drescher CW, Peters W III, Roberts JA: The role of endocervical curettage in a colposcopy clinic. Obstet Gynecol 62:343, 1983.
29. Sevin B-U, Ford JH, Girtanner RD, et al: Invasive cancer of the cervix after cryosurgery. Pitfalls of conservative management. Obstet Gynecol 53:465, 1979.
30. Townsend DE, Richart RM, Marks E, et al: Invasive cancer following outpatient evaluation and therapy for cervical disease. Obstet Gynecol 57:145, 1981.
31. Roberts JA: Management of gynecologic tumors during pregnancy. Clinics in Perinatology, 1983, (in press).
32. Van Nagell JR Jr, Parker JC Jr, Hicks LP, et al: Diagnostic and therapeutic efficacy of cervical conization. Am J Obstet Gynecol 124:134, 1976.
33. Boyes DA, Worth AJ, Fidler HK: The results of treatment of 4389 cases of preclinical cervical squamous carcinoma. J Obstet Gynaecol Br Commonw 77:769, 1970.
34. Bjerre B, Sjoberg N, Soberberg H: Further treatment after conization. J Reprod Med 21:232, 1978.
35. Kolstad P, Klen V: Long-term follow-up of 1121 cases of carcinoma-in-situ. Obstet Gynecol 48:125, 1976.
36. Friedell GH: Endometrial surface involvement by carcinoma of the uterine cervix. Obstet Gynecol 12:179, 1958.
37. Javert CT: Pathological classification for staging of squamous cancer of the cervix. Cancer 8:285, 1955.
38. Perez CA, Zivnuska F, Austin F, et al: Prognostic significance of endometrial extension from primary carcinoma of the uterine cervix. Cancer 35:1493, 1975.
39. Rotman M, John M, Boyce J: Prognostic factors in cervical carcinoma: implications in staging and management. Cancer 48:560, 1981.
40. Bosch A, Frius Z, DeValda GC: Prognostic significance of ureteral obstruction in carcinoma of the cervix uteri. Acta Radiol Ther (Stockh) 12:47, 1973.
41. Van Nagell JR, Sprague AD, Roddick JW: The effect of intravenous pyelography and cystoscopy on the staging of cervical cancer. Gynecol Oncol 3:87, 1975.

42. Lifshitz SG, Buchsbaum HJ: Spread of cervical carcinoma. Obstet Gynecol Annual 6:341, 1977.
43. Averette HE, Ford JH, Dudon RC, et al: Staging of cervical cancer. Clin Obstet Gynecol 18:215, 1975.
44. Plentl AA, Friedman EA: Lymphatic System of the Female Genitalia. Philadelphia, WB Saunders, 1971.
45. Pilleron JP, Durand JC, Hamelin JP: Location of lymph node invasion in cancer of the uterine cervix: Study of 140 cases treated at the Curie Foundation. Am J Obstet Gynecol 119:453, 1974.
46. Deale CJC, du Toit JP: Routine investigations in the clinical staging of invasive carcinoma of the cervix. A critical evaluation. S Afr Med J 58: 895, 1976.
47. Shingleton HM, Fowler WC Jr., Koch GG: Pretreatment evaluation in cervical cancer. Am J Obstet Gynecol 110:385, 1971.
48. Van Nagell RJ Jr, Harralson JD, Roddick JW Jr: The effect of examination under anesthesia on staging accuracy in cervical cancer. Am J Obstet Gynecol 113:938, 1972.
49. Van Nagell JR Jr, Roddick JW Jr, Lowin DM: The staging of cervical cancer: Inevitable discrepancies between clinical staging and pathologic findings. Am J Obstet Gynecol 110:973, 1971.
50. Javert CT: The lymph nodes of the pelvis. In Meigs JV (ed): Surgical treatment of Cancer of the Cervix. New York, Grune and Stratton, 1954, pp 83–84.
51. Piver MS, Barlow JJ: Para-aortic lymphadenectomy, aortic node biopsy, and aortic lymphangiography in staging patients with advanced cervical cancer. Cancer 32:367, 1973.
52. Averette HE, Ford JH Jr, Dudan RC, et al: Staging of cervical cancer. Clin Obstet Gynecol 18:215, 1975.
53. Piver MS, Barlow JJ: Para-aortic lymphadenectomy in staging patients with advanced local cervical cancer. Obstet Gynecol 53:544, 1974.
54. Wharton JT, Jones HW III, Day TG Jr, et al: Preirradiation celiotomy and extended field irradiation for invasive carcinoma of the cervix. Obstet Gynecol 49:333, 1977.
55. Belinson JL, Goldberg MI, Averette HE: Paraaortic lymphadenectomy in gynecologic cancer. Gynecol Oncol 7:188, 1979.
56. Averette HE, Dudan RC, Ford JH Jr: Exploratory celiotomy for surgical staging of cervical cancer. Am J Obstet Gynecol 113:1090, 1972.
57. Averette HE, Dudan RC, Ford JH Jr: Exploratory celiotomy for surgical staging of cervical cancer. Am J Obstet Gynecol 113:1090, 1972.
58. Buchsbaum HJ: Extrapelvic lymph node metastases in cervical carcinoma. Am J Obstet Gynecol 133:814, 1979.
59. Buchsbaum HJ: Para-aortic lymph node involvement in cervical carcinoma. Am J Obstet Gynecol 113:942, 1972.
60. Nelson JH Jr, Macasaet MA, Lu T, et al: The incidence and significance of para-aortic lymph node metastases in late invasive carcinoma of the cervix. Amj Obstet Gynecol 113:749, 1974.
61. Berman ML, Lagasse LD, Watring WG, et al: The operative evaluation of patients with cervical carcinoma by an extraperitoneal approach. Obstet Gynecol 50:658, 1977.
62. Ballon SC, Berman ML, Lagasse LD, et al: Survival after extraperitoneal pelvic and paraaortic lymphadenectomy and radiation therapy in cervical carcinoma. Obstet Gynecol 57:90, 1981.
63. Welander CE, Pierce VK, Nori D, et al: Pretreatment laparotomy in carcinoma of the cervix. Gynecol Oncol 12:336, 1981.

64. Vongtama V, Piver SM, Tsukada Y, et al: Para-aortic node irradiation in carcinomas. Cancer 34:169, 1974.
65. Guthrie RT, Buchsbaum HJ, White AJ, et al: Para-aortic lymph node irradiation in carcinoma of the uterine cervix. Cancer 34:166, 1974.
66. Lepanto P, Littman P, Mikuta J, et al: Treatment of paraaortic nodes in carcinoma of the cervix. Cancer 35:1510, 1975.
67. Silberstein AB, Aron BS, Alexander LL: Para-aortic lymph node irradiation in cervical carcinoma. Radiology 95:181, 1970.
68. Delgado G, Smith JP, Ballantyne AJ: Scalene node biopsy in carcinoma of the cervix. Cancer 35:784, 1975.
69. Lee RB, Weisbaum GS, Heller PB, et al: Scalene node biopsy in primary and recurrent invasive carcinoma of the cervix. Gynecol Oncol 11:200, 1981.
70. Buchsbaum HG, Lifshitz S: The role of scalene node biopsy in advanced carcinoma of the cervix uteri. Surg Gynecol Oncol 142:246, 1976.
71. Javert CT: The natural history of cancer of the cervix. Am J Obstet Gynecol 82:56, 1961.
72. Morley GW, Seski JC: Radical pelvic surgery versus radiation therapy for stage I carcinoma of the cervix (exclusive of microinvasion). Am J Obstet Gynecol 126:785, 1976.
73. Newton M: Radical hysterectomy or radiotherapy for stage I cervical cancer. A prospective comparison with 5 and 10 year follow-up. Am J Obstet Gynecol 123:535, 1975.
74. Graham H, Graham R, Schultz M: Cancer of the uterine cervix. Am J Obstet Gynecol 89:421, 1964.
75. Averette HE, LaPlatney DR, Little WA: Current role of radical hysterectomy as primary therapy for invasive carcinoma of the cervix. Am J Obstet Gynecol 105:79, 1969.
76. Bean JLM, Whetham JCG, Vernon CP: Results of surgical treatment of carcinoma of the cervix. Am J Obstet Gynecol 103:465, 1969.
77. Park RC, Patow WR, Rogers RE, et al: Treatment of stage I carcinoma of the cervix. Obstet Gynecol 41:117, 1973.
78. Webb MJ, Symmonds RE: Wertheim hysterectomy: a reappraisal. Obstet Gynecol 54:140, 1979.
79. Sall S, Pineda AA, Calanog A, et al: Surgical treatment of stages IB and IIA invasive carcinoma of the cervix by radical abdominal hysterectomy. Am J Obstet Gynecol 135:442, 1979.
80. Underwood PB Jr, Wilson WC, Kreutner A, et al: Radical hysterectomy: a critical review of twenty-two years' experience. Am J Obstet Gynecol 134:889, 1979.
81. Benedet JL, Turko M, Boyes DA, et al: Radical hysterectomy in the treatment of cervical cancer. Am J Obstet Gynecol 137:254, 1980.
82. Lerner HM, Jones HW III, Hill EC: Radical surgery for the treatment of early invasive cervical carcinoma (stage IB): review of 15 years' experience. Obstet Gynecol 56:413, 1980.
83. Symmonds RE, Pratt JH, Welch JS: Extended Wertheim operation for primary, recurrent, or suspected recurrent carcinoma of the cervix. Obstet Gynecol 24:15, 1964.
84. Seski JC, Diokno AC: Bladder dysfunction after radical abdominal hysterectomy. Am J Obstet Gynecol 128:643, 1977.
85. Van Nagell JR Jr, Penny RM Jr, Roddick JW Jr: Suprapubic bladder drainage following radical hysterectomy. Am J Obstet Gynecol 113:849, 1972.
86. Symmonds RE, Pratt JH: Prevention of fistulas and lymphocysts in radical hysterectomy. Obstet Gynecol 17:57, 1961.
87. Green TH Jr: Ureteral suspension for prevention of ureteral complications following radical Wertheim hysterectomy. Obstet Gynecol 28:1, 1966.

88. Parente JT, Silberblatt W, Stone M: Infrequency of metastasis to ovaries in stage I carcinoma of the cervix. Am J Obstet Gynecol 90:1362, 1964.

89. Webb GA: The role of ovarian conservation in the treatment of carcinoma of the cervix with radical surgery. Am J Obstet Gynecol 122:476, 1975.

90. McCall ML, Keaty EC, Thompson JD: Conservation of ovarian tissue in the treatment of carcinoma of the cervix with radical surgery. Am J Obstet Gynecol 75:590, 1958.

91. Surwit E, Fowler WC Jr, Palumbo L, et al: Radical hysterectomy with or without preoperative radium for stage IB squamous cell carcinoma of the cervix. Obstet Gynecol 48:130, 1976.

92. Villasanta U: Combined radium therapy and radical hysterectomy with pelvic lymphadenectomy in treatment of invasive cancer of the cervix. Obstet Gynecol 32:6, 1968.

93. Rampone JF, Klem V, Kolstad P: Combined Treatment of Stage Ib carcinoma of the cervix. Obstet Gynecol 41:163, 1973.

94. Christopherson WM, Parker JE: Microinvasive carcinoma of the uterine cervix. Cancer 17:1123, 1964.

95. Frick HC II, Janovski NA, Gusberg SB, et al: Early invasive cancer of the cervix. Am J Obstet Gynecol 85:926, 1963.

96. Boronow RC: Stage I cervix cancer and pelvic node metastasis. Special reference to the implications of the new and the recently replaced FIGO classifications on stage Ia. Am J Obstet Gynecol 127:135, 1977.

97. Sedlis A, Sall S, Tsukada Y, et al: Microinvasive carcinoma of the uterine cervix: a clinical-pathologic study. Am J Obstet Gynecol 133:64, 1979.

98. Fennell RH Jr: Microinvasive carcinoma of the uterine cervix. Obstet Gynecol Surv 33:406, 1978.

99. van Nagell JR Jr, Donaldson ES, Gay EC: Evaluation and treatment of patients with invasive cervical cancer. Surg Clin North Am 58:67, 1978.

100. Rubio CA, Soderberg G, Einhorn N: Histological and follow-up studies in cases of micro-invasive carcinoma of the uterine cervix. Acta Path Microbiol Scand 82:397, 1974.

101. Piver MS, Rutledge F, Smith JP: Five classes of extended hysterectomy for women with cervical cancer. Obstet Gynecol 44:265, 1974.

102. Yajima A, Noda K: The results of treatment of microinvasive carcinoma (stage IA) of the uterine cervix by means of simple and extended hysterectomy. Am J Obstet Gynecol 135:685, 1979.

103. Savage EW: Microinvasive carcinoma of the cervix. Am J Obstet Gynecol 113:708, 1972.

104. Foushee JHS, Greiss FC, Lock FR: Stage IA squamous cell carcinoma of the uterine cervix. Am J Obstet Gynecol 105:46, 1969.

105. Tunca JC, Dement OE: Simple hysterectomy is inadequate therapy for invasive cervical cancer. W Virg Med J 73:255, 1977.

106. Green TH Jr, Morse WJ Jr: Management of invasive cervical cancer following inadvertent simple hysterectomy. Obstet Gynecol 33:763, 1969.

107. Barber HRK, Pece GV, Brunschwig A: Operative mangement of patients previously operated upon for a benign lesion with cervical cancer as a surprise finding. Am J Obstet Gynecol 101:959, 1958.

108. Andras EJ, Fletcher GH, Rutledge F: Radiotherapy of carcinoma of the cervix following simple hysterectomy. Am J Obstet Gynecol 115:647, 1973.

109. Davy M, Bentzen H, Jahren R: Simple hysterectomy in the presence of invasive cervical cancer. Acta Obstet Gynecol Scand 56:105, 1977.

110. Crawford EJ, Robinson LS, Vaught J: Carcinoma of the cervix: results of treatment by radiation alone and by combined radiation and surgical therapy in 335 patients. Am J Obstet Gynecol 91:480, 1965.

111. Fletcher GH, Rutledge FN, Chau PM: Policies of treatment in cancer of the cervix uteri. Am J Roentgen 87:6, 1962.

112. Nelson AJ III, Fletcher GH, Wharton JT: Indications for adjunctive conservative extra-fascial hysterectomy in selected cases of carcinoma of the uterine cervix. Am J Radiol 123:91, 1975.

113. Rutledge FN, Wharton JT, Fletcher GH: Clinical studies with adjunctive surgery and irradiation therapy in the treatment of carcinoma of the cervix. Cancer 38:596, 1976.

114. Rutledge FN, Fletcher GH, MacDonald EJ: Pelvic lymphadenectomy as an adjunct to radiation therapy in treatment for cancer of the cervix. Am J Radiol 93:607, 1965.

115. O'Quinn AG, Fletcher GH, Wharton JT: Guidelines for conservative hysterectomy after irradiation. Gynecol Oncol 9:68, 1980.

116. Stevenson CS: The combined treatment of carcinoma of the cervix with full irradiation therapy followed by radical pelvic operation. Second progress report on a series now numbering 95 cases. Am J Obstet Gynecol 81:156, 1961.

117. Kelso JW, Funnell JD: Combined surgical and radiation treatment of invasive carcinoma of the cervix. Am J Obstet Gynecol 116:205, 1973.

118. Funnell JW, Kelso JW, Funnell JD: Combined surgical and irradiation treatment of invasive carcinoma of the cervix. J Okla State Med Assn 64:123, 1971.

119. Quigley MM, Knab DR, McMahon EB: Carcinoma of the cervix. A third treatment. Obstet Gynecol 45:650, 1975.

120. Bonar LD: Results of radical surgical procedures after radiation for treatment of invasive carcinoma of the uterine cervix in a private practice. Am J Obstet Gynecol 136:1006, 1980.

121. Churches CK, Kurrle GR, Johnson B: Treatment of carcinoma of the cervix by combination of irradiation and operation. Am J Obstet Gynecol 118:1033, 1974.

122. Perez CA, Breaux S, Askin F, et al: Irradiation alone or in combination with surgery in stage IB and IIA carcinoma of the uterine cervix: a nonrandomized comparison. Cancer 43:1062, 1979.

123. El-Minawa MF, Perez-Mesa CM: Parametrial needle biopsy follow-up of cervical cancer. Int J Obstet Gynecol 12:1, 1974

124. Slater JM, Fletcher GH: Ureteral strictures after radiation therapy for carcinoma of the uterine cervix. Am J Radiol 61:269, 1971.

125. Brunschwig A: Complete excision of pelvic viscera for advanced carcinoma. A one-stage abdominoperineal operation with end colostomy and bilateral ureteral implantation into the colon above the colostomy. Cancer 1:177, 1948.

126. Buchsbaum HJ, White AJ: Omental sling for management of the pelvic floor following exenteration. Am J Obstet Gynecol 117:407, 1973.

127. Lifshitz S, Johnson R, Roberts JA: Intestinal fistula and obstruction following pelvic exenteration. Surg Gynecol Obstet 152:630, 1981.

128. Brunschwig A, Daniel W: Evaluation of pelvic exenteration for advanced cancer of the cervix. Surg Gynecol Obstet 103:337, 1956.

129. Bricker EM, Butcher HR, McAfee A: Results of pelvic exenteration. Arch Surg 73:661, 1956.

130. Bricker EM: Functional results of small intestinal segments as bladder substitutes following pelvic evisceration. Surgery 32:372, 1952.

131. Symmonds RE, Pratt JH, Welch JS: Exenterative operations. Experience with 118 patients. Am J Obstet Gynecol 101:66, 1968.

132. Symmonds RE, Pratt JH, Webb MJ: Exenterative operations: Experience with 198 patients. Am J Obstet Gynecol 121:907, 1975.

133. Rutledge FN, Smith JP, Wharton JT, et al: Pelvic exenteration: analysis of 296 patients. Am J Obstet Gynecol 129:881, 1977.
134. Morley GW, Lindenauer SM: Pelvic exenterative therapy for gynecologic malignancy. An analysis of 70 cases. Cancer 38:581, 1976.
135. Morley GW: Pelvic exenterative therapy and the treatment of recurrent carcinoma of the cervix. Seminars in Oncology 9:331, 1982.
136. Lagasse LD, Berman ML, Watring WG, et al: The gynecologic oncology patient: restoration of function and prevention of disability. In McGowan L (ed): Gynecologic Oncology. New York, Appleton-Century-Crofts, 1978.

4 | Radiation Therapy in the Management of Invasive Cervical Carcinoma

Kwang N. Choi
Marvin Rotman

Cervical carcinoma spreads in a slowly progressing predictable pathway from the cervix through surrounding lymphatics to the pelvic lymph nodes. It tends to confine itself to the pelvis for a substantial period of time thus making it amenable to the locoregional therapeutics of irradiation. Interestingly, almost half the patients (45 percent) with cervical carcinoma present with the disease only in the cervix and an additional 43 percent of these patients have tumor confined to the true pelvis. Disease outside the pelvis at the time of presentation exists in 11 percent of cases.[1]

Prior to 1960 survival results seemed to have reached a plateau, with improvement coming primarily through refinement of surgical and/or radiotherapeutic techniques. In the past two decades, much effort has been directed towards understanding the biological behaviour of the tumor and the disease spread in the lymphatics. It has been the continued appreciation of the prognostic significance and treatment of the primary and its lymphatic pathways that accounts for the major improvements in survival over these past 20 years. Much of the material in this chapter has been modified from previous publications of the second author.

LYMPHATICS

Excellent summaries of the anatomy of the cervix and its lymphatic drainage are available elsewhere.[2] However, information from anatomic texts and surgical dissections is both incomplete and misleading. It is evident that the disease spreads from a complex intra-cervical network through the para-cervical lymphatics to the pelvic and para-aortic lymph nodes. Its proclivity for any particular group or groups of lymph nodes is uncertain. Information gleaned from surgical dissection is subject to the variability of surgical techniques, the accessibility or ease of dissection, and the proficiency of the surgical pathologist. Thus, the true significance of collected statistics of pelvic lymph node involvement in early disease can be unreliable and difficult to assess. Further, tumor blockage of lymphatics or surgical disruption can lead to embolization of malignant cells through unrecognized collateral channels. Conversely, groups of nodes previously unobserved can become identifiable in areas perfused by tumor emboli. For example, the intercalary nodes of Henricksen lying within the vesico-vaginal and recto-vaginal septum are rarely described.[3] This is underscored by the reported differential incidence of parametrial and para-cervical lymph nodes ranging between 2 and 35 percent.[2] What needs to be appreciated is that the distribution of positive lymph nodes and lymphatic channels in the diseased state is unpredictable and does not necessarily follow the previously described, so-called normal anatomic pathways.

Anatomic features that inexplicably remain unidentified in large surgical series relate to 3 major lymphatic networks that (1) posteriorly invest the rectum and interconnect with an ureteral sheath (2) form a plexus that covers the posterior wall of the bladder, and (3) anastomose with the plexus surrounding the uterine fundus and its adnexa.

This leads to the belief that the failure to control disease locally, even in the early stages may be a direct consequence of our underestimating the complexities of lymph node and lymphatic distribution, as well as the difficulty of surgical identification and dissection of certain groups of these nodes.

PATTERNS OF INFILTRATION

From the study of biopsy sections, Miller et al.[4] divided infiltrative characteristics into three types: (1) the expansile type with outpouching or budding of neoplastic process, (2) the diffuse type with spread disseminated in the section and characterized by cells present throughout the stroma, (3) a thromboembolic type in which tumor cells are found in the lymphatics and blood capillaries.

The expansile type of invasion spreads slowly mainly by continuity. In the diffuse infiltrative type the tumor insinuates through the interstitial tissue spaces. Thromboembolic spread is self-explanatory. Here the tumor spreads to lymph nodes and distant organs and also locally disseminates.

The traditional concept that the cervical cancer characteristically confines itself at first to the cervix, and later involves regional lymphatics in a progressive and systemic fashion incorrectly suggests that cancer cells lodge only in the cervix or the

Table 4-1. Factors Influencing Prognosis in Stage 1 Carcinoma of the Cervix

	Local Recurrence	5 Year Survival
Pelvic Node		
Positive	18–45%	62–68%
Negative	6–8%	90–92%
Size of Primary		
>2 cm.	44%	58% (2–12 yrs.)
<2 cm.	9%	94%
Quadrants Involved		
3–4	29%	73%
Depth of Invasion		
11–15 mm	31%	72%
<11 mm	4%	96%
Vascular Invasion		
Positive	25–34%	69–73%
Negative	5–8%	93–94%
Corpus Extension		
Positive	56%	50–55%
Negative	3%	84–95%

draining lymph nodes. However, cancer cells that infiltrate through tissue planes, anastomose with lymphatic plexuses that envelope pelvic organs. Thus, the entire pelvic contents can be at risk, due to lymphatic infiltration, even in the early stages of the disease. Recent observations suggest that treatment failures in the early stage may be attributed to the inadequacy of localized therapy because of lymphatic spread when certain morpho-histologic tumor features exist (Table 4-1). By modifying treatment techniques for this substrata of patients a significantly improved survival can result.[21,34]

EVOLUTION OF TREATMENT

Brachytherapy

During the first five decades, the techniques of the radiation treatment of cervical cancer with radium brachytherapy evolved empirically. Soon after the discovery of radium by Marie Curie in 1896, Becquerel unintentionally produced the first known erythematous skin reaction on his chest skin by carrying a tube of radium in his vest pocket. Noting this, Pierre Curie became our first clinical dosimetrist by deliberately inducing a similar reaction on his arm.[5]

Radium's application to medicine was suspected as early as 1903, and some cases of cancer were reported cured.[6] Beginning in the early 1920's, two methods of brachytherapy were developed and continued relatively unchanged for the next 30 years. The first, practiced in Stockholm, utilized high intense radiation over a short period of time. This technique was fundamentally experimental in development deriving data from the personal experiences of Forsell and Heyman. It consisted of a 20–24 hours intra-uterine and vaginal application of radiation filtered by 3 mm of lead, 50 to 60 mg were in the intra-uterine tandem, and 80 to 100 mg were in the vaginal applicators. A second similar application was performed 3 weeks later. Supplementary external therapy was also given, although its value was underestimated. 4,600 patients were treated between 1914 and 1941.[7,8]

The second, the so-called Paris technique, used smaller amounts of radium, 60 mg, over a longer period of time. This treatment lasted 96 hours to 120 hours and as long as 200 hours. The packing and radium were removed frequently at which time the radium was cleansed and replaced immediately with fresh packing. This technique was developed at the Curie Institute based on the radiobiologic low dose rate treatment experiments of Regaud and Lacassagne. Their results showed a commendable Stage I survival rate of 70.4 percent.[9,10]

It was during the 1930's that a third method of treatment of carcinoma of the cervix was established; a system that was to influence the techniques, dosimetry and general philosophy of the treatment of carcinoma of the cervix for the next 30 years. This Manchester system of treatment originally described by Tod and Meredith was a modification of the Paris method and introduced the concept of a predetermined dose to a standard anatomical point, the classical point A.[11,12]

The Manchester philosophy essentially stated that intracavitary radium was to be regarded as the mainstay of treatment and was unlikely to be successfully replaced by any presently, then available form of external radiation and that for Stage I and II, the addition of external radiation made no appreciable differences to results. There were two radium insertions at one week intervals each lasting for about 3 days, the overall treatment time being 10 days. In Stage III, radium was inserted initially, followed by external therapy. It was felt that an attempt to treat the primary growth plus the whole of the potentially invaded lymph node territory by external treatment alone, even if only up to the hypogastric and external iliac node areas, called for the radiation of such a large volume of tissue that lethal dose levels could not possibly be achieved.

In the 1940's through the 1960's although the premises of the Stockholm, Paris, and Manchester techniques were accepted, a number of different treatment policies were formulated. A variety of contrasting methods were used for various reasons at different times. Study of the results helped to weed out the unsatisfactory and emphasize the more valuable elements in each method.

External Therapy

External x-ray initially used in treatment of cervical cancer was of such low energy that it had to be directed to the cervix and uterus through a vaginal speculum in the treatment of pruritis vulvae, uterine myomate, and bleeding uterus. By 1918, the first teletherapy radium machine was installed at Memorial Hospital in New York. With the use of more energetic external radiation, radiation therapy showed early signs of sophistication in treatment planning. Dose quantitation became better defined when external therapy was employed. Because the lower energies concentrated most of the radiation dose in the skin such expressions as the threshold, erythema, tolerance and lethal skin dose became part of the daily vocabulary of the radiation therapist. During the 1930's there developed a more critical awareness of the complications attributable to radiation therapy in large measure due to the death of M. Curie from aplastic anemia and the lytic lesions seen in the radium dial worker. Care was taken to avoid over dosage to the urinary bladder and rectum, and the concept of a therapeutic ratio was born.

Following World War II, there began a world wide installation of teletherapy and other supervoltage units. Supervoltage radiation therapy began to show advantages such as an increased tolerance by normal tissues, skin sparing, better penetration so that greater depth doses could be achieved, no preferential bone absorption, and less side radiation scatter. Obese people received greater depth dosage with less bowel and bladder irradiation. Radiation sickness was reduced due to the decreased scatter, and with more accurate treatment planning and techniques there was a 15 percent increase in dose delivered to tumor bearing tissues without significant untoward effects and survival increased in advanced stages. External treatment soon proved to be of prime importance and the significance of the regional lymphatics became apparent.

Megavoltage irradiation showed that a cancerocidal dose of radiation could be delivered to the pelvic nodes, a concept previously unappreciated if not disbelieved. It was during the 1950's that external therapy was shown to sterilize regional disease and significantly improve survival statistics.[13] A comparison of survival rates in stage I and II cervical cancer illustrated that the survivals were superior (approximately 20 percent) in four leading institutions where external irradiation was added to the standard Manchester radium only insertions.[14] The concept of combining external and intra-cavitary radiation was further developed by Fletcher, so that each modality was made to fit the extent of the disease, and the local anatomy.[15] For example, in large bulky disease, external therapy prior to intracavitary radium produced shrinkage of tumor which then allowed the intracavitary radium with its rapid fall-off of dose to more efficiently reach the full extent of the remaining cancer. It was emphasized that the radiotherapist must not treat the stage of the disease per se, but rather the disease with its particular spread in the patient. Individualization of treatment was essential and became the cornerstone of the therapeutic management of early and moderately advanced disease, particularly Stage I and II.

RADIOTHERAPEUTICS—GENERAL CONCEPTS

External Beam Therapy

The energy of the commonly used megavoltage units ranges from 1.25 MeV (Cobalt 60 Teletherapy) to 4 to 35 MeV (Linear Accelerator or Betatron). The dose distribution in the pelvis using 1.25 MeV to 6 MeV photons radiation is not as uniform as using 10 to 35 MeV photons. The most widely used field arrangement for the best therapeutic ratio is anterior, posterior, right lateral, and left lateral fields (4 fields, box technique). This arrangement results in reducing so called "hot-spots" of radiation in the surrounding normal tissues, without compromising the dose to the target volume.

Hall et al.[16] Ellis et al.[17] and Stupar et al.[18] elaborated the necessity of treating all fields at every session, directing attention toward the biological effect on the tumor instead of only considering the absorbed dose. The biological homogeneity within the treatment volume is best preserved if all the fields are treated every session. If only one field is treated per day, superficial tissues (subcutaneous tissue, small bowel, urinary bladder, rectum and femoral head) may receive a much higher biological dose than that received by treating all four fields every session, even though the measured absorbed dose at the tumor are equal in both types of treatment. This biological inhomogeneity can be enormously accentuated by treating an obese patient with one field per day using a lower energy machine. The indications for whole pelvic irradiation using external beam are: (1) The tumor extent is beyond effective treatment volume of intracavitary irradiation (involvement of parametrium, or pelvic wall); (2) the possibility of tumor spread to lymph nodes outside of the confinement of intracavitary irradiation; (3) in cases where there is sub-optimal anatomy, preventing an ideal dose distribution with an intracavitary irradiation; (atrophic senile vagina; post-hysterectomy). (4) in order to shrink a large exophytic tumor, and obtain better geometric placement of the intracavitary applicators.

The dose-response relationship observed in treatment of head and neck tumors similarly applies to carcinoma of the cervix.[15] A dose of 4,500 rads delivered in 4½ weeks can sterilize sub-clinical amounts of disease, whereas significantly higher doses up to 7,000 rads are required for gross disease (enlarged pelvic lymph nodes etc).

Intracavitary Irradiation

The success of radiation therapy in the management of cervical carcinoma can be attributed to the location of the cervix in the pelvis and to predictable loco-regional spread of disease. From the anatomical point of view, the female genitalia contain natural vehicles, the uterus and vagina, to carry the radioactive sources. Thus, a high radiation sterilizing dose using brachytherapy can be delivered to the tumor bearing tissues. Few other organs can accommodate radioactive materials by non-invasive procedures.

As early as 1903, Alexander Graham Bell commented that radium in glass tubes should be "inserted into the very heart of a cancer." The various applicators in use today are loosely derived from the historical systems of Stockholm, Paris, and Manchester. They include loose and semi-fixed intra-uterine capsules and tandems, vaginal bombs, radium needles and rubber cork, and steel and plastic colpostats. The most widely used instruments in the U.S. are the ones invented by Fletcher and Henschke. Each system has its advantages and disadvantages. Each requires its own technique and has its own distribution, and most importantly the systems are not interchangeable.

A typical intracavitary system includes a central tandem in the uterine cavity carrying three sources and two vaginal colpostats each carrying one source. This results in the delivery of a high dose of radiation to the tumor bearing area (cervix, corpus, upper vagina, para-cervical and parametrial tissue) which is the equivalent of doing a Schauta's vaginal hysterectomy. Figure 4-1 illustrates the dose distribution in a classical intracavitary system. The radiation dose falls off rapidly as the distance

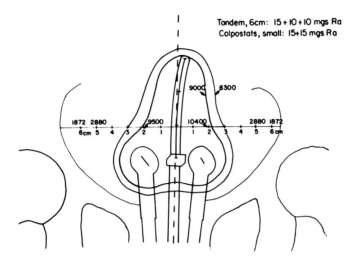

Fig. 4-1. Radiation dose distribution from a standard intracavitary inserion using Fletcher-Suit's tandem and colpostats for approximately 10,000 milligram hours (total of two insertions for 72 hours).

from the radiation sources increases. Thus, the dose to the surrounding normal tissues and distant targets such as pelvic wall lymph nodes is relatively small compared to that to the central area. This form of irradiation is suitable for the control of tumor in and around the cervix and limited in its capabilities to sterilize tumors that extend laterally into the parametria or involve pelvic lymphatics. A 10,000 mg hrs of radium can deliver at the most 2,000 rads to the pelvic wall. Intracavitary irradiation alone is effective in early stages of cervical cancer where there is no risk of disease spread outside of the effective range of intracavitary radioactive sources. It must be used together with external beam irradiation where there is tumor extention or a high risk of lymphatic spread beyond the effective range of the brachytherapy. Not infrequently local tumor extent or vagaries of the anatomy prevent the radiation oncologist from achieving an ideal dose distribution from the intracavitary application, thus requiring the additional use of external irradiation.

After Loading Techniques   Prior to 1960, intracavitary therapy was carried out by inserting radium pre-loaded instruments into the patient in the operating room. Radiotherapists, anesthetists, and scrub nurses were, therefore, exposed to unnecessary amounts of radiation. Speed became the best way to minimize radiation exposure. Henschke, in 1960, introduced the so-called "after loading" technique into radiotherapy, and this allowed the oncologist suffient time to achieve an ideal arrangement using the intracavitary system. In the after loading technique, hollow applicators were first inserted and x-ray films later taken to verify the position of the system and the need for any further manipulation. The radioactive sources were inserted into the hollow instruments when the patient was back in her hospital bed.

Dosimetry of Intracavitary Irradiation   The dosimetry of intracavitary irradiation has some inherent problems. It is not possible to adequately characterize or describe intracavitary irradiation throughout the pelvis due to the rapid dose fall-off and dose anisotropy by using a single measurement. It is also quite difficult if not impossible to integrate the dose delivered by intracavitary irradiation with that from external beam irradiation. Not only is there a variation of 1 to 2 weeks time between the external treatment and the radium insertion or insertions, but there is also a dose rate effect as pointed out by Newall,[19] and Hall.[20] Admittedly relatively vague parameters exist for comparison of the various treatment techniques and their dosimetry. Efforts to try and correlate these techniques (Manchester system and M.D. Anderson system) have been unsuccessful.

Dosimetry in the "Manchester System" (Limitation of the Point A Concept)
The "Manchester System" introduced the concept of the use of a required pre-determined dose delivered to a standard anatomical point, point A. The original definition described point A as being 2 cms lateral to the uterine canal and 2 cms superior to the lateral fornix which corresponds to the crossing of uterine artery and the ureter. Theorectically the dose at this point is representative of the dose to the para-cervical triangle. The para-cervical tissue was regarded as the site of the early extension of cancers. It was also in this tissue that the tolerance was of particular importance for there seemed to be evidence that high doses delivered to this area produced increased morbidity. Thus, the point A came to be representative of the dose required for effective treatment in terms of survival and avoidance of complications. The dose at point B, 3 cms lateral to point A, was representative of the dose delivered to the node bearing areas.

"Tod and Meredith"[11] believed that the optimum dose must be delivered in two sessions to point A: 7,600 rads (8,000 R) for patients under 65 years of age, and for patients over 65 years of age 6,300 rads. When combined with the external beam (3,000R with 250KV), the dose at point A was limited to 6,300 rads. This dose requirement concept remained standard practice for some 50 years.

The serious limitation in the point A concept has been offered by Schwarz[14] and Rotman.[21] Essentially, cancer of the cervix often grows irregularly producing distortion of the local and pelvic anatomy. Hence, a predetermined dose to point A might fall in the center of a tumor, and the rapid fall-off there may lead to delivering inadequate dose to the periphery of the tumor. Furthermore, the nearness of point A to the radium sources may produce appreciable fluctuation in the dose rate by a rather minor variation in either radium placement or the point chosen to represent point A on the dosimetry radiograph.

Rotman et al.[21] believed that the reliance on pre-determined doses may be a major cause of treatment failure as well as the high complication rate. He stated that requirements calling for a predetermined dose to point A preclude individualization of treatment, a necessity in radiation therapy. Fulfilling protocol requirements, delivery of a certain dose to point A, may result in delivering excessively high doses to the rectum and bladder. This becomes particularly true in the use of compact intracavitary systems and applicators that have short source-surface distances. We will discuss this further in the section dealing with complications.

Dosimetry of M.D. Anderson System   With the appreciation of the defect in the Manchester System mentioned above, Fletcher adapted the total milligram hours (mg hrs) and hours of insertion as parameters for the intracavitary insertion. From the M.D. Hospital Experience there developed, a concept of maximum mg hrs and hours of insertions, and "maxima" (total number of mg hrs and external beam rads) for optimal treatment.[22] Fletcher recommended a maximum of 10,000 mg hrs or two applications each of 72 hours with the intracavitary irradiation alone. When external beam irradiation and intracavitary irradiation are combined, then the maxima of 10,000 (the addition of external rads and mg hrs) or maximum hours of insertion (which is attenuated depending on the amount of external beam rads, i.e., 24 hours reduction for each 2,000 rads) are to be used. The two parameters (mg-hrs and hours of insertions) are equally important. The insertion is terminated whenever either one of these two parameters (mg-hrs or hours) is reached first.

Treatment Planning

Combined External Beam and Intracavitary Irradiation   Central to the current treatment of cervical cancer by irradiation is the principle that external and intracavitary irradiation are complimentary rather than competing modalities. Their combination must be individualized for each case to achieve maximum results with minimum complications. Planning of treatment is based on the assessment of the volume and the extent of the primary tumor, the risk of regional lymphatic involvement, and anatomy of the pelvic organs. In general, as tumor size or stage of disease increases, so does the need for larger field size and higher doses. The external radiation causes shrinkage of the tumor and as the malignancy is reduced in size it becomes more vulnerable to the intense radiation delivered by the intracavitary applications (Fig. 4-1).

The increasing use of external beam radiation to larger cervical tumors has led to both improved local control and survival. The survival benefits related directly to the ability of external radiation to sterilize regional lymphatics. Fletcher influenced a major change in treatment philosophy by advocating the need for external irradiation in stage II carcinoma, a departure at the time from the entrenched Manchester technique that relied heavily on intracavitary radiation.

Dose Requirements   The treatment volume—radiation dose relationship first advocated by Fletcher in the treatment of epithelial head and neck and breast tumors has been confirmed and accepted by others as a basic principle in modern radiation oncology. He showed that the probability of tumor control is more than 95 percent using a dose of 4,500 rads to 5,000 rads delivered in 4½ to 5 weeks to microscopic deposits (10^6 cells). This dose is well tolerated by most normal tissues. With increasing tumor size to 2 cm (10^8 cells), the radiation dose necessary to control tumor increases to 6,000 to 6,500 rads delivered in 6 to 6½ weeks which carries a proportionately increased normal tissue injury.[15]

At the present time, for best results it appears that a minimal dose of 4,000 rads in 4 to 4½ weeks should be delivered to the lateral parametrial area and pelvic wall in all patients except those with localized disease. Most radiotherapists deliver 6,000 to 6,500 rads to the lateral parametrium where macroscopic disease exists in regional lymph nodes. The minimal dose delivered to the paracervical triangle in these cases ranges from 8,000 to 9,000 rads.

Field Size   Since the radiation dose required depends on the presence and amount of tumor in each area in the target volume, it is important to accurately determine the extent of disease including areas of possible metastases. The pelvic examination mapping the size of cervical tumor, the extension into the vagina, parametrial involvement and/or pelvic wall fixation determines the field size and dose requirement locally. Other information obtained from I.V.P. lymphangiogram, CAT scan or ultrasonograms give the oncologist the extent of tumor away from the primary site. Recent observations suggest that regional disease spread can be predicted by certain morpho-histologic characteristics (Table 4-1). Once the tumor extent and target volume is determined, the radiation dose to be delivered can be determined, using correct individualized proportions of external beam and intracavitary radiation.

RADIOTHERAPEUTIC MANAGEMENT

Micro-Invasive Cancer

Micro-invasive cancers can be managed either by surgery or intracavitary radiation where control of disease approaches 100 percent with either of these modalities. Surgery offers the possibility of preservation of ovarian function in young women. Since the incidence of pelvic lymph node involvement is practically zero and the risk of involvement of para-cervical lymphatics is rare, intracavitary irradiation may be delivered in two 48 hour applications for a total of 7,000 to 8,000 mg-hrs.

Early Invasive Carcinoma (FIGO Stage IB or IIA)

Stage IB disease has increased in incidence over the last 15 years and has thus assumed more importance. FIGO stage IB lesions range from clinically undetectable invasive carcinoma in a conization specimen to a lesion a number of cms in diameter. In these stages of disease individualization of treatment becomes of prime importance, and the volume irradiated must be tailored to tumor size and other biologic factors that increase the risk of regional lymphatic metastasis.

Intracavitary Irradiation Alone   Selection of patients for intracavitary radiation alone requires some caution and rigid criteria. A recent review by Volterrani of 182 patients of stage IB disease showed a 64.8 percent 5-year survival with the use of intracavitary radiation alone.[23] In his analysis, the local failure was as high as 20 percent, and isolated pelvic failure was noted in 14.2 percent of the cases. Hamberger showed that none of 93 patients with a lesion less than 1 cm had developed local failure. Only four patients developed regional failure. However, three out of 17 patients with lesions larger than 1 cm had regional failure and none had local failure. He concluded that patients with small IB lesions (less than 1 cm) can be treated safely with intracavitary irradiation alone and recommended limiting the dose to 8,000 mg hrs for 1A and 10,000 mg hrs for larger IB lesions.[24] However, the higher failure rate in Volterrani's and Hamberger's series cannot be explained on size alone. As will be shown later, certain morphohistologic factors dictate the need of external beam for ablation of regional lymphatics.

Occasionally, external beam is necessary in early stage IB (smaller than 1 cm) disease, where the pelvic anatomy is unsuitable for an ideal intracavitary insertion. If the patient's vaginal anatomy is very narrow or distorted, the number of mg hrs of insertion must be diminished after an appropriate amount of external irradiation is added.

In summary, stage IB patients who have small volume (less than 1 cm) of tumor without poor prognostic morpho-histologic factors and with normal anatomy can be treated with intracavitary irradiation alone delivering 10,000 mg hrs in two separate insertions spaced 2 weeks apart.

Intracavitary and Parametrial External Irradiation Both intracavitary and external parametrial irradiation is used where the central tumor volume is small but the regional lymphatics are at risk. The combination of modalities treats the primary tumor with the intracavitary therapy and relies on external beam irradiation to sterilize parametrial and pelvic wall lymphatics (Fig. 4-2). Unal et al.[25] analyzed the treatment failure results of 173 patients with IB tumor of limited volume (larger than 1 cm, smaller than 3 cm) treated at M.D. Anderson Hospital. The patients received two intracavitary radium insertions and 4,000 rads parametrial irradiation. The determinant 4-year survival rate was 92.5 percent. Eleven patients died of the disease, 2 patients died of complications. The complication rate was high when total mg-hrs exceeded 9,000 (13 out of 125 patients). Their recommendation was a maximum of 9,000 mg-hrs or 120 hours insertions (whichever comes first) given in two insertions and supplemental parametrial irradiation delivered to the pelvic wall to a total external and intracavitary dose of 5,000 to 5,500 rads.

Intracavitary Irradiation Plus Whole Pelvic Irradiation If the lesion is greater than 3 cms in diameter, the periphery of the tumor is beyond the effective

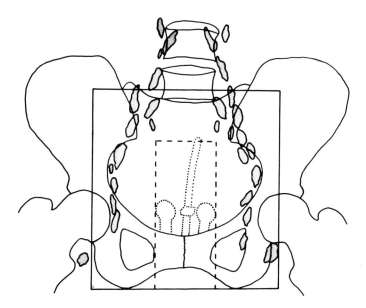

Fig. 4-2. External whole pelvis irradiation is indicated by the solid line. The area inside the broken line is blocked during the parametrial irradiation. This area correponds to the effective dose delivery by the intracavitary application (dotted line).

irradiation volume of the intracavitary insertion and external whole pelvic irradiation is required to shrink the tumor bulk prior to intracavitary irradiation. Depending on the amount of tumor regression the dose of external whole pelvic irradiation varies from 2,000 to 4,000 rads. When patients receive 2,000 rads whole pelvic irradiation they require an additional parametrial boost of 2,000 rads in order to deliver a combined external and intracavitary dose to the pelvic lymph nodes of 5,000 to 5,500 rads. Unal et al.[25] reported an 86 percent five-year survival in 81 patients treated with 2,000 rads whole pelvic irradiation followed by intracavitary irradiation and parametrial irradiation. He recommended that the intracavitary irradiation be limited to a maximum of 7,500 mg-hrs or 100 hrs of insertion (whichever comes first) in two insertions in patients receiving 2000 rads whole pelvic irradiation plus parametrial irradiation. He observed a higher complication rate in patients who had more than 7,500 mg-hrs (0 out of 22 patients vs. 5 out of 54 patients).[25]

Stage IIA

Stage IIA disease is treated the same as I-B lesions depending on the volume of tumor. In general, when there is a significant amount of disease in the vaginal fornix, 4,000 rads whole pelvic irradiation is required to allow for proper placement of the vaginal colpostats.

Stage-IIB and IIIB

Stage II-B cancer of the cervix is a challenging disease for the radiation oncologist both from a diagnostic and a treatment standpoint. Determining tumor extent on pelvic examination requires skill and experience. Disagreement in staging often arises even amongst the most experienced gynecological oncologists, and radiation oncologists.

The presence of paremetrial infiltration of tumor precludes surgical treatment. Because of tumor spread throughout the parametrium and the high incidence of pelvic node metastasis in this stage the use of combined external whole pelvic and intracavitary irradiation is required. The external whole pelvic dose of 4,000/rads in 4 to 4½ weeks is followed by two applications of intracavitary insertions each of 48 hours duration. The initial whole pelvic dose of 4,000 rads will treat the central tumor and pelvic lymphatics. The addition of intracavitary insertion of 6,000 mg-hrs will both raise the central dose enough to control gross disease and contribute an additional 500 to 1,000 rads to the pelvic lymph nodes. This is a conventional treatment approach in most institutions. The survival results in stage II-B disease are summarized in table 4-2.

Bulky disease extending into the lateral parametria requires external whole pelvic irradiation of 4,500 rads to 5,000 rads with an additional 500 rads to the involved side raising tumor dose to at least 6,000 rads. Intracavitary irradiation used for control of central disease should not be omitted. Local disease control is markedly improved with intracavitary insertions despite high doses from the external beam.

Table 4-2. Treatment Results of Carcinoma of the Cervix Using Radiation Therapy (5 Year Survival Rate)

	Stage			
	I	II	III	IV
M.D. Anderson Hospital[26]	91.5	A 83.5	A 45	14
		B 66.5	B 36	
Kottmeier[27]	86.4	60	35	7
Puerto Rico Nuclear Center[28]	88	61	35	19
Cancer Institute Hospital[29]	88.2	68.7	43.1	14.8
Hahnemann Medical College[30]	89	64	52	12
Tufts-New England Med. Ctr.[31]	90.9	A 79	42	23
		B 58		

Stage-IIIA

Although the incidence of this stage of cervical carcinoma is comparatively uncommon, its management calls for additional skill. The infiltration of tumor down the vaginal wall requires higher dose irradiation to be delivered to the related bladder and rectum. Sterilizing doses must be delivered to the entire vaginal mucosa without severely injuring the adajcent bladder and rectum. External radiation is directed to the cervix, vaginal extension, pelvic nodes, and inguinal nodes. Following this, brachytherapy using uterine tandem and intravaginal cylinders rather than colpostats facilitates the delivery of a mucosal dose of 8,000 to 10,000 rads. Localized tumor remaining can be treated with needle implants of radium or radium substitutes. Recently, the concomitant addition of infusion 5-FU to the radiation shows promise of synergistic benefit in reducing large vaginal tumor volume. This will be discussed later in the chapter.

Massive IIIB-Frozen Pelvis

At times massive tumor negates entirely the effectiveness of intracavitary irradiation. Often in very advanced disease the anatomy is so markedly distorted that the proper placement of instruments is practically impossible. In these cases external whole pelvic irradiation is used alone. In order to give meaningful doses of radiation (6,000 to 7,000 rads), a "shrinking field" technique is crucial to reduce the complication rate as much as possible.

Stage IVA

Tumours in this category can be divided into two distinct subgroups. In one, massive tumor extends to both pelvic walls and involves bladder and/or rectum. The management of this group follows the same guidelines as mentioned above for massive stage IIIB disease. In the other group tumour expansion is primarily in an anterior-posterior direction (bladder/rectum), and there is very little, lateral extension (parametrium/pelvic wall). Thus, although the tumor is technically staged as IVA, the volume is relatively much smaller. In these cases following whole pelvic irradiation of 4,000 to 5,000 rads and one intracavitary insertion, the tumour in the bladder and/or rectum is reevaluated. If persistent tumour is found, exenteration is considered. If on the other hand there is tumor clearance, a second intracavitary irradiation will complete all required therapy.

Concomitant infusion of chemotherapeutic agents such as 5FU during whole pelvic external beam may facilitate tumor clearance.

CONTROVERSIES IN MANAGEMENT

Surgery vs. Radiation

At present, surgery, radiation therapy and a combination of these two modalities have been employed successfully to manage early stages (IB & IIA) of the disease. To a great extent, the facility, the experience and beliefs of the personnel involved influence the type of therapy that will be employed.[30] General consensus is that there is little difference in the cure rate of stage I and II-A disease treated by either surgery or radiation therapy. There has not been a large scale prospective randomized study to date, to prove or disprove this belief. However, surgery has superceded radiation therapy in the management of early disease, especially for patients who are young, in good physical condition, relatively thin, and with favorable lesions. The rationale for surgery has been the possibility of preservation of ovarian function in young women and the belief that the remaining vagina provides for better sexual function.

In cases where lymphatic spread in early disease is absent or limited, the results of surgery are rarely compromised. However, when spread through the lymphatics or tissue plane occurs the surgeon's ability to encompass all malignancy becomes severely restricted. Most surgeons recognize difficulties in accomplishing a complete pelvic node dissection not to mention the high probability of cutting through disease leading to a high probability of local recurrence and distal spread. Thus the role of surgery alone is limited to a selected group of women with early disease.

It has, however, become increasingly clear that there exists a significant subpopulation of patients with apparent early disease who are prone to treatment failure, poor survival, and increased local recurrence when managed by radical hysterectomy. Numerous authors have reported the poor prognosis of early stage I-B patients with positive pelvic nodes.[32,33,34] Factors associated with a high incidence of recurrence include size of primary lesion, depth of stromal invasion, vascular invasion, and corpus extension (Table 4-1).[33–38] Patients with these poor prognostic factors require adjuvant treatment after radical hysterectomies. Theoretically post-operative irradiation would destroy microscopic disease in the pelvis. However, there remains the question as to whether post-operative pelvic irradiation can accomplish this to the fullest extent. Radical surgery disrupts normal lymphatic flow creating a "mechanical" collateralization and possible tumour embolization. The surrounding tissue environment and its micro-vasculature is impaired. There is increased fibrosis and scarring within which radioresistant hypoxic tumor cells are embedded. In treating the head and neck area or breasts, an additional dose of 1,000 rads beyond the post-operative basic dose of 5,000 rads is required to overcome this altered hypoxic tissue environment. This requirement is difficult to repeat in the pelvis. Following radical hysterectomy the pelvic organs and fixed loops of bowel are intolerant to doses higher than 4,000 rads. Further, it is difficult to clearly delineate tumor containing areas that might require supplemental irradiation. In addition a number of cases will require post-operative irradiation because of unfavorable prognostic factors. Thus a not small proportion of those early patients with cervical cancer will have radical surgery and intensive radiotherapy and of course the resultant increase in complications.

Brady,[30] in a review of treatment results of surgery and radiation therapy in stages I & II at leading institutions, showed comparable end results. However, in his own series he had a complication rate of 6 percent from radiation therapy, primarily proctitis and cystitis, and about a 10 to 20 percent complication rate from radical surgery, namely lymphedema of the lower extremity, lymphocyst, bladder, or ureteral injury. Eisert analyzed the Kottmeier's annual report on the result of treatment of the cervix with regards to the institutional treatment policies.[39] Ninty-five institutions treated 8,457 patients with favorable medically acceptable stage I disease with surgery and the remainder of 8,343 patients with radiation therapy alone. The overall 5 year survival was 80.7 percent. Fourteen institutions treated all patients with stage IB disease (1,640 patients) with radiotherapy alone with 5-year survival of 77.1 percent. This result is fairly comparable to that of institutions treating surgically the most favorble stage I cases.

Table 4-2 shows the treatment results of early stage disease with radiation alone.

Bulky (Barrel Shaped) Endocervical Carcinomas

Cervical tumors arising from the endocervical canal tend to expand the cervix in concentric fashion, creating a distinct clinical presentation known as the "barrel shaped" cervix. Attention was first paid to the entity by Durrance who analyzed the rate of central recurrence in 1,341 patients with stage I and II cancer of the cervix. The central failures in stage I and II were 1.9 percent and 5.6 percent respectively.[40] In the overall group, many of the central failures were directly related to problems of "geometry" in placing the radium sources around tumor and by slippage of the tandem and colpostats. Further sifting of the material showed that many central failures in stage II occurred in patients who had endocervical bulky disease. This higher local failure rate in barrel shaped cervix cases led to the post-irradiation use of the extra fascial hysterectomy. A later analysis of the 423 patients with barrel shaped cervix at that same institution revealed that patients with lesions 6 cms or less in diameter did not show a statistically significant difference in the incidence of central recurrences with this hysterectomy (4 percent vs. 6 percent) whereas patients with lesions greater than 6 cms benefitted by hysterectomy (2 percent vs. 15.9 percent). However, there was no difference in survival between the groups, as one would have anticipated. Complications were minimal since treatment consisted of 4,000 rads whole pelvis plus a dose reduced one 72 hours radium insertion (limited 5,000 mg hrs) followed by hysterectomy 6 weeks later. Only 1 patient out of 102 patients developed a vesicovaginal fistula, and 1 patient had a small bowel obstruction.[15] Results of other small series prompted a resurgence in post-radiation surgery extending the criteria to all bulky barrel-shaped disease presentations. Instead of limiting this combined modality therapy to cervical lesions over 6cms it created a Pandora's box where additional surgery was performed in all bulky stage IB through II cases.

A retrospective study by Rotman et al. refuted the use of the combined approach. He found that in patients treated with the combined surgical-radiation approach for bulky, exophytic, and barrel-shaped tumors, there was no evidence of disease in the surgical specimen in over 90 percent of the cases. Among patients receiving radiation and surgery, there was an increased incidence of severe gastrointestinal (15 percent fistulization) and urinary complications including a significantly higher incidence of a varying degree of obstructive uropathy. However, the radiation only treatment in his study for barrel shaped disease was more intense and included the use of 4,000 to 5,000 rads whole pelvic irradiation in 5 to 6 weeks and two or three intracavitary radium insertions (4,500 to 6,000 mg-hrs).[41] The RTOG and GOG are attempting to answer the question of the need of conservative surgery following radiation in prospective randomized controlled trials.

Attempts to predict radiation sterilization of cervical carcinoma have gone on for several decades. Recently Hardt and Van Nagell resurrected the concept of radiation induced tumor regression as a prognostic factor.[42] In a retrospective analysis of 200 patients with cervical cancers, the extent of tumor response to radiation evaluated 1 month after completion of therapy was well correlated with the recurrence rate. Thus the rate of tumor regression during the radiation treatment can be used as a parameter in determining the necessity for an additional conservative hysterectomy. It should be kept in mind that an analysis of central regression is incomplete unless poor radium geometry due to poor placement is ruled out. Further, the rate of tumor regression may be entirely misleading from a radiobiological standpoint. A logical therapeutic sequence based on the discussion presented suggests individualization of treatment is necessary. For example, following 4,000 rads whole pelvic irradiation and one or two radium insertions totalling 4,000 to 4,500 mg hrs, if residual tumor can be included within the effective intracavitary irradiation volume (probably less than 4 cms in diameter) the treatment can be continued with irradiation alone. Whereupon, a total of 6,000 mg hrs is delivered using up to three radium insertions. If the tumor is still large the chance of control with radiation alone becomes doubtful. In this case an extra fascial hysterectomy should be done without further radiation therapy (tumors originally larger than 8 cms will usually fall into this group).

Para-Aortic Irradiation

The ability to encompass and sterilize lymphatics by external radiation therapy has improved 5 year survival over techniques that concentrated only on the primary site.[43] More recent attempts to improve these statistics by concentrating therapeutics only to the pelvic region have had little impact on survival but instead have increased the incidence and severity of complications.[43,44] The incidence of pelvic disease recurrence in patients with less than Stage III disease treated by radical radiation therapy is minimal.[15] In the majority of patients who fail, disease is found outside the pelvic confines. This pattern of failure has not been altered by the addition of systemic chemotherapeutic and immunological treatments.

Para-aortic nodal involvement increases progressively with the stage of disease. It rises from less than 10 percent of patients with stage IA-IB disease to 15 to 46 percent in stages II-IIIB.[45-47] It should be recognized that statistical reports of nodal involvement are often based on random samplings from relatively small numbers of patients, and consequently should be considered minimal estimates. Microscopic foci of tumor are often missed both in the operating room and in the surgical pathology examination. The value of the lymphangiogram in identifying nodal metastasis is controversial. Even its most avid supporters admit that important nodes are not opacified, that metastases must have a minimum size to be visible, and that benign alterations may be misinterpreted leading to a 25 to 50 percent disparity between clinical and surgical staging.[45,46] Radiation oncologists recognizing the pathophysiologic spread of cervical cancer have extended radiation portals to encompass the para-aortic nodes in an attempt to improve survival. No doubt enthusiasm for this approach was tempered by early reports of increased complications. Analysis of the data showed that unacceptable morbidity resulted from the empirically chosen high total dose and the techniques utilized.[47,48] Attempts to ablate disease in the para aortic region have been made therapeutically or prophylactically.

Therapeutic Para Aortic Irradiation   Exploratory celiotomy followed by extended field irradiation was based on the premise that (1) tumor extent can be accurately assessed and (2) that reduction of tumor volume to subclinical amounts would require only limited irradiation for tumor control. Tewfik reported the treatment results of 23 patients who received 5,000 to 5,500 rads to the para-aortic area for histologically proven metastases. Five patients (21.7 percent) are alive and well more than 45 months later. Three out of 5 survivors developed late bowel complications.[49] Still the results of therapeutic para-aortic irradiation are rather disappointing not withstanding a higher complication rate. The reason for poor results may be related to the tumor burden and its higher dose requirements or possibly of disease spread at time of surgery beyond the irradiated areas. One of the dilemmas in the therapeutic irradiation of these nodes is that the radiation dose required for more than microscopic aggregates (more than 4,500 rads) results in increasing late complications. Surgical debulking to reduce tumor volume to microscopic status may decrease the required radiation dose but at the same time it decreases tissue tolerance. In fact the question must be raised as to whether partial lymphadenectomy may result in (1) blood born spread of tumor cells during the surgical procedure (2) formation of collateral channels of lymphatics forcing tumor outside normal pathways or (3) lymphatic reflux of tumor cells away from the treated areas.

Intraoperative electron beam therapy directed to the para-aortic area at the time of exploratory laparotomy, prophylactically or therapeutically, may eliminate or reduce the above mentioned limitations of therapy. The aluminum and plastic collimators allow visualization of treatment areas and keep the bowel out of the treatment beam. The precise beam alignment reduces the morbidity because uninvolved tissue is retracted out of the radiation field. However, radiobiologic tolerance of normal tissue and the tumor control dose of a single electron beam treatment require further evaluation.[50]

Extended field techniques following positive lymphangiography at M.D. Anderson Hospital are based on the lymphangiographic evidence of nodal metastasis as well as the clinical stage of the disease.[51] Their 5 percent false positive rate using lymphangiograms results from the strict criteria adopted by Wallace et al.[52] In patients with favorable pelvic disease the fields are extended to cover the next tumor free echelon of nodes. Usually, a dose of 4500 rads is delivered at 180 rads per day to the nodal areas. An additional 1000 to 1500 rads is later directed through smaller fields to the positive nodes. In patients with more extensive pelvic disease requiring at least 5000 rads, fields are extended 3 cm above the highest positive node seen on the lymphangiogram and no boost treatment is given to positive nodes.

Prophylatic Para-aortic Irradiation   The rationale for prophylactic irradiation of the para-aortic lymph nodes includes: (1) the lack of acceptable and accurate diagnostic methods of detection of clinical para-aortic disease; (2) the documented increase in morbidity with combination radiation and surgery; (3) the large percentage of ultimate treatment failures with distant metastases due to clinically undetected micrometastatic disease in the para-aortic nodes. Rotman et al.[53] reported a retrospective study of 78 patients, followed for a minimum of 2 years. The patients who received para-aortic irradiation had a statistically increased survival over patients treated only to the pelvis (79 percent vs. 53.8 percent in stage II-B). The dose employed was 4500 rads in 4½ to 5 weeks. Using multiple field techniques, they demonstrated that extended field irradiation was well tolerated. The value of para-aortic irradiation is being evaluated currently by randomized prospective clinical trials.

COMPLICATIONS

The art of radiation therapy lies in the ability to judge the optimal dose required to achieve maximum therapeutic benefit. This requires consideration of the probability of tumor control versus the risk of corresponding complications.

While newer multidisciplinary approaches to the treatment of oncologic disease have increased survival, consistent refinements in treatment methods have been required to prevent increases in short- and long-term morbidity. Attempts to evaluate and avoid complications have, at times, only underlined our basic inability to quantitate the insults of combined therapy.

Classification

Radiation complications are predominantly related to bladder, ureter, rectosigmoid, and small bowel injuries.[54,55] Acute reactions which commonly develop during treatment include bowel or urinary symptoms of diarrhea, tenesmus, frequent urination, or dysuria. These reactions although frequent are more or less transient and easily managed by conservative diet or oral medications. The problematic complications are those that appear some 6 to 24 months after the completion of therapy. In the bowel these include persistent symptoms of enteritis, proctitis, and sigmoiditis as well as bowel obstruction, hemorrhage, and fistula. Similar symptom complexes are found in the bladder ranging from mild cystitis to hemmorrhage or fistulization. They vary in intensity from mild symptoms and minimal changes in mucosa (Grade I), to mucous discharge and bleeding (Grade II), necrosis, ulceration, pain and moderate stenosis, and finally to stenosis requiring colostomy, perforation or fistula formation (Grade III).[56] Obstructive uropathy varies in degree from mild (Grade I), through moderate (Grade II), and severe (Grade III), to non-visualization (Grade IV).[57]

Pre-Disposing Factors

Inherent   Anemia, systemic diseases such as hypertension and diabetes, poor nutritional status (lower economic groups), advanced age and higher clinical stage of disease lend themselves to decreased tolerance of radiation treatment.[55] Localized inflammatory processes including colitis, diverticulitis, pelvic inflammatory disease, tubo-ovarian abscess and peritonitis all significantly add to complications.[25,55] The above inherent factors also affect survival either directly i.e., anemia and hypoxia, or indirectly by causing treatment interruption and delay.

Extrinsic

Radiation and Surgery

1.   Biopsies for suspected recurrent disease following radical radiation therapy is a major cause of fistula formation.[58]

2.   Laparotomy: a disruption of the peritoneal lining results in adhesions and fixation of bowel loops and an increase in bowel complications by a factor of 2.6.[59] Where exploration is necessary for diagnostic evaluation of nodal disease, a retroperitoneal approach is preferred.

3.   Radical hysterectomy and lymphadenectomy has been reported to increase the incidence of complications by a factor of 4.[41,58,60] A retrospective study by Rotman of 41 patients with Stage IIB carcinoma of the cervix treated with radiation alone, versus radiation and radical hysterectomy, showed an increased incidence of severe complications when radical surgery was used. There was a higher incidence of fistula formation and, interestingly a 60 percent incidence of prolonged unilateral or bilateral obstructive uropathy in patients undergoing surgery in addition to radiation.

Radiation Alone   Moderate to severe bowel damage becomes evident 6 to 18 months following initial radiation. Severe lesions are usually localized in the anterior rectal wall immediately behind the cervix. In cases where the intrauterine radium dosage has been considerably increased, damage may appear higher up in the rectum or even the lower sigmoid.[56]

Bladder complications other than cystitis become symptomatic later than bowel occurring up to several years following irradiation. At that time differentiation between injury and tumor recurrence may be difficult as biopsy in these cases should be avoided.

Technical factors affecting normal tissue tolerance include daily and total dose, time-dose factors, beam energy and size and separation of fields. With higher energies (20 MeV), larger fields with larger separations are better tolerated. The need to treat all fields during each session has assumed greater importance in recent years because of the higher doses and larger field sizes required to encompass and sterilize nodal disease, i.e., common iliac and para-aortic nodes.[16,17,18]

It is well documented that whole pelvic irradiation of more than 5,000 rads increases complication significantly. Treatment portals should be reduced to 12×12 cms after 5,000 rads, and further reduced to 10×10 cms after 6,000 rads. With this shrinking field technique, only 5 percent of 104 patients who were treated by external radiotherapy (5,000 rads to 7,000 rads) developed severe sigmoiditis.[61]

The high rate of complications associated with extended field irradiation relates to the upper limit of the field, total dose, and daily dose. The field extended above the second lumbar vertebra includes a significant proportion of stomach and small intestine. Anterior and posterior parallel opposing field arrangement with low megavoltage radiation throughout the whole course of treatment produces hot spots in the superficially located organs (GI tract and spinal cord). In a recent analysis of complications in extended field irradiation, Senoussi and Fletcher concluded that a total of 4,500 rads at the rate of 900 rads per week is all that can be given safely.[62] If higher doses are required, reduced field size and multiple protals may safely deliver an additional 500 to 1,000 rads.

Generally, complications are not greatly influenced by the amount of radiation delivered by intracavitary radiation as compared to external therapy. However, under certain circumstances, the incidence of complications is directly proportional to the dose given by intracavitary radiation. The parameters involved in these instances include the type of applicator and the arrangement of radioactive sources, the geometry of the application, and its isodose distribution.[22,25] For example (1) a protruding vaginal source was a major cause of rectal ulcers in 60 percent of 32 patients with fistulas in Strockbine's series.[22] (2) A tandem deviated to the side creates a hot spot in the acute angle between the deviated tandem and the colpostats. This produces ureteral strictures at the ureteral vesical junction, obstructing sigmoditis, and fistulas. (3) An anteriorly or posteriorly flexed tandem delivers a high dose to the base of bladder anteriorly or sigmoid colon posteriorly. (4) Structural shortcomings of applicators as reported by Rotman give up to a 9 percent incidence of fistulas. The Ernst applicator used in his series had inherent structural design deficiencies resulting in severe complications.[63] He pointed out that gauze used as packing in a vagina when wet flattens out leading to a 26 percent increase in the dose delivered to the rectal mucosa. In his series there was a 4-fold increase in the incidence of fistulae in these patients as compared to cases treated later using other applicators.

The proliferation in recent years of numerous types of intracavitary applicators demands a cautious approach prior to their adoption. A long-term study of new instruments with established apparatus comparing their ability to control disease while avoiding complications is required.

FUTURE MODALITIES

The radioresistance of hypoxic tumor cells and the concept of tumor burden are foremost amongst the factors blamed for failure of disease control. Hypoxic cells are $2\frac{1}{2}$ times resistant to the effects of radiation compared to well oxygenated cells. The term tumor burden was coined to encompass characteristics such as tumor size, virulence of the neoplastic cells, lymphatic involvement with reference to the number and size of involved nodes, and the hypothesized influence of various little known immune factors.

Hypoxic cell sensitizers, high L.E.T. (Linear Energy Transfer) radiation, infusional chemotherapy, and hyperfractionation are the new therapeutics being evaluated to enhance radiation response.

Heavy Particle Radiation

Unlike the low L.E.T. gamma radiation in widespread clinical use today, high L.E.T. or heavy particle radiation does not afford the same protection to hypoxic tumors cells. Therefore, it is logical to assume that the latter radiations would be more effective in bulky locally advanced tumors with their large hypoxic fraction than the low L.E.T. radiation in current use.

Neutrons

Recent trials conducted by the RTOG have compared neutron irradiation vs. neutron and photon mixed beam irradiation. Analysis of the results to date have not demonstrated any significant difference between the two arms.

Hypoxic Cell Sensitizers

These drugs sensitize hypoxic tumor cells. Their effect is analogous to the enhanced radiosensitivity imparted by oxygen at the cellular level. Misonidazole (RO-07-0582), the drug most extensively investigated to date, belongs to the group of electron affinic drugs, which are the most effective hypoxic cell sensitizers. Metronidazole (Flagyl), the well-known trichomonacide, also belongs to this group. There are dose related neurotoxic and central nervous system effects including sensory polyneuropathy, confusion, lethargy, and coma observed during the use of these drugs. However, when the dose of misonidazole does not exceed 12 gm/m^2 the toxicity is negligible and transient.

Misonidazole is presently being intensively studied in treatment of stage IIIB and IV. There has been no statistical advantage observed thus far in treatment of either stage.

Infusional Chemotherapy and Radiation

The concomitant use of infusional 5-fluorouracil (5-FU) and radiation has exciting potential as a therapeutic modifier. Dramatic tumor responses have been obtained in the treatment of squamous cell and adenocarcinomas of the anus, esophagus, and rectum.[64,65] The benefits of such a combination following 5-FU were demonstrated by Heidelberger.[66] Later Bagshaw showed a synergistic cytocidal response when cells exposed to 5-FU were irradiated.[67] Viettie confirmed the synergism of 5-FU plus radiation and also showed that this synergism was strongly dependent on the time of administration of the drug and x-rays.[68] 5-FU is a pyrimidine analog which blocks the enzyme thymidilate synthetase, thus preventing the conversion of deoxyuridylic acid to thymidilic acid: a percursor for DNA synthesis. 5FU also blocks the pathway for RNA synthesis thus preventing or slowing down the protein synthesis necessary for radiation repair pathways. Byfield found that 5-FU continuous infusion (up to 9 hours), as compared to conventional intravenous bolus administration, was synergistic and significantly less myelotoxicity.[64]

Although acute small and large bowel reactions have not appreciably increased with the combined technique, it is prudent to maintain the daily fractionation below 200 rads to reduce the incidence of long term bowel complications. The treatment of cases with advanced cervical carcinoma using an 120 hour (five day) infusion of 5FU (25 mgm/kgm body weight) with daily radiotherapy is expected to greatly facilitate tumor control with minimal increase in morbidity.

Fractionation

Much effort has been directed to the fractionation of radiation to improve the therapeutic ratio. Multifractionated daily treatment schedules seems to have the potential benefit of increasing the therapeutic ratio, probably by utilizing the different biological behavior of tumors and normal tissues to fractionated courses of radiation (repair of sublethal damage, regeneration and redistribution of tumor cells etc). A time gap of 3 to 4 hours between each session of treatment should provide enough time for normal tissue to repair sublethal damage whereas this is not the case for the tumor cells. There are two different techniques where more than one fraction per day is given.

Hyperfractionation delivers more than one radiation treatment fraction per day in a conventional over-all treatment time. Consequently, a larger number of smaller size fractions are used in this technique. By doing so, the probability of radiation acting on the more sensitive phases within the tumor cell cycle increases, leading to increased cell kill. Further, the smaller dose per fraction is tolerated better by normal tissues thereby reducing late complications.

Accelerated fractionation is the technique in which the overall treatment time is reduced but not the total dose by delivering more than one fraction per day. The fraction size is similar to that used in conventional therapy. The strategy of shortening the overall treatment time is to upset the tumor regeneration which would occur during a protracted course of conventional radiation therapy in rapidly proliferating tumors. Thus multifractional treatment per day may hold promise for sterilization of a large or rapidly progressing tumor without increase of complications.

REFERENCES

1. Recent Trends in Survival of Cancer Patients. U.S. Department of Health, Education and Welfare, 1974.
2. Plentl AA, Friedman EA: Lymphatics of the cervix uteri. In Lymphatic System of the Female Genitalia. Philadelphia, WB Saunders Co., 1971, 75–93.
3. Henriksen E: The lymphatic spread of carcinoma of the cervix and the body of the uterus. Am J Obstet Gynecol 58:925, 1959.
4. Miller NF, Hinerman DL, Riley GM, et al: The nature of cervix cancer. Obstet Gynecol 14:703, 1959.
5. Beclere A: The use of radium in medicine. Smithsonian Institute, Annual Review, 201–202, 1924.

6. Anonymous: Radium, cure of cancer. Current Literature 35:348, 1903.

7. Heyman J: Radiological or operative treatment of cancer of uterus. Acta Radiol 8:363, 1927.

8. Kottmeir HL: Studies of dosage distribution in pelvis in radium treatment of carcinoma of uterine cervix according to the Stockholm Method. J Fac Radiol 2:312, 1951.

9. Baud J: Carcinoma of the cervix (Stage I) treated intracavitarily with radium alone. J Am Med Assoc 138: 1138, 1948.

10. Lacassagne A: Results of the treatment of cancer of the cervix uteri. B Med J 2:912, 1932.

11. Tod M, Meredith WJ: Treatment of cancer of cervix uteri: A revised "Manchester Method: Br J Radiol 26:252, 1953.

12. Tod M, Meredith WJ: Dosage system for use in treatment of cancer of uterine cervix. Br J Radiol 11:809, 1938.

13. Rutledge FN, Fletcher GH, MacDonald EJ: Pelvic lymphadenectomy as an adjunct to radiation therapy in treatment for carcinoma of the cervix. Am J Roentgenol 93:607, 1965.

14. Schwarz G: An evaluation of the Manchester System of treatment of the cervix. Am J Roentgenol 105:579, 1969.

15. Fletcher GH: Textbook of Radiotherapy. ed 3. Philadelphia, Lea and Febiger, 1980, pp. 720–773.

16. Wilson CS, Hall EJ: On the advisability of treating all fields at each radiotherapy session. Radiology 98:419, 1971.

17. Ellis F, Sorensen A, Lesorenier C: Radiation therapy schedules for opposing parallel fields and their biological effects. Radiology 111:701, 1974.

18. Stupar TA, Bahr GK, Elson HR, et al: Generation of iso-TDF maps: considerations for radiation therapy planning, Radiology 126:773, 1978.

19. Newall J: Intracavitary applicators for cervical carcinoma: their present status. Int J Rad Oncol Biol Phys 4:1115, 1978.

20. Hall EJ: Radiation dose rate: a factor of importance in radiobiology and radiotherapy. Br J Radiol 45:81, 1972.

21. Rotman M, John M, Boyce J: Prognostic factors in cervical carcinoma: Implications in staging and management. Cancer 48:560, 1981.

22. Strockbine MF, Hancock JE, Fletcher GH: Complications in 831 patients with squamous cell carcinoma of the intract uterine cervix treated with 3,000 rads or more pelvis irradiation. Am J Roentgenol 58:293, 1970.

23. Volterrani F, Lombardi F: Long term results of radium therapy in cervical cancer. Int J Rad Oncol Biol Phys 6:565, 1980.

24. Hamberger AD, Fletcher GH, Wharton JT: Results of treatment of early stage I carcinoma of the uterine cervix with intracavitary radium alone. Cancer 41:980, 1978.

25. Unal A, Hamberger AD, Seski JC, et al: An analysis of the severe complications of irradiation of carcinoma of the uterine cervix: treatment with intracavitary radium and parametrial irradiation. Int J Rad Oncol Biol Phys 7:999, 1981.

26. Fletcher GH: Cancer of the uterine cervix, Janeway lecture-1970. Am J Roentgenol 111:225, 1971.

27. Kottmeier HL: Classification and staging of malignant tumors in the female pelvis. J Int Fed Gynecol Obstet 9:172, 1971.

28. Marcial VA: Carcinoma of the cervix: Present status and future. Cancer 39:945, 1977.

29. Masubuchi K, Tenjin Y, Kubo H, et al: Five-year cure rate for carcinoma of the cervix uteri. Am J obstet Gynecol 103:566, 1969.

30. Brady LW: Surgery or radiation therapy for Stage I and IIA carcinoma of the cervix. Int J Rad Oncol Biol Phys 5:1877, 1979.

31. Tak WK, Munzenrider JE, Mitchell GW: External irradiation and one radium application for carcinoma of the cervix. Int J Rad Oncol Biol Phys 5:29,1979.

32. Disaia PJ: Surgical aspects of cervical cancer. Cancer 48:548, 1981.
33. Boyce J, Fruchter RG, Nicastri A, et al: Lesion size, extent of disease and outcome in stage I carcinoma of the cervix. J Gynecol Oncol 12:154, 1981.
34. Chung CK, Nahas WA, Stryker JA, et al: Analysis of factors contributing to treatment failure in Stage IB and IIA carcinoma of the cervix. Am J Obstet Gynecol 138:550, 1980.
35. Van Nagell JR, Donaldson ES, Wood EG, et al: The significance of vascular invasion and lymphocytic infilitration in invasive cervical cancer. Cancer 41:228, 1978.
36. Perez CA, Zivnuska F, Askin F, et al: Mechanisms of failure in patients with carcinoma of the uterine cervix extending into the endometrium. Rad Oncol Biol Phys 2:651, 1977.
37. Boyce J, Fruchter R, Nicastri A, et al: Vascular invasion in Stage I carcinoma of the cervix. Cancer (in press).
38. Van Nagell JR, Donaldson ES, Parker JC, et al: The prognostic significance of cell type and lesion size in patients with cervical cancer treated by radical surgery. Gynecol Oncol 5:142, 1977.
39. Del Regato JA, Spjut HJ: Cancer. 5th ed. In Cervix. St Louis, CV Mosby, 1977.
40. Durrance FY, Fletcher GH, Rutledge FN: Analysis of central recurrent disease in Stage I and II squamous cell carcinoma of the cervix in the intact uterus. Am J Roentgenol 106:831, 1969.
41. Rotman M, John MJ, Moon SH, et al: Limitations of adjunctive surgery in carcinoma of the cervix. Int J Rad Oncol Biol Phys 5:327, 1979.
42. Hardt N, Van Nagell JR, Hanson M, et al: Radiation induced tumor regression as a prognostic factor in patients with invasive cervical cancer. Cancer 49:35, 1982.
43. Rutledge FN, Fletcher GH: Transperitoneal pelvic lymphadenectomy following supervoltage irradiation for squamous cell carcinoma of the cervix. Am J Obstet Gynecol 76:321, 1958.
44. Rutledge FN, Wharton JT, Fletcher GH: Clinical studies with adjunctive surgery and radiation therapy in the treatment of carcinoma of the cervix. Cancer 38:596, 1976.
45. Minutes: Gynecology Oncology Group Meeting: Los Angeles, California, Los Angeles, California. 1977, pp. 294–297.
46. Averette HEe, Ford Jr JH, Dudan RC, et al: Staging of cervical cancer. Clin Obstet Gynecol 18:215, 1975.
47. Nelson JH, Boyce J, Maccasaet M, et al: Incidence, significance, and follow-up of para aortic lymph node metastasis in late invasive carcinoma of the cervix. Am J Obstet Gynecol 128:336, 1977.
48. Piver MS, Barlow JJ, Krishnamsetty R: Five-year survival (with no evidence of disease) in patients with biopsy-confirmed aortic node metastasis from cervical carcinoma. Am J Obstet Gynecol 139:575, 1981.
49. Tewfik HH, Buchsbaum HJ, Latourette HB, et al: Para-aortic lymph node irradiation in carcinoma of the cervix after exploratory laparotomy and biopsy-proven positive aortic nodes. Int J Rad Oncol Biol Phys 8:13, 1982.
50. Goldson AL, Delgado G, Hill L: Intraoperative radiation of the para-aortic nodes in cancer of the uterine cervix. Obstet Gynecol 52:713, 1978.
51. Hamberger AD, Fletcher GH: Is surgical evaluation of the para-aortic nodes prior to irradiation of benefit in carcinoma of the cervix? Int J Rad Oncol Biol Phys 8:151, 1982.
52. Wallace S, Jing BS, Zornoza J, et al: Is lymphangiography worthwhile? Int J Rad Oncol Biol Phys 5:1873, 1979.
53. Rotman M, Moon S, John M, et al: Extended field para aortic irradiation in cervical carcinoma: The case for prophylactic treatment. Int J Rad Oncol Biol Phys 4:795, 1978.
54. Roswit B, Malsky SJ, Reid CB: Radiation tolerance of the gastrointestinal tract. Frontiers Rad Therapy Oncol 6:160, 1972.

55. Rubin P, Casarett GW: Clinical Radiation Pathology, Vol 1. WB Saunders Co, 1968.
56. Kottmeier HC, Gray MJ: Rectal and bladder injuries in relation to radiation dosage in carcinoma of the cervix. A five year follow-up. Am J Obstet Gynecol 82:74, 1961.
57. Butcher HR Jr: Ileal conduit method of ureteral urinary diversion. Ann Surg 156:682, 1962.
58. Boronow RC, Rutledge F: Vesico-vaginal fistula, radiation and gynecologic cancer. Am J Obstet Gynecol 111:85, 1971.
59. Powell-Smith C: Factors influencing the incidence of radiation injury in cancer of the cervix. J Canada Ass Radiol 16:132, 1967.
60. Rafla S: Surgery after high dose radiotherapy. Radiology 114: 131, 1972.
61. Castro JR, Issa P, Fletcher GH: Carcinoma of the cervix treated by external irradiation alone. Radiology 95:163, 1970.
62. Senoussi MAE, Fletcher GH, Borlase BC: Correlation of radiation and surgical parameters in complications in the extended field technique for carcinoma of the cervix. Int J Rad Oncol Biol Phys 5:927, 1979.
63. Rotman M, John M, Roussis K, et al: The intracavitary applicator in relation to complications of pelvic radiation—The Ernst System. Int J Rad Oncol Biol Phys 4:951, 1978.
64. Byfield JE, Barone R, Medelsohn J, et al: Infusional 5 fluorouracil and x-ray therapy for non-resectable esophageal cancer. Cancer 45:703, 1980.
65. Seifert P, Baker LD, Reed MS, et al: Comparison of continously infused 5 fluorouracil with bolus injection in treatment of patients with colorectal adenocarcinoma. Cancer 36:123, 1975.
66. Heidelberger C, et al: Studies of fluorinated pyrimidines II. Effects on transplanted tumors: Cancer Res 3:305, 1958.
67. Bagshaw MA, et al: Possible role of potentiators in radiation therapy. Am J Roentgenol 85:822, 1961.
68. Vietti T, et al: Combined effect of x-irradiation and 5 fluorouracil on survival of transplanted leukemic cells. J Nat Ca Inst 47:865, 1971.

5 | Cervical Cancer: Role of Chemotherapy

Arlene A. Forastiere
Gary A. Schnur

Carcinoma of the uterine cervix will be the cause of approximately 6800 deaths in American women in 1984.[1] This reflects a greater than 50 percent reduction in the annual death rate from cancer of the cervix over the past 30 years. This impressive gain represents the results of a shift to the diagnosis of earlier stage invasive and in-situ disease due to the widespread use of the Papanicolaou cytologic screening test. Advances in radiation therapy, surgical techniques, and improvements in post-operative care for those patients undergoing radical pelvic surgery have also improved the outlook for women with cervical cancer. However, when one looks at survival of women with invasive cervical cancer, on a stage for stage basis, there has, in fact, been little improvement in cure rates.[2] Forty to 50 percent of patients eventually manifest persistent or recurrent cervical cancer and as few as 6 percent survive 3 years from the time of recurrence.[3] Thus, as the Pap smear has become more widely used, the identification of more effective treatment for patients with (1) recurrent disease following local-regional treatment and (2) a high risk for recurrence after primary curative local treatment have become the major challenges confronting medical, gynecologic and radiation oncologists treating this disease.

The magnitude of the problem becomes further apparent when one looks at the patterns of spread and sites of failure. The predilection for this tumor to invade local structures within the pelvis is reflected in the clinically defined staging system discussed in other chapters. The risk of lymphatic spread to pelvic and para-aortic nodes

Partially supported by PHS Grant #5T32 CA09357-03 awarded by the National Cancer Institute, DHHS and hematogeneous dissemination through the venous plexus of the paracervical veins is related to tumor volume or stage at diagnosis. Tumor spread is initially into the vaginal mucosa, the myometrium and paracervical lymphatics with secondary spread to the common iliac, hypogastric, and para-aortic nodes. The incidence of metastases to para-aortic nodes ranges from 6 to 22 percent for stage IB and II lesions, 30 to 40 percent for stage III disease and 50 to 60 percent for stage IV disease.[4-7]

Eighty percent of treatment failures occur within 24 months of primary therapy. Reported pelvic recurrence rates, by stage, are: stage IB 6 percent, stage II 12 to 19 percent, stage III 36 to 47 percent, IVA-68 to 75 percent. Distant metastases develop in up to 14 percent of stage IB patients, approximately 25 percent of IIA + B patients, 40 percent of stage III and 65 percent of stage IVA patients.[3,8-10] Lung, mediastinal and supraclavicular lymph nodes, bone and liver are the most common sites.[10-12] Hence, although great strides have been made in the earlier diagnosis of carcinoma of the cervix, there remains a significant population of poor prognosis patients who will have persistent or recurrent disease despite aggressive primary treatment with radical surgery and/or irradiation.

Since the mid-1970's chemotherapy has been used to treat patients with recurrent or persistent disease who are not candidates for salvage surgery or radiotherapy. Prior to that time experience with chemotherapy was minimal.[13,14] In general, both single agents and combination chemotherapy regimens have had little impact on prolonging survival in this patient population. The identification of active treatment regimens has been slow and difficult for several reasons. Most patients have previously been heavily irradiated resulting in limited bone marrow reserve. Hence, the maximally tolerated dose of chemotherapy may indeed be suboptimal to observe a therapeutic response to a potentially active agent. Poor renal function due to ureteral obstruction will limit the use of renally excreted drugs. Disruption of the vascular supply to the tumor bed by prior surgery and radiotherapy may limit the concentration of drug delivery achievable by the systemic route. Persistent disease in the pelvis may consist of tumor masses with necrotic and hypoxic centers containing a low growth fraction, resistant cell population. For squamous tumors, in particular, the likelihood of observing significant disease regression in this setting is small. Other problems arise in evaluating response of disease in a previously irradiated field since a significant component of the observed disease may represent fibrotic tissue. Although the CT scanner has greatly improved our ability to "visualize" pelvic masses, evaluation of percent regression of actual tumor is likely to be inaccurate.

In spite of these obstacles, chemotherapy has the potential to significantly contribute to the primary management of invasive disease as an adjunct to local treatment modalities in the poor prognosis patient. The limitations of local treatment modalities in effecting cure in patients with stages III and IV disease, bulky endocervical lesions, or para-aortic node involvement have been well defined. In addition to its use as a systemic form of therapy for recurrent disease, the role of chemotherapy as a radiosensitizer and for regional perfusion of pelvic disease is being explored. The current results of systemic chemotherapy and alternative therapeutic strategies for squamous cell carcinoma of the cervix will be the focus of this discussion.

SYSTEMIC THERAPY OF RECURRENT DISEASE

Single Agents

Numerous cytotoxic drugs have been tested in patients with recurrent disease. Table 5-1 details those with reported activity. With the exception of more recent trials such as those evaluating cisplatin[24–32] and phase II new drug trials (Table 5-2), response rates are difficult to interpret. Much of the data generated from trials prior to 1976[15] employed non-uniform response criteria and a variety of doses and schedules with small numbers of patients in any one study. Never-the-less some degree of activity generally ranging from 10 to 25 percent has been observed with multiple alkylating agents, antimetabolites, and antibiotics. Nearly all responses are partial and of brief duration. Those historically reported to be the most active are cyclophosphamide, bleomycin, Adriamycin, and mitomycin-C although it is difficult to find data from more recent, carefully controlled trials to support this conclusion.

Piver et al.[21] evaluated Adriamycin in doses of 60 to 90 mg/m^2 every 3 weeks.

Table 5-1. Activity of Single Agents

Agent	No. of Trials	Evaluable Patients	% Responding (range)	Reference
Alkylating Agents				
Cyclophosphamide	7	241	14% (5–23%)	14,15,16
Chlorambucil	2	44	25% (22–27%)	15
Melphalan	1	20	20%	15
Thiotepa	1	6	17%	15
Carmustine (BCNU)	1	7	14%	15
Lomustine (CCNU)	2	63	5% (3–20%)	15,17
Semustine (methyl-CCNU)	2	94	7% (5–13%)	15,17
Antimetabolites				
5-Fluorouracil	7	350	14% (0–33%)	14,15
Methotrexate				
Conventional dosage	7	85	15% (8–21%)	15,18
High dose with				
leukovorin	1	7	29%	
Antibiotics				
Bleomycin				
Intermittent dosing	6	172	10% (0–17%)	15
Continuous infusion	1	32	25%	19
Porfiromycin	4	78	22% (7–33%)	15,20
Mitomycin-C	2	23	22% (20–22%)	15
Adriamycin	5	115	10% (5–25%)	15,16,18,21
Other				
Vincristine				
Weekly	2	44	23% (8–29%)	15
Continuous infusion	1	11	0	22
Dacarbazine (DTIC)	1	12	25%	15
Hexamethylmelamine	4	56	21% (5–38%)	15,16
Cytembena	1	35	20%	23
Cisplatin	10	492	27% (0–100%)	24–32

Table 5-2. New Agents in Cervical Cancer Tested by the GOG

Agent	Dose & Schedule	Eval. Pts.	% CR + PR	Reference
Maytansine	1.2 mg/m² IV q 3 wks	29	3%	33
ICRF-159	2.5 gms/m² IV q wk	28	18%	34
Baker's Antifol	500 mg/m² q wk	32	16%	35
VP-16-213	100 mg/m² d 1,3,5 q 4 wks	30	0	36
Dianhydrogalactilol	60 mg/m² IV q wk	36	19%	37
Piperazinedione	9 mg/m² q 3 wks	43	5%	38

Of 50 patients with recurrent disease there were 2 complete and 1 partial response for a 6 percent response rate. Cavins et al.[18] reported only 1 of 18 patients (5.5 percent) who had prior radiotherapy responding to Adriamycin, 60 mg/m² every 3 weeks. A randomized prospective comparison of hexamethylmelamine, Adriamycin, or cyclophosphamide as single agent firstline treatment for recurrent squamous cell carcinoma of the cervix was reported by Freedman and colleagues[16] from the MD Anderson Hospital. A total of 59 patients were randomized, 37 of which were considered easily evaluable. Complete and partial responses were observed in 23 percent (3/13) of patients treated with cyclophosphamide compared to 0 percent (0/14) with hexamethylmelamine and 20 percent (2/10) with Adriamycin. Malkasian et al.[14] observed significant disease regression using strictly defined criteria in 20/208 or 9.6 percent of patients treated with 5-fluorouracil and 2 of 40 or 5 percent of patients treated with cyclophosphamide. These investigators did not observe any responses to second-line chemotherapy. Bleomycin administered by continuous infusion at a dose of 0.25 mg/kg/day resulted in 2 complete and 8 partial responses in 32 patients.[19] This suggests that this cell cycle phase specific agent is more effective administered by continuous infusion than intermittent dosing.[15] Thus prior to the identification of cisplatin there was clearly a lack of highly active drugs with which to treat carcinoma of the uterine cervix.

Cisplatin is the single most active drug in the treatment of squamous cell carcinoma of the cervix. Total doses of 50–120 mg/m² every 3 to 4 weeks result in major responses in approximately 30 percent of patients for approximately 6 months (Table 5-3). Responders live longer than non-responders[24,28] and in general a higher response rate is achievable in patients previously untreated with chemotherapy. There does not appear to be any significant difference in response rates of pelvic and extrapelvic sites of disease.[24,25]

Trials conducted by the Gynecologic Oncology Group (GOG) (Table 5-3) have addressed two questions. In the first trial results were analyzed to assess the influence of prior chemotherapy and site of disease. Thigpen et al.[28] treated 34 patients with recurrent squamous cell carcinoma of the cervix with 50 mg/m² of cisplatin every 3 weeks. Among 12 patients previously treated with chemotherapy 2 responses were observed compared to 11 responses in 22 patients without prior exposure to cytotoxic drugs. The difference was statistically significant (17 percent vs. 50 percent, p = 0.059). However response was not related to disease location: 7 of 20 patients with pelvic disease and 6 of 14 patients with extrapelvic disease responded. Responders had a median survival time of 9 months compared to 6 months for non-responders (p = 0.05).

Table 5-3. Single Agent Cisplatin Trials

Investigator	Treatment	Eval. Pts.*	CR	% CR + PR	MDR (mos)
Bonomi [24]	50 mg/m^2 q 3 wks	122 (PU)	15	23%	3.8
(GOG)	100 mg/m^2 q 3 wks	138 (PU)	16	27%	4.4
	20 mg/m^2/day × 5 q 3 wks	121 (PU)	9	24%	3.7
Lira-Puerto [25]	100 mg/m^2 q 3 wks	19 (PU)	1	47%	3–6 +
Hall [26]	60 mg/m^2 q 3 wks	22 (PU)	0	9%	—
Cohen [27]	3 mg/kg q 3 wks	3 (PU)	1	100%	—
Thigpen [28]	50 mg/m^2 q 3 wks	22 (PU)	3	50%	6
(GOG)		12 (PT)	0	17%	6
Rossof [29]	75 mg/m^2 q 3 wks	7 (PT)	0	0%	—
(SWOG)					
Hayat [30]	100 mg/m^2 q 3 wks	11 (6 PU)	1	27%	—
Cohen [31]	120 mg/m^2 q 3 wks	11 (7 PU)	—	42%	4 +
Stehman [32]	50 mg/m^2 q 3 wks	3 (2 PU)	0	33%	—

*PU = previouly untreated with chemotherapy
PT = prior treatment with chemotherapy

The subsequent GOG single agent cisplatin trial reported by Bonomi [24] (Table 5-3) addressed dose and scheduling. Patients with no prior chemotherapy were randomized to receive low dose (50 mg/m^2), high dose (100 mg/m^2), or divided dose cisplatin (20 mg/m^2/day for 5 days) every 3 weeks. There was no difference in response rate, median duration of response or survival time. The low dose regimen was associated with the least toxicity.

In addition to cisplatin, the GOG has systematically evaluated 6 other agents in advanced or recurrent squamous cell carcinoma of the cervix (Table 5-2). [33–38] ICRF-159, Baker's Antifol and dianhydrogalactilol had moderate activity with resonse rates of 18 percent, 16 percent, and 19 percent respectively. [34,35,37] Maytansine, VP-16-213, and piperazinedione had no significant activity. [33,36,38] Results of preliminary testing in phase I-II trials of the vinca alkaloid vindesine and the Adriamycin analog 4' epi-Adriamycin suggest that these agents are active in cervical cancer [39,44] and should undergo further phase II disease-oriented evaluation (Table 5-4).

Combination Chemotherapy

For the most part combination chemotherapy for advanced or recurrent squamous cell carinoma of the cervix has consisted of two to four drugs. Most combina-

Table 5-4. New Agents Tested in Cervical Cancer

Agent	Dose & Schedule	Eval. Pts.	% CR + PR	Reference
Vindesine	3 mg/m^2 IV q wk	2	100%	39
Detorubicin	120 mg/m^2 IV q 4 wks	16	6%	40
Dibromodulcitol	8 mg/kg/day × 10q 4 wks	14	7%	25
m-AMSA	90 mg/m^2 IV q 3 wks	25	4%	41
	120 mg/m^2 IV q 3 wks	16	13%	42
Yoshi 864	2.0 mg/kg/day × 5 IV q 6 wks	18	0	43
4'epi-Adriamycin	75 mg/m^2 q 3 wks	3	33%	44
Spirogermanium	80–120 mg/m^2 qod	14	0	45

tions have been Adriamycin or cisplatin-based or have explored the addition of agents to the two drug combination of bleomycin + mitomycin-C.

Bleomycin-Mitomycin Combination Chemotherapy

The sequential use of bleomycin and mitomycin-C initially reported by Miyamoto et al.[46] produced an 88 percent response rate (65 percent complete regressions) in 30 women, all of whom had prior radiation therapy to pelvic disease. None had received prior chemotherapy and the majority had extrapelvic sites of disease. Toxicity consisted of myelosuppression (27 percent of patients with WBC<2000 cells/ul or platelets<75,000 cells/ul) and pulmonary fibrosis in 7 percent. To improve the brief median duration of response (4.5 months) patients were maintained on an oral mitomycin-C analog, carboquone. With maintenance chemotherapy the relapse rate was reduced from 100 percent (7/7) to 12.5 percent (1/8).

Although the identical regimen has been evaluated by other investigators the response rate has not been reproduced (Table 5-5). These differences have been attributed to variations in the patient population in any one study. Disease limited to previously irradiated pelvic sites and resistance to prior chemotherapy characterize many patients entered into these trials.[47–49,52]

Boice et al.[52] treated 23 patients with a maximum of 5 courses of bleomycin-mitomycin-C. Maintenance chemotherapy was with cyclophosphamide. Sixty-one percent (14/23) of patients had recurrent disease within a previously irradiated port. There were 6 responses, 4 of these in patients with extrapelvic sites of disease; there was no difference in survival for responders and nonresponders. Trope et al.[48] reported only a 36 percent response rate in 33 patients, 2 with adenosquamous histology. Fifty percent of patients with distant metastases were responders compared to 25 percent of patients with central pelvic recurrences. Four of the 5 complete responses (Table 5-5) were observed in patients who had not had prior radiation therapy to the recurrent disease and the lesion was less than 3 cm in size. Krebs et al.[50] observed a similar correlation between bulk of tumor and response. The one complete

Table 5-5. Bleomycin-Mitomycin Combination Chemotherapy Trials*

Investigator	No. Evaluable Patients	CR	CR + PR (%)	MDR (mos)	MST (mos)†
Miyamoto[46]	30	17	26 (88%)	4.5	—
Leichman[47]	19	1	3 (16%)	—	—
Trope[48]	33	5	12 (36%)	CR-12	CR-28+
				PR-6	PR-10.5
Krebs[49]	20	1	8 (40%)	3	6
Pitrilli[50]	9	2	2 (22%)	3.5	—
Greenberg[51]	18	0	4 (22%)	3.4	PR-8.5
					NR-4.0
Boice[52]	23	2	6 (26%)	—	R-8+
					NR-5+
Majima[53]	10	5	7 (70%)	—	—

*Bleomycin 5 mg IV days 1–7 and Mitomycin-C 10 mg IV day 8; cycle repeated every 14 days.
†NR = Non-responder

response occurred in a pelvic lesion 2 cm in diameter, and the 7 partial responses were all reported to be in tumors weighing less than 100 gms.

Pulmonary fibrosis secondary to bleomycin occurred in 5 to 10 percent of patients in several studies.[46,48,49,51] Mucositis and myelosupression were the other major, although manageable, toxicities. The results of these studies demonstrate a 42 percent (68/162) total response rate to this combination. Details of individual studies suggest that response is more frequent in less bulky disease, in unirradiated, and extrapelvic sites.

The addition of vincristine to mitomycin and bleomycin has been evaluated in an initial pilot study by Baker et al.[54] and by the Southwest Oncology Group (Table 5-6).[55] Based on studies demonstrating that vincristine could increase the mitotic index of cells, the sequence of vincristine followed in 6 to 12 hours by bleomycin was explored by Baker.[54,56] Of 27 patients treated as outlined in Table 5-6, there were 2 complete and 11 partial responses. Median duration of response was 4 months. Twenty-five patients had received prior radiotherapy and one had received prior chemotherapy. All patients had metastatic disease. Responses occurred mainly in unirradiated soft tissue and visceral metastases. Toxicity consisted of myelosupression, pulmonary fibrosis in 1 patient, and peripheral neuropathy.

The Southwest Oncology Group observed a 60 percent response rate (16 percent complete) in 50 patients treated with this same MOB combination (Table 5-6).[55] Median duration of response was 9 weeks and median survival time 23 weeks. In a subsequent trial patients were randomized to treatment regimens 2 + 3 outlined on Table 5-6. In an attempt to reduce toxicity, in regimen 2 bleomycin was administered as a 96-hr continuous intravenous infusion (CIVI) and in regimen 3 vincristine and bleomycin were given by bolus injection weekly. The results indicated that the twice weekly schedule (arm 1 in Table 5-6) resulted in significantly more responders than either CIVI bleomycin or the weekly schedule, $p = 0.01$. However, the infusion schedule produced less leukopenia ($p < 0.025$) and response duration tended to be longer, 16 weeks compared to 9 weeks with the twice weekly schedule and 11 weeks with the

Table 5-6. Mitomycin-Vincristine (Oncovin)-Bleomycin (MOB) Regimen

Investigator	Regimen	CR + PR/Eval. Pts. (%)
Baker[54]	M—20 mg/m² IV day 2 q 6 wks O—0.5 mg/m² IV biw × 12 wks B—6 u IM biw, 6–12 hrs after 0, × 12 wks	13/27 (48%)
Baker[55] (SWOG)	1. MOB, same as above	30/50 (60%)
	2. M—20 mg/m² IV day 2, then 10 mg/m² IV q 6–8 wks O—0.5 mg/m² IV biw × 12 wks B—30 u/day, CIVI × 4 days × 2 cycles only	16/41 (39%)
	3. M—20 mg/m² IV q 6 wks O—0.5 mg/m² IV q wk × 24 wks B—6 u/m² IV or IM, 6 hrs after 0, q 6 wks	6/24 (25%)

weekly schedule. The median survival time was significantly better for both infusion and twice weekly schedules (26 weeks and 23 weeks) compared to the weekly schedule (7 weeks), $p<0.01$. Responding patients lived longer than non-responders, median survival time 30 weeks vs 14 weeks, $p<0.01$.

In summary, response and survival appeared to correlate with bleomycin dose, continuous infusion and twice weekly bleomycin being clearly superior. However, response durations were brief and toxicity considerable.

Cisplatin-Containing Combination Chemotherapy

Although the superiority of the MOB regimen over the 2 drug bleomycin-mitomycin-C combination has not been established in a prospectively randomized trial, several investigators have proceeded to add cisplatin to this regimen or a variation of it: MOB + Cisplatin[57,58] or VBMP[59] or BOMP.[60] Because of the well-established activity of cisplatin it was hoped that the addition of this agent would not only improve the overall response rate but in particular prolong the brief duration of response observed with non-cisplatin containing regimens.

Alberts and Surwit at the University of Arizona have reported on two pilot trials using the MOB-Cisplatin regimen (Table 5-7).[57,58] Based on results of the SWOG MOB trial, a reduced dose of mitomycin C (10 mg/m^2) and bleomycin by continuous infusion were utilized. The 14 evaluable patients had either stage IVB and/or recurrent squamous cell carcinoma of the cervix. There were 4 complete responders (29 percent) with a median response duration of 35 months. Disease sites were pulmonary metastases and pelvic masses. Two patients had partial responses lasting 1.5 months. Median survival for all patients was 9 months. The dose limiting toxicity was thrombocytopenia which was severe or life-threatening in 36 percent of patients. In the second trial reported in preliminary form by this group,[58] essentially the same response rate was observed, 47 percent (8/17; 4 CR + 4 PR). The median survival time was 11 months. Again most complete responders demonstrated a substantially prolonged remission duration varying from 5 to 46+ months. Toxicity was similar with thrombocytopenia occurring in 41 percent of patients.

The EORTC has evaluated the VBMP regimen as outlined on Table 5-7.[59] All patients had distant metastases; seven also had previously irradiated local disease. Responses occurred in lung, bone, and soft tissue metastases. Eighty-two percent of patients with only lung and lymph node metastases responded. Those with brain, liver, and previously irradiated sites of disease did not respond. Median duration of response was 20 weeks. Median survival for all 22 patients was 7 months compared to 12 months for responders. Cummulative hematologic toxicity occurred but was manageable.

Vogl reported a 78 percent (10/13) response rate to the BOMP regimen. Assessing only patients with fully evaluable disease the response rate was 63 percent and duration of response 4.0 months.[60] Toxicity to the BOMP regimen was mild and well-tolerated.

Of these 3 treatment regimens the BOMP regimen employed by Vogl appeared to have the least associated toxicity. Overall one would expect about 50 percent of recurrent disease patients to respond to any of these regimens. Whether response to

Table 5-7. Mitomycin-Vincristine (Oncovin)-Bleomycin-Cisplatin Combination Chemotherapy

Investigator	Regimen	CR + PR/Eval. Pts. (%)
Alberts[57]	M—10 mg/m^2 IV day 2 O—0.5 mg/m^2 IV biw B—30 u/day, CIVI × 4 days × 2 cycles only P—50 mg/m^2 day 1 & 22 Recycle every 6 weeks	6/14 (43%)
Surwit[58]	same as above	8/17 (47%)
Vermorken[59] (EORTC)	V—1.4 mg/m^2 day 1 B—15 mg/day, CIVI × 2 days M—6 mg/m^2 day 3 P—50 mg/m^2 day 4 Recycle every 4 weeks	11/22 (50%)
Vogl[60]	B—10 u IV day 1 O—1 mg/m^2 IV day 1,8,15,29 M—10 mg/m^2 IV day 1 P—50 mg/m^2 IV day 1 & 22 Recycle every 6 weeks	10/13 (78%)*

*Includes 2 patients without prior treatment.

these 4 drugs in combination is significantly better than one could achieve using either single agent cisplatin or bleomycin-mitomycin remains to be determined. Toxicity is definitely enhanced without any benefit in prolonging the remission duration. Results of these small pilot studies do suggest that the achievement of complete disease regression which occurred in about 25 percent of patients does impact on survival. However, the numbers of patients entered into these trials are too small to draw further conclusions.

The Southwest Oncology Group initiated a randomized trial addressing the question of multidrug cisplatin containing combination chemotherapy versus single agent cisplatin (Table 5-8). After 68 patients had been randomized there was no difference in response rate among the 3 treatment arms. Arm 3 (single agent cisplatin) was dropped from the trial. Preliminary analysis to date demonstrates no significant differences in response rate, duration, or toxicity between the two remaining drug combinations.[61]

Other cisplatin-containing combination chemotherapy regimens are detailed in Table 5-9. Response rates tend to be in the 30 to 40 percent range, and response durations remain brief with the exception of those patients achieving complete disease regression. Results of these trials further confirm the conclusion from other trials cited in this review that distant disease responds better than local, previously irradiated disease. Several of these studies warrant further comment.

Fine et al.[63] from the Princess Margaret Hospital in Toronto reported a 12 percent (2/17) response rate in patients with local recurrence compared to 55 percent (16/29) response rate in patients with distant disease treated with low dose methotrexate, Adriamycin, and cisplatin. Of note, 5 patients presenting with small cell carcinoma of the cervix responded to this regimen given prior to radiation or surgery. An additional patient with recurrent small cell carcinoma had a complete response to chemotherapy lasting 11 months.

Table 5-8. SWOG Randomized
Trial

1. M—10 mg/m² day 2 & 44
   O—0.5 mg/m² day 2,4,44,46
   B—30 u/day CIVI × 4 days
   P—50 mg/m² IV day 1,22,43,64
2. M—12 mg/m² q 6 wks
   P—50 mg/m² q 3 wks
3. P—50 mg/m² q 3 wks

The GOG[65] reported the preliminary results of a pilot study evaluating cisplatin 100 mg/m² and cyclophosphamide 1,000 mg/m² IV every 3 weeks. This combination was well-tolerated and would seem to warrant further comparative testing in large numbers of patients.

Vogl et al.[66] evaluated the combination of methotrexate 50 mg/m² IV days 1 and 15, cisplatin 50 mg/m² IV day 5 and bleomycin 10 u day 1,8,15. Eighty-nine percent (8/9) of patients responded; all had been treated with prior radiotherapy. However, median duration of response and survival was brief and there were no complete responses. Toxicity was prohibitive with severe stomatitis and myelosuppression occurring in 63 percent. Enhanced toxicity was attributed to delayed excretion of methotrexate because of ureteral dysfunction. Hence, although a high order of response was observed, these investigators recommended replacing methotrexate with other active agents to reduce toxicity. This approach has been explored by Natale et al.[69,70] at the University of Michigan. This group combined cisplatin (70–100 mg/m² day 1 every 4 weeks) with dichloromethotrexate, a dihalogenated methotrexate analog excreted predominantly by the hepatic route. In a preliminary report, a 75 percent (6/8) response rate was achieved.[60] A more recent update indicates a 63 percent (10/16) response rate (6 CR, 4 PR). Complete responses are durable with median duration of 13 months; median survival time has not been reached.[70] Toxicity was manageable with mucositis and myelosuppression predominating. It would be reasonable to test this promising regimen in a comparative trial with larger numbers of patients.

Two trials have evaluated the combination of cisplatin and bleomycin in recurrent carcinoma of the cervix. Daghestani et al.[67] tested high dose cisplatin (120 mg/m²) and continuous infusion bleomycin (10 u/m²/day × 5–7 days), a regimen with dem-

Table 5-9. Non-Bleomycin-Mitomycin Containing Cisplatin Regimens

Drug Combination*	Eval. Pts.	CR	CR + PR (%)	MDR (mos)	MST (mos)	Reference
CAP	16	1	5 (31%)	CR-6 PR-4 +	—	62
Mtx + AP	48	0	18 (38%)	5	—	63
Dianhydrogalactilol + P	18	2	7 (39%)	5	9	64
CP	12	2	5 (42%)	6	—	65
Mtx + BP	9	0	8 (89%)	4	8	66
PB (CIVI)	24	0	13 (54%)	3.5	—	67
PB (bolus)	13	2	2 (15%)	11,26	—	68
P + Dcm	16	6	10 (63%)	CR-13 PR-6	—	69,70

*C = Cyclophosphamide,   A = Adriamycin,   P = Cisplatin,   Mtx = Methotrexate,   B = Bleomycin
Dem = Dichloromethotrexate

onstrated activity in other squamous cell tumors, notably head and neck, and esophageal malignancies. Eighteen patients had recurrent squamous cell carcinoma, 9 were classified as adeno or adenosquamous histology and 3 as anaplastic carcinomas. Thirteen (54 percent) partial responses were observed. Duration of response was brief with no survival benefit for responders compared to non-responders. Surprisingly, 90 percent of patients with non-squamous histologies responded compared to 29 percent of squamous cell patients ($p<0.004$). Responses occurred in 36 percent of patients with previously irradiated disease as the indicator lesion compared to a 57 percent response rate for patients with non-irradiated extra-pelvic disease. Toxicity to this regimen was significant with nausea, vomiting, inanition, and nephrotoxicity being most troublesome. Two patients developed creatinine elevation greater than 5 mg/dl resulting in delayed excretion of bleomycin, severe mucositis and sepsis. Since lower doses of cisplatin may be as effective as high doses these investigators are currently using a reduced cisplatin dose (75 mg/m^2) in combination with CIVI bleomycin as adjuvant treatment for stage IB poor prognosis patients (see Adjuvant Chemotherapy).[71]

In contrast to these results, only 2 of 13 patients responded to low dose cisplatin (50 mg/m^2) and bolus bleomycin (10 u/m^2) repeated every 4 weeks as reported by Sidorowicz et al.[68] These authors concluded that this dose and schedule did not warrant further study because of this low order of activity.

Adriamycin-based Combination Regimens

Adriamycin has most commonly been combined with alkylating agents, such as cyclophosphamide or the nitrosoureas with or without 5-fluorouracil (Table 5-10). Alternatively Adriamycin plus methotrexate has been evaluated in a variety of doses and schedules (Table 5-11). The response rates in most studies have not exceeded

Table 5-10. Adriamycin Combination Chemotherapy

Regimen*	CR + PR/Eval. Pts. (%)	MST (mos)	Reference
A—40 mg/m^2 IV day 1 C—200 mg/m^2 P.O. days 3–6 q 3–4 weeks	1/10 (10%)	—	72
A—50 mg/m^2 IV C—500 mg/m^2 IV q 3–4 weeks	6/20 (30%)	R-13.2 NR-7.2	73
A—60 mg/m^2 day 1 C—200 mg/m^2 IV days 1–5 F—200 mg/m^2 IV days 1–5 q 4 weeks	6/34 (16.5%)	CR-24 R-8.5 all pts. 4.5	74
A—45 mg day 1 C—100 mg/m^2 P. O. days 1–14 F—500 mg/m^2 day 1 & 8 V—1.4 mg/m^2 day 1 & 8 q 28 days	18/31 (58%)	CR-14 PR-11 NR-2.5	75

A—60 mg/m^2 day 1
  45 mg/m^2 day 21
MeCCNU—175 mg/m^2 P.O. day 1
  q 6 weeks
	14/31 (45%)	CR-14
		PR-8
		Prog-7
			76

*A = Adriamycin, C = Cyclophosphamide, F = 5-fluorouracil, V = Vincristine

Table 5-11. Adriamycin-Methotrexate Combination Chemotherapy

Regimen	CR + PR/Eval. Pts. (%)	MST (mos)	Reference
A—50 mg/m² day 1	4/22 (18%)	R-21	77
Mtx—20 mg/m² days 1 & 8		Stable 11.5	
q 3–4 weeks		Prog-3.0	
A—50 mg/m² day 1	7/24 (29%)	—	78
Mtx—20 mg/m² days 1 & 8			
q 3 weeks			
A—50 mg/m² day 1	39/59 (66%)	R-14	79
Mtx—20–40 mg/m² days 1 & 8		NR-5	
± leucovorin			
A—20–30 mg/m²	2/16 (12.5%)	—	80
Mtx—12.5–20 mg/m²			
q 3 weeks			
A—30 mg/m²	5/24 (21%)	R-10	81
Mtx—2.5 mg P.O. bid × 5 days		Prog-5	
q 3 weeks			

those expected from single agent Adriamycin. Those studies reporting more promising results warrant further comment.

Chan et al.[75] evaluated the combination of Adriamycin, cyclophosphamide, 5-fluorouracil, and vincristine in 31 patients (Table 5-10). Both complete and partial responders (58 percent) had significantly prolonged survival compared to nonresponders. All responses occurred within 2 cycles of treatment and all responders had a performance status of 0 to 2 (ambulatory more than 50 percent of waking hours). Day et al.[76] combined Adriamycin and methyl-CCNU. There were 9 complete responses (29 percent) and 5 partial responses (16 percent). Although the high CR rate was encouraging, myelotoxicity was severe, particularly in patients who had received extensive prior irradiation. Moderate to severe nausea and vomiting, anorexia, and weight loss occurred in all patients.

The first 3 Adriamycin-methotrexate regimens detailed in Table 5-11 are nearly identical in drug dose and schedule.[77–79] The highest response rate was reported by Guthrie and Way.[79] These investigators evaluated 5 variations of methotrexate, administering 20 or 40 mg/m² on day 1 and 8 or day 8 only with or without leucovorin. Individual trials had 11 or 12 patients in each and response rates varied from 50 to 83 percent. The least toxicity occurred when methotrexate was administered in the lowest dose (20 mg/m²) on day 1 and 8 repeated every 3 to 4 weeks. Papavasiliou et al.[78] administered this exact regimen to 24 patients but failed to confirm Guthrie's results. A response rate of only 29 percent was observed even though 10 newly diagnosed patients who subsequently received radiation were included in the trial. Somewhat lower response rates were reported in the two trials by Haid[80] and Trope[81] in which lower doses of both drugs were employed (Table 5-11).

In summary, the results of some of the Adriamycin plus alkylating agent regimens and the Adriamycin plus methotrexate regimens suggest that more complete responses can be achieved with combinations than single agents. However, high response rates have not been reproducable and in some trials toxicity appeared to outweigh potential therapeutic benefit. The methotrexate combinations in particular, warrant close monitoring of renal function to minimize toxicity.

Table 5-12. Randomized Trials

Investigator	Treatment*	CR	CR+PR/ Eval. Pts. (%)	MDR (mos)	MST (mos)
Wallace [82] (GOG)	1. A 60 mg/m² IV	7	12/61 (20%)	3.3	5.9
	2. A 60 mg/m² IV V 1.5 mg/m² IV	1	9/54 (17%)	3.4	5.5
	3. A 50 mg/m² IV C 500 mg/m² IV All drugs recycled every 3 weeks	3	7/39 (18%)	3.9	7.3
Malkasian [83]	1. F 450 mg/m² day × 5 days V 1.5 mg/m² day 1 & 5 IV Recycle every 5 weeks	0	1/20 (5%)	2.3	7
	2. A 60 mg/m² IV q 3 wks	0	4/19 (21%)		
Omura [84]	1. A 50 mg/m² day 1 V 1.4 mg/m² day 1 & 8 F 500 mg/m² day 1 & 8	1	3/31 (10%)	—	7.6
	2. C 1100 mg/m² IV day 1	0	2/30 (7%)	—	6.5
Greenberg [85]	1. A 30 mg/m² esc. to 60 mg/m² q 3 wks	0	5/9 (55%)	—	4.3
	2. A (same as 1) B 10 mg/m² q wk	0	0/11 (0%)	—	4.0

*See tables 5-9 and 5-10 for abbreviations

Randomized Trials

In an effort to further define the value of single agents several comparative trials have been conducted (Table 5-12). The GOG compared Adriamycin + cyclophosphamide and Adriamycin + vincristine with single agent Adriamycin. There was no significant difference in response rate, duration, or survival among the three treatment regimens. The response rate of 20 percent and brief duration (less than 4 months) further defined the low-order of activity for single agent Adriamycin in recurrent disease patients.

Malkasian et al.[83] compared 5-fluorouracil and vincristine to single agent Adriamycin. Only 1 patient responded to the combination. This was not statistically different from the 21 percent response rate to Adriamycin.

Omura et al.[84] compared Adriamycin, vincristine, and 5-fluorouracil to single agent cyclophosphamide. Results showed no benefit for the combination (10 percent vs 7 percent response rate). The poor response rate to both treatments further emphasized the need to identify new active agents to treat cervical cancer.

Greenberg et al.[85] compared Adriamycin + bleomycin to single agent Adriamycin. The numbers of patients in each arm were small. All responses were in extra-pelvic sites of disease. The disproportionate response rate for arm 1 (Table 5-12) may have been due to the fact that none of the 9 patients in that arm had only pelvic disease compared to 5 of the 11 patients receiving the combination.

Results of several other trials comparing combinations have been published (Table 5-13). These trials were conducted in patients with advanced or recurrent carcinoma of the cervix. Histology was primarily squamous. DePalo et al.[86] randomized 34 patients to treatment with either Adriamycin and bleomycin or cyclophosphamide and vincristine. The results, 20 percent and 10 percent CR + PR, indicate that neither

Table 5-13. Randomized Trials Comparing Combination Chemotherapy Regimens

Investigator	Treatment*	CR	CR + PR/ Eval. Pts. (%)	MDR (mos)	MST (mos
DePalo[86]	1. A 75 mg/m² IV day 1 B 15 mg/m² IV day 1 & 8	1	3/15 (20%)	7.5	—
	2. C 1.2 gm/m² IV day 1 V 1.4 mg/m² IV day 1 & 8	1	2/19 (10%)	7.2	—

Wheeler[87]	1. B 20 u/day CIVI×4 days
	   O 2.0 mg IV day 1
	   M 15–20 mg/m² IV q 8 wks
	   Mtx 20–30 mg/m² q wk
		0	2/5 (40%)	11	—

	2. BOM, doses as per arm 1	0	1/3 (33%)	11	—
Scarborough[88] (COG)	1. B 0.5 u/kg IV biw CCNU 130 mg/m² PO day 1	0	2/9 (22%)	3	4.5

	2. B 0.5 u/kg IV q wk
	   A 0.4 mg/kg day 1,2,3 then
	   0.6 mg/kg IV q wk
	   Recycle every 6 weeks
		0	1/7 (14%)	2.5	6.5

*M = Mitomycin-C, O = Oncovin, others as per tables 5-9, 5-10.

combination is superior and suggest little benefit over single agents. This trial was designed with a cross-over to the alternate regimen once patients progressed or were judged to be nonresponders. Of 10 evaluable patients crossed over to the Adriamycin + bleomycin arm there were 2 partial responses (20 percent); none of the 3 patients crossed over to cyclophosphamide + vincristine responded with greater than 50 percent disease regression.

Wheeler et al.[87] evaluated the combination of bleomycin, vincristine, and mitomycin-C with or without methotrexate (BOMM vs BOM) in patients with squamous cell carcinomas. Eight patients with recurrent cervical carcinoma were randomized. Response rates (40 percent vs 33 percent) and duration (11 months) were similar in each arm. Nineteen percent of all 42 squamous cancer patients entered on this study developed pulmonary toxicity which proved fatal in 4 of the 8 patients. Thus, with the brief duration of response achievable the risk of pulmonary toxicity from the combination of bleomycin and mitomycin-C appeared to outweigh potential therapeutic benefit.

Scarborough reported the results of bleomycin and CCNU compared to bleomycin plus Adriamycin conducted by the Central Oncology Group (COG) in various squamous cell tumors.[88] Of the 16 evaluable cervical cancer patients randomized there was no significant difference in response rate, median duration of response, or survival time.

In summary, the management of the patient with recurrent squamous cell carcinoma remains difficult despite the myriad of cytotoxic drug trials which have been reported. In selecting drug therapy the physician must carefully consider the patient's pulmonary and renal function to avoid increased risk of toxicity to these organs and potentiation of other drug toxicities. Nephrotoxic agents such as cisplatin and methotrexate must be used with caution and careful monitoring of creatinine clearance. Bleomycin and mitomycin-C not infrequently cause pulmonary fibrosis, and therefore doses of bleomycin in particular should be limited to avoid cummulative toxicity. Prior abdomino-pelvic radiotherapy may leave a patient with poor bone marrow reserve and hence life-threatening myelosuppression may attend the administration of optimal doses of Adriamycin, mitomycin-C or the nitrosoureas.

Considering these general guidelines in selecting specific cytotoxic agents and initial dosage, the following conclusions can be drawn from the current literature regarding cytotoxic drug therapy for recurrent or advanced squamous cell carcinoma of the uterine cervix.

1. Cisplatin is clearly the most active and reliably tested single agent. Responses, the majority of which are partial, occur in 25 to 30 percent of patients. Low dose (50 mg/m^2) appears to be as effective as high dose (100 mg/m^2) cisplatin.

2. Multiple other single agents have demonstrated activity in the 10–25 percent range. No trials using standardized response criteria have confirmed any consistent superiority of one agent compared to another.

3. Significant improvement in survival correlates with complete disease regression. Complete response rates of 20 to 30 percent have generally been observed with cisplatin-containing and other combinations cited although complete response rates of up to 65 percent have occasionally been reported. These results offer promise for chemotherapy to have a major impact on the natural history of this disease.

4. Distant or extrapelvic metastases are more responsive to chemotherapy than previously irradiated sites of disease. Thus, characteristics of the patient population will influence the apparent observed activity of any one drug or combination tested. For this reason, confirmation of promising results of any one trial has been difficult, i.e., bleomycin-mitomycin-C combination chemotherapy.

5. Comparative trials have not identified a superior combination regimen or confirmed the superiority of combination over single agent chemotherapy using complete response and survival as endpoints. However, more recently reported combinations piloted in single institutions which appear to have significant activity, i.e., MOB-cisplatin, cisplatin-dichloromethotrexate, have yet to undergo comparative testing in large numbers of patients.

REGIONAL CHEMOTHERAPY

Since advanced or recurrent cervical carcinoma is frequently confined to the pelvis, the use of regional therapy has intrinsic appeal. Further impetus for regional treatment studies has stemmed from the limited success of conventional chemotherapy regimens.[89] Regional chemotherapy offers several theoretical advantages. Depending on pharmacokinetic characteristics (primarily total body clearance) and regional blood flow, regional treatment may result in local drug exposures 100–1000 fold greater than systemic exposure.[90] This increases the likelihood of response while allowing for lower systemic toxicity. These factors may be paramount in cervical carcinoma, where chemotherapeutic failure is often ascribed to decreased pelvic blood flow or altered vasuclar permeability following surgery or irradiation.[91] Despite these theoretical advantages, clinical studies have failed to demonstrate a consistant benefit from intra-arterial therapy.

Trussell and Mitford-Barberton, in 1961, generated initial enthusiasm for intra-

Table 5-14. Intra-Arterial Therapy for Advanced or Recurrent Cervical Carcinoma

Regimen	Evaluable Patients	Responses (%)	Complete Responses	Reference
Methotrexate +/−				
Vincristine	14	3 (21)	0	89
Bleomycin	20	3 (15)	0	93
Mitomycin C, Bleomycin,				
Vincristine	20	3 (15)	0	94
Cis-Platinum	9	3 (33)	0	91
	2	2 (100)	0	95

arterial methotrexate, after reporting responses in 14 of 14 previously untreated patients with advanced cervical carcinoma.[92] Patients underwent operative placement of internal iliac catheters, with daily methotrexate (50 mg) and concurrent leucovorin, until leukopenia developed. Although tolerated fairly well, responses were transient with only one complete responder. Lifshitz et al. employing intra-arterial methotrexate (60 to 200 mg over 48 hours) and leucovorin, with or without vincristine, had considerably less success in patients with recurrent carcinoma.[89] He noted only 3 responses (2 MR, 1 PR) in 14 patients treated, with significant catheter related morbidity (arterial occlusion, bleeding and catheter related sepsis). Morrow, utilizing a portable infusion pump to deliver continuous intra-arterial bleomycin (20 mg/m^2/week, to a maximum total dose of 300 mg), noted only 3 responses in 20 patients, again with significant morbidity.[93] Swenerton, using a combination of intra-arterial vincristine (2mg), bleomycin (90mg) and mitomycin C (20 mg/m^2), had similar results, again with responses in only 3 of 20 patients.[94] It is interesting to note, that although objective response rates were quite low, some authors[89,91] reported significant pain palliation in the majority of patients following treatment. This has been ascribed to local neurotoxic effects of the chemotherapy. The results of these studies are summarized in Table 5-14.

Intra-arterial therapy with cisplatin has had slightly more encouraging results. Laboratory studies demonstrating a high degree of cisplatin binding to ovarian and uterine tissue, coupled with a short serum half-life (20 to 30 minutes) make this drug theoretically attractive for intra-arterial therapy.[91,95] In a phase I–II study by Calvo et al.[95] partial remissions were seen in 2 of 2 patients with cervical carcinoma. Carlson, employing a cisplatin dose of 120 mg/m^2 delivered through percutaneously placed internal iliac artery catheters, noted partial remissions in 3 of 9 patients, with subjective responses in 5 of 9 patients.[91] Overall toxicity was acceptable, with mild neuropathy, mild transient renal dysfunction, and treatment associated nausea and vomiting. Catheter related problems were not as prevalent as in earlier reports.

Upon reviewing these reports, it becomes apparent that these studies suffer from many of the same limitations of systemic trials in cervical carcinoma: non-randomized design, relatively small numbers of patients, and non-uniformity in treatment regimens and response criteria. Although the exact role of intra-arterial therapy in cervical carcinoma remains to be established, its use at present remains investigational. Preliminary results suggest that randomized comparisons with systemic therapy, employing cisplatin and other agents, is warranted before broader recommendations can be made.

RADIOSENSITIZERS AND COMBINED RADIOTHERAPY-CHEMOTHERAPY

Although radiotherapy remains the treatment of choice for advanced cervical carcinoma, its overall effectiveness is relatively poor. Five year survival following radiotherapy for stage IIIB disease is in the 25 to 40 percent range, with less than 10 percent of stage IV patients alive at 5 years.[96] A commonly cited reason for radiotherapy failure in bulky solid tumors is the presence of central necrotic areas, with associated hypoxic zones.[97] Since lethal effects of radiation are 2.5 to 3.0 times greater in the presence of oxygen as opposed to hypoxic conditions, these hypoxic or "radioresistant" cells may account for radiotherapy failures. Agents used to increase the effectiveness of radiotherapy may be divided into two major categories. One approach concentrates on potentiating radiolethality by providing higher oxygen concentrations or alternative compounds capable of free radical generation. The other approach utilizes additive chemotherapy, for either cell cycle synchronization or independant, additive cytotoxicity.

Radiosensitizers

Trials using hyperbaric oxygen have been employed since 1957.[98] Results in cervical carcinoma have been conflicting, with little to suggest significant benefit. Watson et al.[99] reported a randomized trial of 320 patients with stage IIB–IVA cervical carcinoma treated in hyperbaric oxygen or air. Significant 5-year survival advantage was confined to patients with stage III disease, primarily in the 45 to 54 year old age range. Although there was an approximate 20 percent decrease in local recurrence, this was confined to the same group with little or no benefit to older patients or those with more advanced disease. Additionally, statistical significance was obtained only by pooling results of several institutions, without a standardized radiotherapy regimen. In 1977, Fletcher reported a randomized trial involving 233 patients receiving radiotherapy in hyperbaric oxygen or air.[98] His results showed no survival advantage in either group at 2 years follow-up.

Diffusion of oxygen into tissue is limited by its consumption by respiring cells within 10 cell layers.[97] This has led to the search for chemical agents that possess oxygen-like effects without being metabolized. Oxygen enhanced radiosensitivity is ascribed to its ability to cause free radical formation.[100] Similarly, compounds which have a high electron affinity also increase free radical formation. Nitroimidazoles, including metronidazole and misonidazole, have been identified as possible radiation sensitizers. Although metronidazole is well-tolerated, no therapeutic advantage to its use has been demonstrated.[96] Misonidazole, with its higher electron affinity, should have a theoretic advantage. Phase I studies have shown it to be tolerated, with dosage limited by neurotoxicity.[101,102] A phase III study of radiotherapy, with or without misonidazole, conducted by the Radiation Therapy Oncology Group is ongoing.

Combined Radiotherapy-Chemotherapy

Accompanying interest in hyperbaric oxygen and high electron affinity compounds have been trials of radiotherapy combined with more conventional agents. Perhaps the most studied is hydroxyurea (HU). Sinclair, in 1968, demonstrated that preincubation of Chinese hamster cells in HU made them more sensitive to the lethal effects of radiation.[103] Presumably, this was due to hydroxyurea's cytotoxic effect on cells during the S phase, and blockage of cells from proceeding from G_1 to S phase. The resultant "synchronized" cell population is more sensitive to the effects of radiation. Piver reported a randomized trial in 130 patients with stage IIB–III cervical carcinoma, of placebo vs. Hydroxyurea, 80 mg/kg p.o. q 3 days for 12 weeks starting on day one of radiotherapy.[104] Although more leukopenia was observed in hydroxyurea treated patients, there was a significant (p<.01) increase in 5 year disease free survival (74 percent vs. 43 percent) in patients with IIB disease who received HU. A similar trend in IIIB patients (52 vs. 33 percent) did not reach significance, but may have been obscured by variations in radiotherapy technique. A similar study by Hreshchyshyn, using the same regimen in 192 patients with stage III–IV disease demonstrated comparable results (Table 5-15).[105] Complete response rates were 68 percent vs. 48 percent in HU treated patients vs. placebo recipients, with overall median survival times of 19.5 and 10.7 months respectively (p<.05). Although nearly 50 percent of his patients were inevaluable for a variety of reasons (staging errors, protocol violation, etc.) these results suggest that combined HU and radiation may have a role for treatment of the patient with advanced disease.

A variety of other regimens have been tried with mixed results. Goolsby reported a non-randomized series of 22 patients treated with concurrent 5-FU and radiotherapy.[106] Although toxicity was mild, results were not better than anticipated from radiotherapy alone. Smith combined radiotherapy with intra-arterial 5-FU or methotrexate in 26 patients.[107] Although he demonstrated that combined therapy could be tolerated, patient numbers and responses were insufficient to draw meaningful conclusions. Kalra et al.[108] treated 10 patients with advanced or recurrent cervical carcinoma with mitomycin-C (10 mg/M^2) and continuous intravenous infusion of 5-FU (1 gm/m^2 per day for 5 days) and concurrent pelvic radiotherapy (3000 R). Chemotherapy was repeated once for residual disease. Six of 10 patients had complete responses, two had partial responses and two had no response. Although results are suggestive of a highly effective regimen, median follow-up is only 7 months.

One particularly interesting study was that performed by Sugimori et al.[109] com-

Table 5-15. Hydroxyurea Combined with Radiation Therapy for Advanced Cervical Carcinoma

Author	Stage	Response RT + Hydroxyurea	RT Alone
Piver[104]	IIB	20/27 (74%)*	17/39 (45%)
	III	12/12 (52%)	9/27 (33%)
Hreshchyshyn[105]	III + IV	32/47 (68%)**	21/43 (48%)

*Response defined as no evidence of disease at 2 years.
**Response defined as complete tumor regression.

bining radiation with hormonal therapy. They theorized that estrogens should increase uterine blood flow and hence oxygen delivery, thereby enhancing radiosensitivity. In a non-randomized study, 147 patients were maintained on exogenous estrogen during radiation treatment. Only stage III patients demonstrated a 5-year survival advantage compared to the control group (55 percent vs. 34 percent, p<.01). In other stages, estrogen treatment appeared to offer an advantage, but results did not reach statistical significance.

Disappointment with chemotherapy following radiation-induced vascular changes has led some investigators to propose using chemotherapy before radiotherapy is administered. This induction or "neo-adjuvant" use of chemotherapy has had some interesting results. Mathew treated 251 patients with stage I–IV cervical carcinoma with mitomycin-C, 10 mg IV every 4 days (total dose 30 to 80 mg) before standard radiotherapy.[110] Although toxicity was increased (nine patient deaths), overall results were encouraging, with 2½ year disease free survivals of 72 percent and 25 percent in Stage III and IV patients, respectively. These results compare favorably with historical control rates of approximately 40 percent and 14 percent. Surwit et al. described treating seven patients with advanced disease (stage IIIB) with mitomycin-C, vincristine, bleomycin, and cisplatin (MOB + plat) for two 6 week cycles, followed by conventional radiotherapy and continued cisplatin treatments.[58] There was one complete remission and four partial remissions prior to radiotherapy, for an overall response rate of 71 percent. Radiotherapy was well tolerated without significant myelosuppression. Their preliminary report does not include long term, post-radiotherapy follow-up. Kavenough et al. have recently described a protocol of intravenous vincristine with intra-arterial mitomycin-C, bleomycin, and cisplatinum for patients with advanced disease (IIIB–IVA) accepted for radiotherapy with curative intent.[111] Three cycles are delivered prior to re-evaulation for planned radiotherapy. To date, six of 10 patients have had a greater than 50 percent reduction of tumor bulk, two patients have stable disease post-chemotherapy and treatment is ongoing in two additional patients. Although encouraging, toxicity (primarily myelosuppression) was substantial, with 25 percent of patients requiring hospitalization for treatment related complications.

Review of the literature suggests significant potential for the combination of chemotherapy and radiotherapy in the treatment of advanced cervical carcinoma. Unfortunately, the relative number of patients so treated is too small to draw firm conclusions regarding specific treatment recommendations. Clearly the need for additional pilot studies and prospective comparative trials exists. At present, efforts should be directed at entering appropriate patients into protocol studies when available. Current data would support consideration of combined therapy in those patients with advanced disease (stage III–IV) and low likelihood of cure with radiotherapy alone.

ADJUVANT CHEMOTHERAPY

Adjuvant chemotherapy has historically played little or no role in the treatment of cervical carcinoma. This may relate to a number of factors, including the relatively recent recognition of active agents, high cure rates with surgery or radiotherapy alone in early tumors, and prior disappointments treating patients with advanced or recurrent disease. Remarkably few adjuvant trials have been published.

Hakes et al. reported a series of 20 patients with stage IB or IIA disease who were found to have either positive para-aortic nodes at the time of radical hysterectomy or were felt to have advanced disease on the basis of large primary size (>4cm.).[71] Postoperatively, they received bleomycin 20 u/m^2 I.V. bolus, then a continuous infusion of 20 u/m^2 daily for 3 days, in addition to cisplatin 75 mg/m^2. Following 2 cycles of chemotherapy, 4000–4200 rads of external beam radiotherapy were delivered. With a median follow-up of 16 months, only one recurrence has been noted. Kardinal reported considerably less success, treating thirteen patients with stage IIB or III cervical carcinoma with melphalan 0.15 mg/kg qd for 5 days every 6 weeks for 1 year after conventional radiotherapy.[112] Eight of thirteen recurred within eighteen months, with only five patients disease free at 32 months. Survival curves were identical to historical controls. These conflicting results underscore the need for further studies prior to making specific treatment recommendations. At present, there is a dearth of experience in adjuvant chemotherapy in cervical carcinoma. Experience in other tumor types and the theoretical advantage of increased chemotherapeutic response with decreased tumor burden suggest that this approach warrants further attention.

FUTURE DIRECTIONS

The identification of new active agents is clearly needed and therefore should be a primary focus of single institution and cooperative group treatment programs for recurrent carcinoma of the cervix. Moreover, promising combinations need to be further tested in comparative trials with large numbers of patients, using complete disease regression and survival time as major endpoints.

However, significant improvements in survival and enhanced cure rates are likely to occur only with new and innovative approaches to the initial management of patients at high risk for recurrence. The identification of cisplatin as an agent with significant activity and the promising results from cisplatin-based combination chemotherapy in the treatment of recurrent disease have opened the way to explore the earlier use of chemotherapy in combined modality or adjuvant settings. Hence, the use of chemotherapy prior to definitive local treatment to reduce tumor bulk and improve local control rates as has been done in other squamous cell tumors, i.e., head and neck cancer, needs to be evaluated. Similarly, a more traditional adjuvant approach for high risk groups identified at the time of initial surgical and/or radiotherapeutic treatment needs investigation.

The use of radiosensitizers clearly has tremendous potential to augment local control and cure rates. Regional perfusion of pelvic disease with intra-arterial chemotherapy as a single modality or combined with radiation therapy would appear to be a more rational approach to treating localized disease which is not surgically curable. The delivery of high concentrations of drug while avoiding systemic toxicity is certainly appealing.

Thus, although invasive carcinoma of the cervix has proved difficult to control, particularly in advanced stages, exciting new directions in the application of chemotherapy offer an optimistic future for improved cure rates and prolonged survival.

REFERENCES

1. Silverberg E: Cancer Statistics, 1984 Ca-A Journal for Clinicians 34:7, 1984.
2. Kottmeier HL (ed): Annual report on the results of treatment in gynecological cancer, Vol 17. Stockholm, 1979.
3. Van Nagell JR, Rayburn W, Donaldson ES, et al: Therapeutic implications of patterns of recurrence in cancer of the uterine cervix. Cancer 44:2354, 1979.
4. Lagasse LD, Creasman WT, Shingleton HM, et al: Results and complications of operative staging in cervical cancer: Experience of Gyencologic Oncology Group. Gynecol Oncol 9:90, 1980.
5. Beyer FD Jr, Murphy A: Patterns of spread of invasive cancer of the human cervix. Cancer 18:34, 1965.
6. Chism SE, Park RC, Keys HM: Prospects for para-aortic irradiaton in treatment of cancer of the cervix. Cancer 35:1505, 1975.
7. Emami B, Watring WG, Tak W, et al: Para-aortic lymph node radiation in advanced cervical carcinoma. Int J Radiat Oncol Biol Phys 6:1237, 1980.
8. Marcial VA, Amato DA, Mark RD, et al: Split-course versus continuous pelvis irradiation in carcinoma of the uterine cervix: A prospective randomized clinical trial of the Radiation Therapy Oncology Group. Int J Radiat Oncol Biol Phys 9:431, 1983.
9. Perez CA, Breaux S, Madoc-Jones H, et al: Radiation therapy alone in the treatment of carcinoma of the uterine cervix. Analysis of tumor recurrence. Cancer 51:1393, 1983.
10. Thur TL, Million RR, Daly JW: Radiation treatment of carcinoma of the cervix. Seminars in Oncology 9:299, 1982.
11. Carlson V, Delclos L, Fletcher GH: Distant metastases in squamous cell carcinoma of the uterine cervix. Radiology 88:961, 1967.
12. Badib AO, Kurohara SS, Webster JH, et al: Metastases to organs in carcinoma of the uterine cervix; influence of treatment on incidence and distribution. Cancer 21:434, 1968.
13. DeVita VT Jr, Wasserman TH, Young RC, et al: Perspectives on research in gynecologic oncology. Cancer 38:509, 1976.
14. Malkasian GD, Decker DG, Jorgensen ED: Chemotherapy of carcinoma of the cervix. Gynecol Oncol 5:109, 1977.
15. Wasserman TH, Carter SK: The integration of chemotherapy into combined modality treatment of solid tumors: VIII Cervical Cancer. Cancer Treat Rev 4:25, 1977.
16. Freedman RS, Herson J, Wharton JT, et al: Single agent chemotherapy for recurrent carcinoma of the cervix. Cancer Clin Trials 3:345, 1980.
17. Omura GA, Shingleton HM, Creasman WT, et al: Chemotherapy of gynecologic cancer with nitrosoureas: A randomized trial of CCNU and methyl-CCNU in cancers of the cervix, corpus, vagina, and vulva. Cancer Treat Rep 62:833, 1978.
18. Cavins JA, Greisler HE: Treatment of advanced, unresectable, cervical carcinoma already subjected to complete irradiation therapy. Gynecol Oncol 6:256, 1978.
19. Krakoff IH, Cvitkovic E, Currie V, et al: Clinical pharmacologic and therapeutic studies of bleomycin given by continuous infusion. Cancer 40:2027, 1977.
20. Panettiere FJ, Talley RW, Torres J, et al: Porfiromycin in the management of epidermoid and transitional cell cancer: a phase II study. Cancer Treat Rep 60:907, 1976.
21. Piver MS, Barlow JJ, Xynos FP: Adriamycin alone or in combination in 100 patients with carcinoma of the cervix or vagina. Am J Obstet Gynecol 131:311, 1978.

22. Jobson V, Jackson D, Homesley H, et al: Treatment of recurrent gynecologic malignancies with prolonged intravenous vincristine (VCR) infusion. Proc Am Soc Clin Oncol 2:149, 1983.

23. Hyat M: A phase II clinical trial of cytembena. Biomedicine 26:392, 1977.

24. Bonomi P, Bruckner HW, Cohen C, et al: A randomized trial of cisplatin regimens in squamous cell carcinoma of the cervix. Proc Am Soc Clin Oncol 1:110, 1982.

25. Lira-Puerta V, Tenorio F, Wernz J, et al: Phase II study of cisplatin or dibromodulcitol (DBD) for carcinoma of the cervix. Proc Am Soc Clin Ocnol 1:111, 1982.

26. Hall DJ, Diasio R, Goplerud DR: Cis-platinum in gynecologic cancer: II Squamous cell carcinoma of the cervix. Am J Obstet Gynecol 141:305, 1981.

27. Cohen CJ, Deppe G, Castro-Marin CA, et al: Treatment of advanced squamous cell carcinoma of the cervix with cis-platinum (II) diamminedichloride (NSC-119875). Am J Obstet Gynecol 130:853, 1978.

28. Thigpen T, Shingleton H, Homesley H, et al: Cis-platinum in treatment of advanced or recurrent squamous cell carcinoma of the cervix: a phase II study of the Gynecologic Oncology Group. Cancer 48:899, 1980.

29. Rossof AA, Talley RW, Stephens R, et al: Phase II evaluation of cis-dichlorodiammine platinum II in advanced malignancies of the GU or Gyn organs: A Southwest Oncology Group study. Cancer Treat Rep 63:1557, 1979.

30. Hayat M, Bayssas M, Brule G, et al: Cis-platinum-diammino-dichloro (CPDD) in chemotherapy of cancer. Phase II therapeutic trial. Biochimie 60:935, 1978.

31. Cohen CJ, Castro-Martin A, Deppe G, et al: Chemotherapy of advanced recurrent cervical cancer with platinum II. Proc Am Assoc Cancer Res 19:401, 1978.

32. Stehman FB, Ballon SC, Lagasse LD, et. al: Cis-platinum in advanced gynecologic malignancy. Gynecol Oncol 7:349, 1979.

33. Thigpen T, Ehrlich C, Blessing J: Phase II trial of maytansine in treatment of advanced or recurrent squamous cell carcinoma of the cervix: A Gynecologic Oncology Group study. Proc Am Assoc Cancer Res 21:424, 1980.

34. Conroy J, Blessing J, Lewis G, et al: Phase II trial of ICRF-159 in treatment of advanced squamous cell carcinoma of the cervix. Proc Am Assoc Cancer Res 21:423, 1980.

35. Arseneau JC, Bundy B, Dolan T, et al: Phase II study of Bakers Antifol (Triazinate, TZT, NSC 139105) in advanced squamous cell carcinoma of the cervix. Amer J Clin Oncol 5:61, 1982.

36. Slayton RE, Creasman WT, Pethy W, et al: Phase II trial of VP-16-213 in the treatment of advanced squamous cell carcinoma of the cervix and adenocarcinoma of the ovary. A Gynecologic Oncology Group study. Cancer Treat Rep 63:2089, 1979.

37. Blom J, Blessing J, Mladineo J, et al: Dianhydrogalactitol (DAG) in the treatment of advanced gynecologic malignancies. Proc Am Assoc Cancer Res 21–416, 1980.

38. Thigpen JT, Homesley H, Perm K, et al: Phase II trial of piperazinedione in the treatment of advanced squamous cell carcinoma of the cervix. Proc Am Assoc Cancer Res 19:162, 1978.

39. Stambaugh JE: Vindesine (DVA) in the treatment of patients with advanced neoplastic disease. Proc Am Assoc Cancer Res 21:344, 1980.

40. EORTC Clinical Screening Group: Preliminary results of a phase II trial on solid tumors of detorubicin, a new anthracycline. Cancer Clin Trials 3:115, 1979.

41. Bonomi P, Blessing JA, Sedlack TV, et al: Phase II trial of AMSA in patients with advanced or recurrent squamous cell carcinoma of the cervix: A Gynecologic Oncology Group study. Cancer Treat Rep 67:197, 1983.

42. Brenner DE, Garbino C, Kasdorf H, et al: A phase II trial of m-AMSA in the treatment of advanced gynecologic malignancies. Am J Clin Oncol 5:291, 1982.

43. Slavik M, Muss H, Blessing JA: Phase II clinical study of Yoshi 864 in squamous cell carcinoma of the uterine cervix. Cancer Treat Rep 67:195, 1983.
44. Hurteloup P, Mathe G, Hayat M: A phase II trial of 4'-Epi-Adriamycin (4"EA) for advanced solid tumors. Preliminary results (meeting abstract). UICC conference on Clinical Oncology, October 28–31, 1981. Lausanne, Switzerland. International Union Against Cancer, 1981.
45. Brenner D, Forastiere A, Rosenchein N, et al: A phase II study of spirogermanium in patients with advanced carcinomas of the ovary and cervix. Proc Am Soc Clin Oncol 1:115, 1982.
46. Miyamoto T: Recent results in the treatment of a metastatic cervical cancer with a sequential combination of bleomycin and mitomycin-C. In Carter SK, Crooke ST (eds): Mitomycin C: Current Status and New Developments. Academic Press, New York, 1979, pp. 163–171.
47. Leichman LP, Baker LH, Stanhope CR, et al: Mitomycin-C and bleomycin in the treatment of far-advanced cervical cancer. A Southwest Oncology Group Pilot Study. Cancer Treat Rep 64:1139, 1980.
48. Trope C, Johnson J, Simonsen E, et al: Bleomycin-mitomycin-C in advanced carcinoma of the cervix—a third look. Cancer 51:591, 1983.
49. Krebs HB, Girtanner RE, Nordqvist SRB, et al: Treatment of advanced cervical cancer by combination of bleomycin and mitomycin-C Cancer 46:2159, 1980.
50. Petrilli ES, Castaldo TW, Ballon SC, et al: Bleomycin-mitomycin-C therapy for advanced squamous carcinoma of the cervix. Gynecol Oncol 9:292, 1980.
51. Greenberg BR, Hannigan J, Gerretson L, et al: Sequential combination of bleomycin and mitomycin-C in advanced cervical cancer. An American Experience: A Northern California Oncology Group Study. Cancer Treat Rep 66:163, 1982.
52. Boice CR, Freedman RS, Herson J, et al: Bleomycin and mitomycin-C (BLM-M) in recurrent squamous uterine cervical carcinoma. Cancer 49:2242, 1982.
53. Majima H: Combination chemotherapy of disseminated cervix carcinoma with bleomycin (BLM) and mitomycin-C (MMC) Proc Am Soc Clin Oncol 18:320, 1977.
54. Baker LH, Opipari MI, Izbicki RM: Phase II study of mitomycin-C, vincristine, bleomycin in advanced squamous cell carcinoma of the uterine cervix. Cancer 38:2222, 1976.
55. Baker LH, Opipari MI, Wilson H, et al: Mitomycin-C, vincristine and bleomycin therapy for advanced cervical cancer. Obstet Gynecol 52:146, 1978.
56. Baker LH: A bleomycin combination for disseminated cervical cancer. In Carter SK, Crooke ST, Umezawa H (eds): Bleomycin: Current Status and New Developments. Academic Press, New York, 1978, pp. 173–183.
57. Alberts DS, Martimbeau PW, Surwitz ON: Mitomycin-C, bleomycin, vincristine and cisplatin in the treatment of advanced, recurrent squamous cell carcinoma of the cervix. Cancer Clin Trials 4:313, 1981.
58. Surwit EA, Alberts DS, Aristizabal S, et al: Treatment of primary and recurrent, advanced squamous cell cancer of the cervix with mitomycin-C + vincristine + bleomycin (MOB) plus cisplatin (Plat). Proc Am Soc Clin Oncol 2:153, 1983.
59. Vermorken JB, Oosterom AT, Ten Bokkel Huinink WW, et al: Phase II study of vincristine (V), Bleomycin (B), Mitomycin-C (M) and Cisplatin (P) in disseminated squamous cell carcinoma of the uterine cervix. Third NCI-EORTC Symposium on New Drugs in Cancer Therapy, October 15–17, 1981, Brussells, Belgium European Organization for Research on Treatment of Cancer, pp. A9, 1981.
60. Vogl SE, Moukhtar M, Calanog A, et al: Chemotherapy for advanced cervical cancer with bleomycin, vincristine, mitomycin-C and cis-diammenedichloroplatinum (11) (BOMP). Cancer Treat Rep 64:1005, 1980.

61. Baker LH: Personal Communication.
62. Araujo CE, Simone R, Tessler J: Cyclophosphamide, adriamycin and cis-dichlorodiam-mineplatinum (II) combination chemotherapy treatment of squamous cell carcinoma of the cervix. UICC Conference on Clinical Oncology, October 28–31, 1981, Lausanne, Switzerland. International Union Against Cancer, 1981.
63. Fine S, Sturgeon JFG, Gospodarowicz MK, et al: Treatment of advanced carcinoma of the cervix with methotrexate, Adriamycin and cisplatin. Proc Am Soc Clin Oncol 2:154, 1983.
64. Vogl SE, Seltzer V, Camacho F, et al: Dianhydrogalactilol and cisplatin in combination for advanced cancer of the uterine cervix. Cancer Treat Rep 66:1809, 1982.
65. Jobson VW, Muss HB, Thigpen JT, et al: Chemotherapy of advanced carcinoma of the cervix with cyclophosphamide and cisplatin.—A pilot study of the Gynecologic Oncology Group. Proc Am Assoc Cancer Res 22:475, 1981.
66. Vogl SE, Moukhtar M, Kaplan BH: Chemotherapy for advanced cervical cancer with methotrexate, bleomycin, and cis-dichlorodiammuneplatinum (II). Cancer Treat Rep 63:1005, 1979.
67. Daghestanian AN, Hakes TB, Lynch G, et al: Cervix carcinoma: Treatment with combination cisplatin and bleomycin. Gynecol Oncol (in press).
68. Sidorowica E, Hand R, Popkin D: Cis-platinum and bleomycin in advanced carcinoma of the cervix. Proc Amer Soc Clin Oncol 2:148, 1983.
69. Natale RB, Wheeler RH, Ensminger W, et al: Cisplatin + dichloromethotrexate (DCM): A pharmacologically rational combinaton with high activity. Proc Amer Assoc Cancer Res 24:166, 1983.
70. Natale RB: Personal communication.
71. Hakes TB, Daghestani AN, Nori D, et al: Adjuvant chemotherapy for poor risk stage IB/IIA cervix carcinoma patients—a pilot study with cisplatin/bleomycin (CP/B). Proc Amer Soc Clin Oncol 2:154, 1983.
72. Alberts DS, Ignoffo R: Adriamycin-cyclophosphamide treatment of squamous cell carcinoma of the cervix. Cancer Treat Rep 62:143, 1978.
73. Hanjani P, Bonnell S: Treatment of advanced and recurrent squamous cell carcinoma of the cervix with combination doxorubicin and cyclophosphamide. Cancer Treat Rep 64:1363, 1980.
74. Piver MS, Barlow JJ, Dunbar J: Doxorubicin, cyclophosphamide and 5-fluorouracil in patients with carcinoma of the cervix or vagina. Cancer Treat Rep 64:549, 1980.
75. Chan WK, Aroney RS, Levi JA, et al: Four drug combinaton chemotherapy for advanced cervical carcinoma. Cancer 49:2437, 1982.
76. Day TG, Wharton JT, Gottleib JA, et al: Chemotherapy for squamous carcinoma of the cervix; Doxorubicin-methyl-CCNU. Am J Obstet Gynecol 132:545, 1978.
77. Von Maillot K, Ranger IM: Chemotherapy for advanced, recurrent carcinoma of the cervix. A report on the treatment of 22 patients. Arch Gynecol 231:253, 1982.
78. Papavasiliou C, Pappas J, Aravantinos D, et al: Treatment of cervical carcinoma with adriamycin combined with methotrexate. Cancer Treat Rep 62:1387, 1978.
79. Guthrie D, Way S: The use of adriamycin and methotrexate in carcinoma of the cervix, the development of a safe, effective regimen. Obstet Gynecol 52:349, 1978.
80. Haid M, Homesley HL, White DR, et al: Adriamycin-methotrexate combination chemotherapy of advanced carcinoma of the cervix: A Second Look. Obstet Gynecol 50:103, 1977.
81. Trope C, Jonnson JE, Grundsell H, et al: Adriamycin-methotrexate combinaton chemotherapy of advanced carcinoma of the cervix. A Third Look. Obstet Gynecol 55:488, 1980.
82. Wallace HJ, Hreshchyshyn MM, Wilbanks GD, et al: Comparison of the therapeutic ef-

fect of adriamycin alone versus adriamycin plus cyclophosphamide in the treatment of advanced carcinoma of the cervix. Cancer Treat Rep 62:1435, 1978.

83. Malkasian GD, Decker DG, Green SJ, et al: Treatment of recurrent and metastatic carcinoma of the cervix: Comparison of doxorubicin with a combinaton of vincristine and 5-fluorouracil. Gynecol Oncol 11:235, 1981.

84. Omura GA, Velez-Garcia E, Birch R: Phase II randomized study of doxorubicin, vincristine, and 5-fluorouracil versus cyclophosphamide in advanced squamous cell cancer of the cervix. Cancer Treat Rep 65:901, 1981.

85. Greenberg BR, Kardinal CG, Pajek TF, et al: Adriamycin versus adriamycin and bleomycin in advanced epidermoid carcinoma of the cervix. Cancer Treat Rep 61:1383, 1977.

86. DePalo GM, Bajetta E, Beretta G, et al: Adriamycin plus bleomycin versus cyclophosphamide plus vincristine in advanced carcinoma of the uterine cervix. Tumor 62:113, 1976.

87. Wheeler RH, Liepman M, Baker SR, et al: Bleomycin, vincristine and mitomycin-C with or without methotrexate in the treatment of squamous cell carcinoma. Cancer Treat Rep 64:943, 1980.

88. Scarborough JP, Metter GE, Moseley HS, et al: Adriamycin, bleomycin, and CCNU as effective induction chemotherapeutic agents in advanced squamous cell carcinoma (COG Protocol 7333). J Surg Oncol 10:501, 1978.

89. Lifshitz S, Railsback L, Buchsbaum H: Intra-arterial pelvic infusion chemotherapy in advanced gynecologic cancer. Ob Gyn 52(4):476, 1978.

90. Ensminger W, Gyves J: Regional chemotherapy of neoplastic disease. J Pharm Ther (in press).

91. Carlson J, Freidman R, et al: Intra-arterial cis-platinum in the management of squamous cell carcinoma of the cervix. Gyn Onc 12:92, 1981.

92. Trussell R, Mitford-Barkerton G: Carcinoma of the cervix treated with continuous intra-arterial methotrexate and intermittent intramuscular leucovorin. Lancet 1:971, 1961.

93. Morrow P, DiSaia P, Mangan C, et al: Continuous pelvic arterial infusion with bleomycin for squamous carcinoma of the cervix recurrent after irradiation therapy. Cancer Treat Rep 61(7):1403, 1977.

94. Swenerton K, Evers J, White G, et al: intermittent pelvic infusion with vincristine, bleomycin, and mitomycin C for advanced recurrent carcinoma of the cervix. Cancer Treat Rep 63(8):1379, 1979.

95. Calvo D, Patt Y, Wallace S, et al: Phase I–II trial of percutaneous intra-arterial cis-diamminedichloroplatinum (11) for regionally confined malignancy. Cancer 45:1278, 1980.

96. Perez C, Knapp R, Young R: Gynecologic tumors. In Devita V, Hellman S, Rosenberg S (eds): Cancer: Principles and Practice of Oncology. Philadelphia, JB Lippincott, 1982, PR. 823–849.

97. Chapman J: Hypoxic sensitizers-implications for radiation therapy. N Eng/J Med 301 (26):1429, 1979.

98. Fletcher G, Lindberg R, Caderno J, et al: Hyperbaric oxygen as a radiotherapeutic adjuvant in advanced cancer of the uterine cervix. Cancer 39:617, 1977.

99. Committee for Radiation Oncology Studies: Radiation Sensitizers. Cancer 37(4 suppl):2062, 1976.

100. Watson E, Halran K, et al: Hyperbaric oxygen and radiotherapy: a medical research council trial in carcinoma of the cervix. Br J Rad 51:879, 1978.

101. Wasserman T, Stetz J, Phillips T: Radiation therapy oncology group clinical trials with misonidazole. Cancer 47:2382, 1981.

102. Thomas G, Rauth A, et al: A phase I study of misonidazole and pelvic irradiation in patients with carcinoma of the cervix. Br J Cancer 45:860, 1982.

103. Sinclair W: The combined effect of hydroxyurea and x-rays on chinese hamster cells in vitro. Cancer Res 28:198, 1968.
104. Piver M, Barlow J, Vongtama V, et al: Hydroxyurea as a radiation sensitizer in women with carcinoma of the uterine cervix. Am J Obstet Gynecol 129:379, 1977.
105. Hreshchyshyn M, Aron B, Boronow R, et al: Hydroxyurea or placebo combined with radiation to treat IIIB and IV cervical cancer confined to the pelvis. Radiation Onc Biol Phys 5:317, 1979.
106. Goolsby C, Daly J, Skinner O, et al: Combination of 5 fluorouracil and radiation as primary therapy of carcinoma of the cervix. Ob Gyn 32(5):674, 1968.
107. Smith J, Randall G, Castro J, et al: Hypogastric artery infusion for advanced squamous cell carcinoma of the cervix. Am J Roen Rad Ther Nuc Med 114(4):110, 1972.
108. Kalra J, Cortes E, et al: Effective multimodality treatment for advanced epidermoid carcinoma of the female genital tract. Proc Am Soc Clin Onc 2:152, 1983.
109. Sugimori H, Taki I, Koga K Adjuvant hormone therapy to radiation treatment for cervical cancer. Acta Obst et Gynaec Jap 23(2):77, 1976.
110. Mathew CD: Mitomycin-C combined with radiotherapy in the management of carcinoma cervix. Ind J Cancer 13:39, 1976.
111. Kavenough J, Wallace S, Delclos L, et al: Induction intra-arterial (IA) chemotherapy for advanced squamous cell carcinoma of the cervix. Proc Am Soc Clin Onc 2:154, 1983.
112. Kardinal C, Wyckoff D, Canoy N: Evaluation of melphalan as a post-irradiation adjuvant in stage IIB and III carcinoma of the uterine cervix: a negative study. Proc Am Assoc Cancer Res 20:345, 1979.

6 | Ovarian Cancer: Diagnosis and Surgical Management

Hugh R. K. Barber

Deaths from cancer of the ovary have slowly increased over the last 40 years, and the rate is now two and one half times that of 1930. It is anticipated that 1.4 percent or one of every 70 newborn girls will develop ovarian cancer at some time during their lives. In 1984 the projected figure for new cases of cancer of the ovary is 18,000 and the death rate is 11,400. Cancer of the ovary is the leading cause of death from gynecologic cancer. The dramatic figure is that ovarian cancer constitutes only 25 percent of gynecologic cancers, but accounts for half of all deaths from cancers of the female genital tract.

Unfortunately, progress in curing ovarian cancer has been disappointingly slow. More than 100,000 women died of this disease in the past decade, and ovarian cancer continues to increase as a major gynecologic disease in the United States. Currently, the optimal treatment for each stage of the disease is not even known. The results of therapy were no better in 1983 than had been achieved in the previous two decades. Current methods of management are helping these women live longer and hopefully more comfortably, but at present the dismal five year survival rate has not been improved.[1]

The incidence of ovarian cancer starts to rise at age 40 with an annual rate of 10 per 100,000, increases to a peak at about age 80 where the rate is about 52 per 100,000 women and then drops after age 80, but the rate continues throughout the remainder of their life at about 45 per 100,000. It is obvious that the ovary get too old to function, but never gets too old to develop a cancer. It is essential that these figures and the distribution of the incidence be kept in mind when making the decision whether to retain the ovaries at the time of hysterectomy in women over age 40.

119

Since the incidence of ovarian cancer is on the increase in highly industrialized nations, an effort must be made to achieve earlier diagnosis than has been possible in the past, or to practice prophylaxis by removing ovaries at the time of pelvic surgery in women over age 40.[2]

Ovarian cancer is one of the most frustrating problems in gynecology. For those patients not cured, death is often prolonged, with repeated bouts of intestinal obstruction. The cancer spreads over the surface of the bowel, and, although the lumen of the bowel is not totally obstructed, the end result is the same as though it were. Segments of the bowel are so coated with cancer that the gut is paralyzed and is unable to respond with peristalsis. Patients develop inanition and malnutrition, and literally vomit themselves to death. It is unfortunate that these individuals remain alert up until the moment of death. They often become ravenously hungry, and after digesting food or liquid, begin to vomit. It is a dismal clinical picture of a women who not only is terminally ill, but also is being tormented by her hunger and thirst. The pathology described as carcinomatosis ileus is one of the few indications for the intermittent use of a nasogastric tube as definitive therapy to decompress the bowel. Responsible physicians should be well-versed in gastroenterology and the surgery of gastroenterologic disorders. Those therapeutic nihilists who plead that the patient should be left to die with dignity must face a dilemma when forced to apply their philosophy to the case of a woman dying with advanced ovarian cancer.

CLINICAL MANIFESTATIONS

It is usually stated that there are no early manifestations of ovarian cancer. This in itself is considered a major contributing factor to the poor therapeutic results. The usual manifestations of abdominal swelling, pain, and a mass as recorded in hospital charts, are associated with an advanced stage of the disease.[3]

The earliest symptoms are usually insidious and include vague abdominal discomfort, dyspepsia, indigestion, gas with concommitant distension, flatulance, gastrointestinal unrest, feeling of fullness after a light meal, slight loss of appetite, and other mild digestive disturbances. Although the specific manifestations are certainly not specific, such gastrointestinal complaints are not uncommon. They are suggestive of ovarian cancer when encountered in the proper clinical setting and may signal difficulty. Unfortunately, such complaints are usually not considered important.

The gastrointestinal symptoms may precede other symptoms by months. It is imperative to rule out ovarian cancer in women over age 40 who present with gastrointestinal symptoms that cannot definitely be diagnosed. Elderly women without pelvic complaints, but with complaints referable to the intestinal tract, are more apt to consult their internists or family doctor for their extrapelvic complaints. Such clinicians have a great opportunity to diagnose ovarian cancer at an early stage.

The following triad may be an aid in diagnosis of ovarian cancer: (1) A woman 35 years of age or over has a significant risk because of her age. With advancing age, the ovary ceases to function but remains at risk for the development of ovarian cancer. (2) In a patient over 40 years of age, persistent gastrointestinal symptoms which cannot be definitely diagnosed; (3) A long history of ovarian imbalance and malfunction, including increased premenstrual tension, heavy menstruation with marked breast tenderness, dysfunctional bleeding, tendency for spontaneous abortion, infertility, nulliparity, as well as an early menopause should alert the physician to the possibility that ovarian cancer may be present. The ovary is like a cam running off center.

In the triad of a woman over age 35 with ovarian dysfunction and gastrointestinal symptoms, it is important to consider the possibility of ovarian cancer, and systematically carry out all diagnostic measures as outlined below. Unfortunately, there are no specific diagnostic measures for early ovarian cancer, but a high index of suspicion and education of the public as well as the medical profession will help achieve an earlier diagnosis, and occasionally an early diagnosis.

DIAGNOSIS

A knowledge of the cause of death from any cancer is helpful in understanding the natural history of that particular cancer. The cause of death in ovarian cancer is often difficult to identify. Some patients hemorrhage from break down of tumor, others have sepsis, and most have an ovarian cachexia caused by interference with alimentary function. Widespread disease undoubtedly causes cellular metabolic imbalances and deranges cellular enzymatic processes. Most ovarian cancers in the advanced stages have sepsis and many also have an autoimmune disorder.

The early diagnosis of ovarian cancer is a matter of chance and not a triumph of the scientific approach. One cubic centimeter contains 10^9 or a billion cells with the power to metastasize. By any known method available including clinical examination or any x-ray examination it is almost impossible to detect the presence of this small amount of tumor. Therefore, methods of early detection are extremely limited. In the majority of cases, the finding of a pelvic mass is the only available diagnostic sign, with the exception of functional tumors, which may manifest endocrine activity with minimal ovarian enlargement. In some cases, pelvic findings may be uncertain, even late in the disease. Pain in the early stages is associated with a complication, such as torsion, or perforation or hemorrhage. Later, pain occurs when adjacent organs or nerve sheaths are infiltrated by tumor.

Menstrual disorders may result from hormone producing tumors. In the menopausal patient, vaginal bleeding may occur. This has been attributed to the functioning stroma in a malignant ovary. Ascites with malignant cells is a sign of advanced disease.

In terms of function, it must be also emphasized that a variety of endocrine effects, such as hypercalcemia, hypoglycemia, and Cushing's syndrome, as well as disorders such as hemolytic anemia, may occasionally be related to the presence of an ovarian tumor. The diagnosis of an ovarian cancer should be included in the differential diagnosis when dealing with the paraendocrine syndrome.

The pelvic findings are often inconclusive even later in the disease. The tumor may be deep in the pelvis, the patient may be obese, heavy muscled, and uncooperative. The elderly patient may have an inelastic conical vagina, complicated by marked atrophy. Occasionally, there may be widespread metastasis with minimal pelvic findings. The usual signs and symptoms, as well as the physical findings, associated with ovarian cancer, all represent an advanced cancer of the ovary. Abdominal mass or distension or both are the most common diagnostic features reported in most hospital charts. However, ovarian cancer seldom gives symptoms until it grows to a size of 15 cm. The ovaries cannot be palpated abdominally until they achieve this size. Ascites with positive cells is a sign of advanced disease, and the 5-year survival rate is reported to be less than 8 percent in these patients.[4]

Routine pelvic examination will detect about one cancer in 10,000 examinations of asymptomatic women. Pelvic findings are often minimal, and are not helpful in making a diagnosis, often even though the patient has advanced disease. However, combined with a high index of suspicion, the findings on pelvic examination may help alert the physician to the diagnosis. The most helpful pelvic findings suggesting the presence of an ovarian tumor are:

1.   A mass in the ovarian area;
2.   Relative immobility due to fixation and adhesion;
3.   Irregularity of the tumor, particularly a difference in the consistency such as one area being cystic and another rubbery, another soft and another very hard. This difference is due to the rapid growth of the tumor as it grows away from its blood supply and there are, therefore, ischemic areas present.
4.   Shotty consistency with increased firmness;
5.   Tumors in the cul-de-sac described as a "handful of knuckles";
6.   Relative insensitivity of the mass;
7.   Increasing size under observation especially if the patient has been followed through one period or is on the contraceptive pill;
8.   Bilaterality (70 percent of ovarian cancer versus 5 percent of benign disease);
9.   In late disease, common findings of nodular hepatomegaly, ascites and palpation of an omental mass.[5]

CYTOLOGY

Some investigators claim good results in detecting ovarian cancer by means of vaginal and cervical cytology but the author's experience with cytology has not been good. This has been confirmed by reports in the literature which state that the Papanicolaou cytologic method for detecting ovarian cancer in the early stages is not reliable. Even in advanced stages cytology is positive in only 10 to 25 percent of women. The Grahams reported that the Pap smear was positive in 40 percent of patients with advanced disease. Cytology is also used to diagnose cells taken from the posterior cul-de-sac by culdocentesis, and this has not been found to be of much benefit in most cases. Not only did the patients find the procedure painful, but in the author's hands the results have not been very reliable. By the time an ovarian cancer spills malignant cells that can be identified in cytologic smears it may no longer be in an early stage of growth. Also, an inflamed mesothelial cell in the smear may look like a malignant cell, in which case surgery is mandatory.

Cytologic diagnosis has limited application. It is valuable in the elderly, poor risk patients in whom there is every evidence of advanced ovarian cancer, including pelvic and abdominal masses and ascites, and in whom laparotomy would be considered dangerous. In these patients the presumptive diagnosis of ovarian cancer may be made on the cells collected by paracentesis. Treatment then can be given.[6]

Fine needle ovarian aspiration biopsy for making a diagnosis of ovarian cancer is not advocated because it ruptures the mechanical barrier which is the capsule of the ovary and may lead to spread of the ovarian cancer. There is also a high false negative rate. Therefore, it must be concluded that cytology has a very limited role in the diagnosis of ovarian cancer.

TUMOR MARKERS

A great number of products of ovarian tumors have been described and in some cases the method described for their measurement in body fluids. For malignant teratomas of the ovary, human chorionic gonadotropin and alpha fetoprotein measurements provide information which is often valuable in management and predicting curability. For the usual common epithelial ovarian cancer, there is at present no universal marker. However, carcinoembryonic antigen, placental alkaline phosphatase, and some newly defined tumor associated antigens may provide useful information to be used to monitor the course of a proportion of the cases.

Ovarian tumor markers can be divided into the following categories: (1) trophoblastic, (2) embryonic, (3) miscellaneous, (4) enzymes, and (5) ovarian antigens.[7–12]

Although carcinoembryonic antigen (CEA), alpha fetoprotein (AFP), and lactic dehydrogenase (LDH) do not help in making the diagnosis, if elevated, they serve to monitor the patient's response to therapy. Some investigators have raised the possibility that lactic dehydrogenase elevation may be valuable as a screening test. In a prospective study the author did not find it useful as a preoperative screening test. Total serum LDH is moderately elevated in most cancer patients with extensive hepatic metastases. The increase is usually associated with minor changes in the isoenzymes pattern, particularly an increase in LDH 3 and LDH 5 (the faster moving isoenzymes. The LDH titer is higher in pleural and peritoneal fluids with malignant cells than it is in the serum. When the association of LDH and advanced ovarian cancer was raised, the review of our data failed to confirm a correlation of the LDH level with the extent of disease. For a period of time, the ovarian cancer project at Lenox Hill Hospital included routine evaluation of the carcinoembryonic antigen in all ovarian cancer patients. However, we have not confirmed the reports that carcinoembryonic antigen has been identified in the plasma of 35 percent of these patients. The author believes that more cases and more time will be required before a definitive statement can be made on the relationship between carcinoembryonic antigen and ovarian cancer. In a study from our laboratory, neither the heterologous nor homologous antibody against the common epithelial ovarian tumors cross reacted with carcinoembryonic antigens. In view of our clinical findings and laboratory data, I doubt that carcinoembryonic antigen will play a significant role as a prognostic screening test. However, in certain patients it may serve to monitor progress during treatment of the cancer. With improved technology there may be a resurgence of interest in the success of the carcinoembryonic antigen in evaluating ovarian cancer.

Serum alpha fetoprotein (AFP) assays have currently gained an important place in the diagnosis of hepatocellular and testicular tumors as well as the endodermal sinus tumors.[13] The observation that AFP may be elevated before tumors are detected by other means has important implications. In addition, successful therapy is associated with the decline in AFP levels to normal and a subsequent rise when the tumor recurs. AFP is known to be a product of the human fetal liver, gastrointestinal tract, and yolk sac. Endodermal sinus tumor which is of vitelline origin invariably gives a positive test for AFP.

Investigators from the National Cancer Institute have shown that malignancies other than trophoblastic disease produce elevated chorionic gonadotropin titers. Significantly, 30 percent of common epithelial ovarian tumors and up to 90 percent or more of the embryonal ovarian tumors are associated with measurable amounts of this hormone using ultrasensitive techniques. Although the finding of these substances does not identify the kind of malignancy—or in some cases whether the patient has a malignancy at all—it clearly indicates high risk and warrants investigation.

In addition to the alpha fetoproteins there are alpha$_2$H-fetoprotein (α_2HF), beta S-fetoprotein and gamma-fetoprotein. Currently these markers play very little role in making an early diagnosis except in certain endodermal sinus tumors, but at present serve as a way to monitor treatment.

Recently Bast and his colleagues[14] have added another assay to monitor the course of epithelial ovarian cancer. The murine monoclonal antibody OC 125 reacts with an antigen, CA 125, common to most nonmucinous epithelial ovarian carcinomas. An assay has been developed to detect CA 125 in the serum. Rising or falling levels of CA 125 correlated with progression or regression of disease in 93 percent of the patients tested.

TISSUE POLYPEPTIDE ANTIGEN (TPA)

TPA has been shown to be a component of the endoplasmic reticulum and plasma membrane.[15] It is a polypeptide with specific antigenic properties which now have been identified in a variety of species. It is a tumor-associated antigen occurring in human placenta, in human cancer tumors, and body fluids of cancer patients. TPA is present in the membrane structures of human cancer cells. It can be detected there by the effects of cytotoxic antibodies or by the localization of fluorescent, nonspecific anti-TPA antibodies. In studies carried out, there is close agreement between TPA levels and the clinical course of patients with metastases from mammary cancer. It has proved to be a good method to monitor the progress of the patient during therapy. In most cases the TPA was reduced to normal levels before remissions were evident from the clinical parameter study.

ENZYMES

There are a great number of enzymes that are being studied in ovarian tumors and identified as markers. These include glycosyltransferases and glycosidases. Other miscellaneous tumor markers that are being studied include pregnancy associated macroglobulin (PAM, PZP) and fibrin-fibrinogen degradation products. Acute phase reactant proteins are under intensive study. The levels of acute phase reactant proteins, complement components, and inhibitors have been measured in sera of patients with Stage IV ovarian carcinoma. A marked elevation of the concentration of the alpha-1-acid glycoprotein, alpha-1-antitrypsin, and haptoglobin, and of C 3 and C 4, C 3PA, and the inhibitors of C 3 (C 3bINA) has been reported compared to a controlled series. Laparotomy and tumor extirpation produced a temporary decrease of the level of all but alpha-proteins. Chemotherapy brought about a decrease in serum level of acute phase reactant proteins and complement components and C3bINA with concomitant rise in total protein level. Measurement of acute phase reactants and complement inhibitors may be an additional tool in evaluating the efficacy of chemotherapy in patients with advanced ovarian ocancer.

REGAN ALKALINE PHOSPHATASE ISOENZYME

The Regan isoenzyme is heat stable, and at least one component of the enzyme has a molecular weight in the 200,000 range. The alkaline phosphatase enzymes are known to occur in serum and are derived from the liver, bones, lung, intestinal tract, and placenta. The placental alkaline phosphatase enzyme does not occur in fetal tissues, blood, or serum but does occur in maternal serum during the third trimester of pregnancy. It is never found in the serum of normal male subjects. The enzyme was first detected in a patient named Regan who had lung cancer. It has been found in association with a variety of cancers. When alkaline phosphatase is present it is a useful method to monitor tumor progression or regression. It can be detected in malignant serosal exudates. In any patient with an elevated serum alkaline phosphatase level found by routine methods, reexamination should be carried out to see if the placental alkaline phosphatase is responsible for the elevation. If it is, a careful evaluation should be carried out to detect or eliminate a latent neoplasm.

Stolbach[16] found the isoenzyme in the serum of 30 to 40 percent of patients with cancer of the ovary and in 50 to 70 percent of malignant fluids from patients with carcinoma of the ovary.

OVARIAN TUMOR ASSOCIATED ANTIGENS

There have been a variety of methods in which heterologous and autologous antibodies have been processed.[17] The current problem is that each antibody is different from the previous one and in absorbing material from it it loses some of its sensitivity. Work with the radioimmunoassay has not been sensitive enough to make a serologic diagnosis. However, work is in progress using the hybridoma method to obtain a monoclonal antibody. One of the most exciting possibilities for monoclonal antibodies is their use in identifying tumor and differentiating antigens on human cells. A crucial benefit of hybridoma technology is that it not only permits whole cells to be used for immunization but also clones out individual antibody forming cells from immunized animals. It is now possible to generate monoclonal antibodies against many antigens. Through hybridoma technology these immunologic reagents can be made available in large quantity and can be regenerated indefinitely. Such tailor made homogeneous antibodies are likely not only to improve the reliability—and reduce the cost of—immunoassays but should also permit the development of new diagnostic procedures and possibly therapeutic modalities in human disease. Combining this with the enzyme linked immunosorbent assay (ELISA) technique there is great potential for making an early diagnosis using a serologic approach.

ULTRASOUND

Ultrasound is being used in many hospitals and physician offices to aid in the detection of ovarian neoplasia and other pelvic pathology. Donald[18] prefers the term "sonar" for "electrosonic diagnostic echography." He has repeatedly emphasized that sonar cannot supplant good, clinical examination but may help materially to reinforce or modify the clinician's findings. Information provided indicates macroscopic appearance only and is concerned with tissue density, distribution, and fluid content. The author stresses that the pictures must therefore be interpreted in the light of clinical knowledge and common sense. Sonar is no substitute for laparotomy and biopsy in a suspected tumor.

Ultrasound is the name given to sound with frequency over 20,000 cycles per second, the upper limits of the human ear.

In most instances it is possible to differentiate ovarian cysts, both malignant and benign, from solid masses. A mass separate from the uterus associated with disorganized internal echoes at normal sensitivity suggests ovarian cancer. Ascites fluid loculation may add to confusion in evaluating suspected masses. Implants in the omentum may be interpreted as masses, especially in serial studies. It is accepted that the efficacy of preoperative evaluation of the primary mass has been adequately documented. More correlation is needed to establish the role that ultrasound will play in the diagnosis and management of the patient with disseminated ovarian cancer.[19]

LAPAROSCOPY

Laparoscopy or peritoneoscopy has been found to be useful in staging suspected ovarian cancer patients and in the follow-up of these patients. It has very limited value as a diagnostic modality in patients with ovarian cancer.[20,21]

Peritoneoscopy has been employed as a tool for the second look in ovarian cancer, and has been performed in patients who have achieved clinical remission with chemotherapy. It can be summarized by saying that a positive finding with biopsy is conclusive but a negative laparoscopy must be followed by an exploratory laparotomy before chemotherapy can be terminated. The role of laparoscopy or peritoneoscopy remains to be evaluated.

COMPUTERIZED AXIAL TOMOGRAPHY (CAT SCAN)

CAT scan has been a valuable tool in identifying and localizing lesions above the pelvic brim. However, its value in diagnosis of early ovarian cancer remains to be determined. High resolution CAT scan, especially of the abdomen, contributes to identifying whether there is disease present or not. It has been helpful particularly in identifying retroperitoneal paraaortic nodes. As each new generation of CAT scanners appear, additional help in identifying pathology in the pelvis and abdomen is achieved. The CAT scan does make a contribution in monitoring effective therapy in patients with disseminated ovarian cancer.

NUCLEAR MAGNETIC RESONANCE (NMR)

In 1946 it was discovered that the partial alignment of some atomic nuclei by an applied static magnetic field could be detected and measured by their response to a second applied magnetic field oscillating at the appropriate radio frequency. This phenomenon known as nuclear magnetic resonance is a consequence of the fact that those atomic nuclei with magnetic moments, that is, those with the A-like magnets, are aligned by a magnetic field, as is a compass needle. The nuclei, however, precess like tops around the direction of their field at a frequency proportional to the magnetic field intensity.

Nuclear magnetic resonance enables a dynamic imaging of the physiologic and pathologic states of the intact human body, including tumor. Measurements of tumors have been made by other staging techniques, but NMR may be not only the safest and best for repeated evaluations, but may also allow earlier diagnosis, even of precancerous stages. Although work with nuclear magnetic resonance technique gives great promise for adding another method for early diagnosis, more work will have to be done before a positive statement can be made.[22]

STAGE GROUPING FOR PRIMARY CARCINOMA OF THE OVARY[23]

Staging is based on findings at clinical examination and/or surgical exploration. The histology is to be considered in the staging, as is cytology as far as effusions are concerned. It is desirable that a biopsy is taken from suspicious areas outside of the pelvis.

Stage I   Growth limited to the ovaries.
  Stage Ia Growth limited to one ovary; no ascites.
        (i) No tumor on the external surface; capsule intact.
        (ii) Tumor present on the external surface or/and capsule ruptured.
  Stage Ib Growth limited to both ovaries; no ascites.
        (i) No tumor on the external surface; capsules intact.
        (ii) Tumor present on the external surface or/and capsule(s) ruptured.
  Stage Ic Tumor either Stage Ia or Stage Ib, but with obvious ascites present or positive peritoneal washings (ascites is peritoneal effusion which in the opinion of the surgeon is pathological and/or clearly exceeds normal amounts).
Stage II   Growth involving one or both ovaries with pelvis extension.
  Stage IIa Extension and/or metastases to the uterus and/or tubes.
  Stage IIb Extension to other pelvic tissues.
  Stage IIc Tumor either Stage IIa or Stage IIb, but with obvious ascites present or positive peritoneal washings.
Stage III Growth involving one or both ovaries with intraperitoneal metastases outside the pelvis and/or positive retroperitoneal nodes.
        Tumor limited to the true pelvis with histologically proven malignant extension to small bowel or omentum.
Stage IV   Growth involving one or both ovaries with distant metastases.
        If pleural effusion is present there must be positive cytology to allot a case to Stage IV.
        Parenchymal liver metastasis equals Stage IV.
        A sub-division of Stage III and also minor modifications of Stages I and II are under discussion.

Ovarian carcinoma is the only gynecological carcinoma that is staged during treatment. The stage can also be changed when the gross and microscopic findings are reported. It is unique in this respect.

SURGICAL MANAGEMENT OF OVARIAN CANCER [24]

When ovarian cancer presents in the form of widespread malignancy, pinhead sized nodules covering all peritoneal surfaces including the bowel, liver, and kidney areas, it is not really a surgical disease. However, surgery is the backbone of therapy and every attempt must be made to excise all tumor and failing in this optimal approach it is important to remove as much tumor as possible. Debulking and significant reductive surgery in many instances convert a patient from the poor prognosis group to a more favorable group. The size of the largest residual tumor mass remaining after surgery is the most important prognostic factor in determining the survival of patients with common epithelial ovarian cancer. In addition, the response to any adjunctive therapy is in inverse proportion to the size of the residual tumor remaining at the end of the surgical procedure.

Surgical excision of ovarian cancer should be approached with a planned, methodical technique. The goal in ovarian cancer surgery is to excise as much tumor as possible and at the same time avoid the possibility of hemorrhage and/or fistula complication.[25–29]

The gynecologic oncologist has come full cycle from a very radical surgical attack to a conservative approach, back to a supraaggressive surgical attack. Why has this come about? In the late 1940's and early 1950's after carrying out a radical surgical operation, oncologists did not have enough knowledge of chemotherapy to control the residual disease; thus recurrence and continued growth of persistent disease was usual. With improved knowledge of fluids and electrolytes as well as the increased use of hyperalimentation and the technology available through the Swan-Ganz catheter to monitor these patients, the morbidity for management of patients undergoing this extensive surgery has been reduced.

INCISION

There is no place for the management of common epithelial ovarian cancer using a Pfannenstiel incision (horizontal, low abdominal incision below the pubic hair line). It is impossible to adequately explore the patient through a Pfannenstiel incision because it is not possible to palpate between the liver and the diaphragm on the posterior peritoneum where millet seed or pinhead areas of cancer may be present. When common epithelial ovarian cancer is understaged, it is undertreated. Reports indicate that only about 20 percent of patients with common epithelial ovarian cancer receive an appropriate type of incision at the time of their original treatment. When the patient is referred to the author for additional treatment for common epithelial ovarian cancer and a Pfannenstiel incision has been made, the patient is considered as a fresh case and needs re-exploration with proper staging and possibly more appropriate surgery. The argument that the Pfannenstiel is cosmetically more attractive and has been requested by the patient violates the rule of professional integrity. The patient looks to a gynecologist for advice, suggestions, and recommendations. It should be carefully explained to the patient why it is necessary to do a vertical incision. She should be told about the consequences of understaging and/or rupturing the tumor by trying to deliver it through an inadequate incision. The patient and the family would much prefer to have a patient who is alive and able to carry out her social and economic responsibilities to herself, to her family, and the community even though the incision rules out wearing a bikini.

TECHNIQUE

To cut down on the possibility of hemorrhage and to hold blood loss to a minimum, a very methodical and planned approach should be used in operating on patients with ovarian cancer. The abdomen must be opened by a vertical incision that extends beyond the upper limits of the mass and is adequate to explore the posterior area between the liver and the diaphragm. Unless this is properly carried out it will be impossible to stage accurately the amount of ovarian cancer present. In addition, a small incision such as a Pfannenstiel may cause an encapsulated cancer to be ruptured, thus converting it from a lesser degree to a stage in which there is spill compromising the cancer and cure.

When the abdomen is opened, any fluid present is collected for cytology and in the absence of fluid, about 50 ml of saline should be instilled into the pelvis and then aspirated for cytologic examination. The abdomen and pelvis should be carefully and thoroughly evaluated to determine the extent of disease. If tissue is readily available for easy biopsy, a frozen section diagnosis is desirable to document the site and type of primary lesion. It is especially important to evaluate the area on the posterior abdominal wall between the liver and the diaphragm. Cancer has been found here in a seemingly stage I cancer of the ovary in about 10 to 15 percent of cases. Of course disease in this area changes the stage from a I to a III.

When one has determined the extent of disease, it is desirable to incise the posterior peritoneum lateral to and just above the pelvic brim, as carried out at the start of radical hysterectomy. This approach exposes the infundibular pelvic ligament and clamping it decreases the blood loss that occurs when ovarian cancer is excised. This procedure permits identification of the ureter, which can be isolated and left attached to the medial peritoneal flap. The ovarian vessels running in the infundibular pelvic ligament can be isolated, clamped, cut, tied, and doubly ligated in toto. As soon as a similar procedure is carried out on the opposite side, a considerable amount of blood is diverted from the ovarian cancer.

With the ureter protected from injury, it is possible by blunt and sharp dissection to incise the peritoneum down to the round ligament and, after it is clamped and ligated, to continue the incision of the peritoneum lateral to the bladder. If the bladder flap of peritoneum is involved with cancer, the incision in the peritoneum should be continued to the pubis. The lateral side of the peritoneum over the bladder can be elevated and dissected by a sharp and blunt dissection from the bladder which is then left denuded. The flap of peritoneum is dissected off the dome of the bladder and left attached to the lower uterine segment and is removed as an en bloc dissection with the uterus. Posteriorly, with the ureter under direct vision, the peritoneum medial to the ureter is incised down over the rectum. This frees up the cul-de-sac from the bowel and leaves it attached to the back part of the uterus. The entire specimen can be removed at the time the hysterectomy is carried out.

With this technique it is possible to remove a large bulk of cancer without an inordinate blood loss. If the tumor involves the rectum and constitutes the only place where macroscopic disease would be left behind, a decision must be made on whether the bowel should be resected to encompass disease. When this is accomplished, the omentum should be removed at the level of transverse colon. Because the appendix is often involved in the tumor mass, and because it is the site of metastases, its removal is recommended.

The operating surgeon should be prepared to resect the small or large bowel if only a segment is involved. Multiple resections are not of value in the management of ovarian carcinoma. At the time of resection it is important to make sure that the bowel that is reanastomosed does not have tumor near the site of anastomosis. The fistula rate is very high among patients who have had anastomosis with tumor within a few centimeters of the anastomosis. Occasionally tumor will be found in the cul-de-sac involving the rectum and it may be necessary to remove this part of the colon in order to debulk the tumor adequately. New stapling instruments permit anastomosis low in the pelvis. The decision of whether a colostomy is indicated must be a clinical judgment made by the operator. In most instances a permanent colostomy should not be performed in the presence of common epithelial ovarian cancer. Griffiths and Fuller have reported improved results employing intensive surgical and chemotherapeutic management of advanced ovarian cancer.

If all macroscopic disease has been removed P^{32} tubes are placed into the abdomen through trocars, which are pushed through the abdominal wall from inside the abdomen to the skin in each lower quadrant. The trocars are directed lateral to the epigastric vessels. Small baby feeding tubes with extra holes cut in them are then threaded into the trocar, and the trocar is withdrawn into the pelvic cavity with the tube. The ends of the tubes remain sealed so that when the P^{32} is instilled it has a watering-can effect. The trocar is removed and the tube is placed along the lateral gutter as high as the diaphragm on the right side and to the liver on the left side. The tubes are sutured into place with black silk sutures. One suture is placed in the opening made by the trocar and left long so that it can be tied in place when the P^{32} tube is removed following instillation of radioactive phosphorus. Phosphorus is instilled within 24 to 48 hours after completion of the surgery.

HOW MUCH IS TOO MUCH?

Physicians do not agree on the amount of tumor that can be excised safely. The author tries to remove as much tumor as possible without inordinate morbidity and mortality and especially the production of gastrointestinal or genitourinary fistula. The success of subsequent chemotherapy or radiation or both is inversely proportional to the amount of tumor left in the abdomen after surgery. Therefore, aggressive surgery is indicated not so much because it is curative, but because it potentiates other forms of treatment. If it is true that the patient is immunized by her own tumors, a point is reached where there is acquired tolerance or excess antigen may stimulate a great number of antibodies which may form complexes around the tumor. These blocking factors result in an immunologic enhancement which protect the tumor from attack by killer lymphocytes. Therefore, the patient's immune response is improved when the volume of tumor has been decreased. Since the tumor is highly immunosuppressive, its removal may convert the patient from being immunoincompetent to being immunocompetent.

SURGICAL TREATMENT OF RECURRENT CANCER OF THE OVARY [30]

With the resurgence of radical surgery as a modality for the treatment of cancer in the 1940's and 1950's attempts were made to aggressively attack recurrent ovarian cancer by surgery. There are ten indications for a radical surgical attack. These include:

1. The tumor is confined to the pelvis.
2. The tumor is surgically resectable.
3. The patient is young enough and in good enough condition to withstand an extensive surgical procedure.
4. All other forms of therapy have been exhausted and there is no other modality of treatment left to offer.
5. The duration of symptoms and the extent of disease as determined by clinical and biopsy examination indicates that metastases out of the pelvis is unlikely.
6. The responsible surgeon and his team must be acquainted with the anatomy and have the technical skill and background to perform the extensive surgery.
7. A thorough knowledge of the natural history of disease is essential.
8. An in-depth knowledge of preoperative and postoperative care is important.
9. An ability to anticipate fluid and electrolyte problems and to correct them in their early stages is necessary.
10. One physician must manage the patient, and although he or she could consult freely, it is their responsibility to give painstaking attention to the most minimal details.

Surgery for recurrent cancer of the ovary is divided into the nonexenterative and exenterative types of surgery. In general there are few indications for extended radical surgical attack and very very few for the exenterative procedure in the management of advanced recurrent cancer of the ovary.

In those patients being treated with nonexenterative radical surgery many presented with far advanced cancer of the ovary. They have often been treated in some fashion or another on one or more occasions and present the clinician with a most frustrating problem. Usually such patients have only a short time to live and immediate relief of symptoms as they evolve is all that is possible. Ironically, many of these patients may still appear to be in fair or even good general condition.

Most of the patients exhibited ascites which in the advanced stages of the disease recurs after previous paracentesis. A large volume of tumor makes it difficult to control the ascites with radioactive substances, external x-ray therapy, or even chemotherapy. If these modalities of treatment do produce a favorable response, it is short-lived in the presence of bulky disease. Debulking the disease usually makes the patient more comfortable, if it can be accomplished without producing inordinate morbidity and mortality. Currently it provides an opportunity to get a second response from chemotherapy and combinations of chemotherapy and immunotherapy.

The extended nonexenterative radical surgery carries high morbidity and mortality. This must be equated against the survival rate. Obviously judgment must be exercised in performing radical excisional surgery in these patients. The patients should not be subjected to an operation if they are debilitated or elderly patients with cancer that has spread beyond the abdomen, or with advanced disease which is not causing, at the moment, particularly acute and distressing symptoms. Resection is considered only when symptoms (gastrointestinal disturbances) are severe enough to warrant attempted relief at the cost of the discomforts and risks of an operation. In the absence of very emphatic contraindications, laparotomy is indicated in selected patients of the type described, as there is always the possibility that the recurrence and/or metastases are localized and macroscopically entirely resectable. With an increased knowledge of chemotherapy and hyperalimentation there is more hope for salvaging many of these patients after their tumor is debulked.

The question is raised about whether exenterative surgery for ovarian cancer is justified.[31] In some instances the growths and their local recurrences appear to be limited to the pelvic structures, and when there is peritoneal involvement of the pelvis, pelvic colon, and bladder, and/or when the cancer has actually penetrated more deeply into these structures, the question of pelvic exenteration arises as a method of dealing with the situation.

All patients operated on by pelvic exenteration were selected by nature, as evidenced by the fact that in one series all survived for more than 1 to 13 years from the initial therapy to the diagnosis of recurrence. These patients were operated upon only if their neoplasms were macroscopically confined to the pelvis and macroscopically completely excisable. In general, ovarian cancer does not lend itself to excision by pelvic exenteration because of its spread to the upper abdomen. However, the series of pelvic exenterations reviewed did not include any endometrioid tumors. These tumors have a lesser tendency to be bilateral and to spread to the upper abdomen compared to other ovarian tumors. In highly selected cases, endometrioid ovarian cancer may be controlled by pelvic exenteration. In summary, it can be stated that the natural history of cancer of the cervix permits a radical surgical attack by pelvic exenteration, while ovarian cancers lend themselves to an exenteration only if they do not have their usual method of spread and, therefore, violate their natural history.[32,33]

SECOND LOOK OPERATION [34,35]

The second look concept has many interpretations. The one followed in this chapter relates to patients who had known disease that could not be adequately removed at the time of surgery, but in whom the tumor regressed after additional therapy so that there is no longer any evidence of disease. The other group of patients in whom a second look has been employed consists of those from whom all disease was removed at the time of the original operation, and in whom prophylactic chemotherapy was then given for a period ranging from 8 to 18 months. At that time, in order to judge whether treatment could be stopped in the absence of any palpable disease, an exploratory laparotomy with multiple biopsies must be carried out. If disease is palpable or detectable by any means prior to surgery, it is not a second look procedure but a planned type of therapy, hopefully to excise all tumor or to relieve complications such as an obstruction, fistula, or abscess. The second look operation has become an established part of the protocol of many centers for patients with common epithelial ovarian tumors or nonepithelial cancers who have received radiation therapy, chemotherapy or a combination of treatments.

The most important question concerning the second look operation is whether it is possible to offer the patient a second chance for cure if disease is present. An attempt will be made to answer this question from personal experience and a review of the literature.[36,37]

The second look operation was popularized, if not introduced, by Wangensteen, for patients who had cancers arising in the stomach and colon and who had a response to treatment and were asymptomatic at the time of the second look operation.

The second look operation gives the surgeon the opportunity to (1) explore the patient and remove all of the residual tumor or to reduce the tumor mass and improve the patient's chances with a new regimen of treatment; (2) to outline the site of the tumor and to determine the status of the residual tumor, and (3) to plan a program of treatment for the patient, and (4) if no disease or positive cytology is found provides confidence in stopping toxic chemotherapeutic drugs. It is obvious that patients with stage I or II disease in whom all disease has been removed, and in whom chemotherapy is given prophylactically will have fewer recurrences than patients in stages III and IV treated therapeutically for residual disease after initial treatment.[38]

There are several reasons for reexploration: (1) The patient may have had a sufficient amount of the drug. (2) The tumor may become more localized and possibly resectable for the first time. (3) The benefit from the drug may be exhausted and it may be time to switch to another drug. (4) The mass may not be suitable for radiation. (5) It may be suspected that the mass that has served as a guide to drug therapy is not cancer as was originally presumed.

The most important factors correlating with second look operations are the stage of cancer, the amount of residual tumor left at the initial operation, and number of courses of chemotherapy administered prior to the second look operation. Survival after second look operations where disease is found vary directly with the volume of tumor remaining at the time of operation and the amount of tumor left behind at the second look operation. Patients who were treated with radiation therapy had a poorer survival rate than those who were treated with chemotherapy when cancer was found at the second look operation.[39]

The technique for second look operations should be planned and meticulously carried out. After the abdomen is opened the pelvis should be washed with saline and then the upper abdomen should receive the same treatment, then both specimens should be sent separately to the laboratory for analysis. The patient should be very carefully explored including an exploration of the diaphragm, the liver and the area between the liver and the diaphragm on the posterior peritoneum. The peritoneum anteriorly and posteriorly, the area over the kidneys, the large and small bowel and their mesenteries, and the paraaortic area should be carefully explored. The pelvis should then be very carefully explored. If no disease is found, it is important to take multiple biopsies and these should be taken from the bladder flap, the cul-de-sac, and the lateral pelvic walls. The posterior peritoneum should be split and both lumbar gutters irrigated and biopsies taken from this area. The retroperitoneal area along the infundibular pelvic ligament should be washed carefully for cytology and biopsies should be taken from this area. This should be followed up to the level where the vessels enter into the vena cava. The paraaortic area should now be exposed and nodes should be dissected from the paraaortic area. Unlike cancer of the cervix that may spread to the nodes just over the promontory it is more common to find nodes if they are present in ovarian cancer at the level of the duodenum and the pancreas. It is therefore very important to obtain cytologic samplings as well as to biopsy any tissue present in this area. The question of how to manage the diaphragm is a difficult one. The author has tried many techniques including the sharp hook pulled on the diaphragm and biopsies taken with the Kavorkian cervical biopsies. This required sutures to be placed and was often technically quite difficult. The other disadvantage is that it represented random sampling. Currently the author is scraping the entire diaphragm and sending the specimen for cytologic examination. This appears to be less traumatic than the method of the biopsy technique and is also more inclusive as far as finding cytology present. However, this must be carried out in a vigorous manner so that if there is any disease present cytology can be obtained for analysis. It is axiomatic that if any disease is present, if possible, it should be resected.

The author believes that a guarded approach must be assumed in reporting on the results of second look operation. It is evident that, although no disease is seen, occasionally there will be unexpected positive cytology on washings and/or unsuspected nests of tumor cells in some of the random biopsies that are taken. It is important to reserve judgment on whether these patients have been cured by waiting 5 or more years. It is devastating to find that in those patients that we have reported as cured that we have merely reduced the volume down to one or a few cells and are really reporting on the time that it takes to regenerate a volume of tumor that is clinically palpable from residual microscopic disease.

SUMMARY

Methods for diagnosing ovarian cancer are reviewed. It is evident that early diagnosis is a matter of chance rather than a scientific approach. However, it is becoming increasingly obvious that with better lay and professional education that earlier diagnoses are being made. The surgical management of the fresh ovarian cancer is reviewed as well as the management of the recurrent ovarian cancer using a nonexenterative and exenterative approach and a discussion of the second look operation is included.

REFERENCES

1. Barber HRK: Ovarian Carcinoma. Etiology, Diagnosis, and Treatment, ed 2. New York, Masson Publishing USA, Inc., 1982.
2. Silverberg E: Statistical and Epidemiological Information on Gynecologic Cancer. American Cancer Society Professional Education Publication, New York City, September 1980.
3. Barr W: Current problems in diagnosis and management. Ovarian Cancer Adv Biosci 26:1, 1980.
4. Graber EA: Early diagnosis of ovarian malignancy. Clin Obstet Gynecol 12:958, 1969.
5. Gusberg SB, Frick HC, II: Corscaden's Gynecologic Cancer. Baltimore, Williams & Wilkins, 1970.
6. McGowan L, Stein DB, Miller W: Cul-de-sac aspiration for diagnostic cytologic study. Am J Obstet Gynecol 96:413, 1966.
7. Stolbach LL, Krant MJ, Fishman WH: Ectopic production of an alkaline phosphatase isoenzyme in patients with cancer. N Engl J Med 281:757, 1969.
8. Shuster J: Immunologic diagnosis of human cancers. Am J Clin Pathol 62:243, 1974.
9. Melnick H, Barber HRK: Cellular immunologic responsiveness to extracts of ovarian epithelial tumors. Gynecol Oncol 3:77, 1975.

10. LoGerfo P, Krupey J, Hansen HJ: Demonstration of an antigen common to several varieties of neoplasia. N Engl J Med 283:138, 1971.
11. Ioachim HL, Dorsett BH, Sabbath M, et al: Antigenic and morphologic properties of ovarian carcinoma. Gynecol Oncol 1:130, 1973.
12. Laurance DJR, Munro N: Fetal antigens and their role in diagnosis and clinical management of human neoplasms: A review. Br J Cancer 26:335, 1972.
13. Vaitukaitis JL: Peptide hormones as tumor markers. Cancer 37:567, 1976.
14. Bast RC, Jr, Klug TL, St. John E, et al: A radioimmunoassay using a monoclonal antibody to monitor the course of epithelial ovarian cancer. N Eng J Med 309 (15):883, 1983.
15. Abelev GI: Alpha fetoprotein in oncogenesis and its association with malignant tumors. Adv Cancer Res 14:295, 1971.
16. Fishman W, Raam S, Stolbach LL: Markers for ovarian cancer: Regan isoenzyme and other glycoproteins. Semin Oncol 2:211, 1975.
17. Dorsett BH, Ioachim HL, Stolbach L, et al: Isolation of tumor-specific antibodies from effusions of ovarian carcinomas. Int J Cancer 16:779, 1975.
18. Donald I: New problems in sonar diagnosis in obstetrics and gynecology. Am J Obstet Gynecol 118:199, 1974.
19. Samuels BI: Usefulness of ultrasound in patients with ovarian cancer. Semin Oncol 2:229, 1975.
20. Rosenoff SH, Young RC, Anderson T, et al: Peritoneoscopy: A valuable tool for the initial staging and "second look" in ovarian carcinoma. Ann Intern Med 83:37, 1975.
21. Rosenoff SH, DeVita VT, Jr, Hubbard S, et al: Peritoneoscopy in the staging and followup of ovarian cancer. Semin Oncol 2:223, 1975.
22. Klimek R, Lauterbur PC, Mendoca Dias H: A discussion of nuclear magnetic resonance (NMR). Gin Pol 52:6, 1981.
23. Report presented by the Cancer Committee to the General Assembly of F.I.G.O., New York, April, 1970. Int J Gynecol Obstet 9:172, 1971.
24. Barber HRK: Surgical management of ovarian cancer. Curr Ob-Gyn Tech 1:6, 1975.
25. Griffiths CT: Surgical resection of tumor bulk in the primary treatment of ovarian cancer. Natl Cancer Inst Monogr. 42:101, 1975.
26. Griffiths CT, Fuller AF: Intensive surgical and chemotherapeutic management of advanced ovarian cancer. Surg Clin North Am 68:131, 1978.
27. Griffiths CT, Parker LM, Fuller AF, Jr: Rule of situ reductive surgical treatment in the management of advanced ovarian cancer. Cancer Treat Rep 63:235, 1979.
28. Hudson CN, Chir M: Surgical treatment of ovarian cancer. Gynecol Oncol 1:370, 1973.
29. Hudson CN: The place of surgery in the treatment of ovarian cancer. Clin Obstet Gynecol 5:700, 1978.
30. Brunschwig A: Attempted palliaton by radical surgery in pelvic and abdominal carcinomatosis primarily in the ovaries. Clin Obstet Gynecol 4:875, 1961.
31. Barber HRK, Brunschwig A: Pelvic exenteration for locally advanced and recurrent ovarian cancer. Review of 22 cases. Surgery 58:935, 1965.
32. Barber HRK: Relative prognostic significance of preoperative and operative findings in pelvic exenteration. Surg Clin North Am 49:431, 1969.
33. Barber HRK, Kwon T: Current status of the treatment of gynecologic cancer by site— Ovary. Cancer 38:610, 1976.
34. Arhelger SW, Jenson CB, Wangensteen OH: Experience with "second look" procedure in the management of cancer of the colon and rectum. Lancet 77:412, 1957.
35. Lewis JL, Jr, Griffiths T, Morrow CP, et al: Managing ovarian cancer. The second look operation. Contemp Obstet Gynecol 12:137, 1978.

36. Wallach RC, Kabakow B, Blinick G: Current status of the second look operation in ovarian carcinoma. Natl Cancer Inst Monogr 42:105, 1974.
37. Wallach RC, Kabakow B, Jerez E, et al: The importance of second look surgical procedures in the staging and treatment of ovarian carcinoma. Semin Oncol 2:243, 1975.
38. Smith JP: Surgery for ovarian cancer. Ovarian cancer. Adv Biosci 26:137, 1980.
39. Schwartz TE, Smith JP: Second look operations in ovarian cancer. Am J Obstet Gynecol 138:1124, 1980.

7 | Ovarian Cancer: Postoperative Management

William T. Creasman
Daniel L. Clarke-Pearson

In the United States ovarian cancer is the most commonly fatal gynecological cancer. At the time of diagnosis only about a third of patients have localized disease capable of complete surgical resection. Ovarian cancer with metastases beyond the true pelvis (Stage III and IV) is the most common finding and the survival for this group of patients at 5 years is no better than 10 percent regardless of subsequent post-surgical therapy.[1]

The surgical management of ovarian cancer is extremely important, not only in making the diagnosis but in thoroughly evaluating the spread of the cancer as well as being able to perform maximum cytoreductive surgery. Fortunately this disease can be surgically staged and it is therefore imperative that this be done thoroughly and completely, as commonly missed metastatic sites such as the diaphragm and lymph nodes must be evaluated. Subsequent therapy can only be given with maximum results when the exact stage and location of the disease is known. A real disservice to the patient is given when a small incision is made followed by inadequate intraperitoneal evaluation and a small biopsy obtained for histological proof of disease. The results of subsequent management are directly related to the amount of tumor that is left behind at the completion of the surgical procedure.[2] In a relatively short period of time the surgeon who is willing to take the time and has the expertise to "debulk" the patient has accomplished what several courses of chemotherapy can do if, in fact, the patient is responsive to the chemotherapeutic agents used. Details of surgical requirements have been detailed in the preceeding chapter, but their importance cannot be overemphasized.

BORDERLINE OR LOW POTENTIAL MALIGNANCY

This diagnosis is being made with an increased frequency in regards to ovarian malignancy. It has been defined by the International Federation of Gynecologists (FIGO) and the World Health Organization (WHO) as ". . . cystadenomas with proliferating activity of the epithelial cells and nuclear abdnormalities, but with no infiltrative destructive growth."[3] It would appear, at least in some institutions, that as many as 15 percent of all ovarian disease are borderline in nature. In contradistinction to the true carcinomas of the ovary about 65 to 70 percent of borderline lesions are Stage I at the time of diagnosis. This speaks to a certain degree to the less aggressive biological activity of the borderline lesions compared with the true carcinomas in that two-thirds of these latter lesions are Stage III or IV at the time of diagnosis. Because of this finding therapy would appear to be less aggressive than for the same stage of the true cancers and at the same time the survival is much better stage for stage.[4]

Treatment for borderline lesions of the ovary is primarily surgical. If a patient has a Stage I lesion, unilateral oophorectomy appears to be adequate treatment. This assumes, of course, that a full surgical exploration has been performed and disease outside of the ovary is undetectable. Subsequent therapy does not appear to be of any benefit in this group of patients. When disease appears to involve both ovaries than a total abdominal hysterectomy, bilateral salpingo-oophorectomy, selective pelvic and para aortic lymph node sampling, partial omentectomy and peritoneal cytology should be obtained. If disease is limited to the ovaries, again surgery is all that is needed. In a recent study by the Gynecologic Oncology Group (GOG) of 55 patients with Stage I borderline lesion who were randomly divided into three categories: surgery only, surgery plus pelvic irradiation, and surgery plus chemotherapy using Melphalan for 1 year, only one patient was said to have developed a recurrence and subsequently died.[5] She had been treated with radiation therapy; however, at the time of surgery the left ovary was enlarged to 34 centimeters in size and disease outside the ovary may have been present but undetected. Data from Norway notes that only 12 of 227 patients with Stage I borderline lesions died from their disease.[6] One hundred ninety of these patients had a Stage IA lesion. These investigators also noted that serous cystadenocarcinomas of low malignant potential had a 5-year life-table survival of 99 percent compared with 89 percent for mucinous lesions. When borderline malignancies are noted to be present beyond the ovaries most investigators will probably treat with adjunctive therapy, using either intraperitoneal radioisotope, external irradiation, or chemotherapy with an alkylating agent. The optimal therapy has not been determined because of the small number of patients with borderline lesions having advanced clinical disease. Even with Stage III disease a 50 percent 5-year survival is noted from collected series in the literature. This compares to less than 10 percent for Stage III true carcinomas. It should be remembered that borderline lesions can have metastasis to lymph nodes and other areas within the peritoneal cavity just as true carcinomas.

The use of conservative surgery for Stage IA carcinoma of the ovary assumes that the patient is young (which is usually the case) and is interested in subsequent fertility. The chances of having bilateral occult disease in this entity probably is less than 10 percent, but the risk is still there. It is probably prudent to remove the other ovary and perform a hysterectomy once childbearing desires have been completed.

TRUE CARCINOMAS

Cancers of the ovaries which histologically fulfill the criteria of true cancers must be treated aggressively with rare exception, if increased survival is to be appreciated. The one exception would appear to be in the young patient interested in future fertility who has a Stage IAi well-differentiated mucinous carcinoma of the ovary. This decision, of course, is based on the fact that proper surgical exploration as previously defined has been completed and disease is truly limited to the one ovary. Some investigators might include all cell types in this category; however, serous cysadeno-carcinomas are said to have a seven-fold increase of having bilateral disease compared to mucinous carcinomas, and some investigators are hesitant to be conservative except when mucinous disease is present histologically. Again, once child bearing desires have been completed it is highly recommended that the other ovary and uterus be removed.

In all other stages, except as noted in the preceeding paragraph, aggressive surgical therapy should be carried out and if possible a bilateral salpingo-oophorectomy, hysterectomy, selective pelvic and para-aortic lymph node sampling, partial omentectomy and peritoneal cytology should be considered the optimal surgical procedure. As previously stated, the amount of disease left behind after surgery is important in regards to not only prognosis but the type of therapy subsequently used.

THERAPY OF OVARIAN CANCER WITH RESECTABLE DISEASE

This situation should apply to all patients with Stage I cancer, the vast majority if not all patients with Stage II, and the occasional Stage III patient. When there is no evidence of clinical gross cancer left behind after the surgical procedure several options are available in regards to adjunctive therapy, and except as noted above for the stage IAi, Grade I mucinous lesions all patients with ovarian cancer should be treated subsequent to their surgery. When surgery only is used for Stage I disease a 60 percent 5-year survival is reported. However, it would appear that the use of adjunctive therapy in this group of patients can increase the 5-year survival to 85 or 90 percent. The options for therapy in this group of patients are radioisotopes, chemotherapy, or radiation therapy.

Radioisotopes

Considerable experience with radioactive gold (198 Au) and phosphorus (^{32}P) in the treatment of ovarian cancer has been reported. Initially 198 Au was used exclusively with reasonably good results but complications from 198 Au appeared to be excessive. The explanation for complications with 198 Au may be attributed in part to its gamma component, the short physical half life, an excessive dose or a combination of these factors.[7] The 198 Au has a short-range radiation component, beta radiation, and a deeply penetrating gamma component. The short half life causes irradiation of tissue at a high rate, which may be responsible for some of the complications. As a result, over the last 20 years or so most investigators have gone to P-32, since there is a higher beta energy resulting in a greater tissue penetration, a longer half-life, and an absence of gamma irradiation. The complications from intraperitoneal P-32 appeared to be minimal and considerably less than were reported for 198 Au. Only recently has intraperitoneal dosage been evaluated in the experimental animal.[7,8] There appears to be both an abdominal distribution and a systemic distribution of P-32. A radioisotope is either absorbed to the peritoneal surface, absorbed by the macrophages lining the peritoneal cavity, or phagocytized by free floating macrophages. The remainder of the radioisotope is then carried to the right diaphragm, where it passes through the diaphragmatic lymphatics and enters the mediastinal lymphatics. It then enters the general circulation, and is rapidly cleared by the liver and to a lesser extent deposited in other tissues such as the lung, kidney, spleen, and bone marrow. Because of this uptake, it would appear that adequate dosage is present in different areas of the peritoneal cavity to be effective in the disease being treated.

Radioisotopes have the advantage, at least theoretically, of covering the entire peritoneal surface of the abdominal cavity. This is extremely important because even in early stage disease one must consider ovarian cancer an intra-abdominal process and not one limited to the pelvis. It has the advantage of being logistically optimal in that only one application is given, the toxicity is minimal and acceptable, and it is relatively inexpensive. At the time of surgery a peritoneal catheter can be left in situ flushed with a saline and heparin solution for patency. A radioisotope can then be instilled within 2 to 3 days postsurgery without difficulty. If the catheter has not been left in place at the time of surgery then a peritoneal dialysis catheter can be placed postoperatively without difficulty. One would like to do this in the immediate postoperative period so that instillation can be performed before adhesions form. At the time of instillation 500 cc's of saline is instilled into the peritoneal cavity to be used as a vehicle for dispursement of the isotope. One millicurie of technetium is then used for scanning to make sure loculations are not present and if good distribution is noted, then the P-32, usually 15 mCi which has been premixed in 500 cc's of saline, is instilled into the peritoneal cavity. The catheter is then removed and over the next 2 to 3 hours the patient is placed in multiple positions, i.e., steep Trendelenburg and rotated 360-degrees, reverse Trendelenburg with the same rotation, and afterwards is allowed to ambulate at will. Contraindications to the use of radioisotopes in this group of patients would be in (1) those individuals with previous surgery resulting in intraperitoneal adhesions, (2) patients in whom metastasis was present in the retroperitoneal space (since P-32 instilled intraperitoneally does not go to the pelvic or para aortic lymph nodes), (3) gross disease present at the completion of surgery, and (4) in patients in whom there is a poor distribution as noted on the technetium scan. Several studies in the literature would suggest that using radioisotopes one should expect an 80 to 90 percent survival in this group of patients.[9,10] A prospective randomized study sponsored by the National Cancer Institute and the GOG is currently ongoing comparing P-32 with Alkeran. Definitive statements concerning comparison of these two modalities is not available at the present time.

Chemotherapy

If chemotherapy is chosen for this group of patients a single agent alkylating drug appears to be the drug of choice. It has the advantage of systemic coverage, the toxicity is relatively low, the drug in most instances is given for a short period of time each month, and the expense is minimal to moderate in amount. Most investigators at the present time would probably advocate a "second look" laparotomy at the completion of the chemotherapy, which in most instances would be at 12 to 18 months after the institution of chemotherapy. If the "second look" laparotomy is negative, then the chemotherapy can be stopped and the patient followed closely. In studies from Norway evaluating chemotherapy in early stage disease, approximately an 80 percent 5-year survival was obtained.

Radiation Therapy

As has already been stated, ovarian cancer is, at least potentially, an intraperitoneal disease, and if adequate therapy is to be given the entire peritoneal cavity must be treated. This applies to radiation therapy as well. Studies of pelvic irradiation in Stage I ovarian cancer have shown the inadequacy of this type of treatment. In a study of Stage I cancer by the GOG in which patients were randomly assigned after their initial surgery to no further therapy, pelvic irradiation, or chemotherapy using Melphalan, patients treated with radiation therapy had the highest recurrence rate (Table 7-1).[11] Because radiation therapy did not appear to improve survival in early stage disease in which radiation was limited to the pelvis, investigators at the M.D. Anderson Hospital appreciated the fact that this disease spreads intraperitoneally and, several years ago, devised a plan to treat the entire abdomen. By using the so-called moving strip technique plus a pelvic boost they were able to obtain a 4-year survival of 81 percent compared to only 55 percent when only pelvic irradiation was used.[12] Because of these results a prospective randomized study was then performed in which abdominal strip plus pelvic boost radiation was compared to Alkeran alone.[13] Although the patients who received chemotherapy had a better survival at 5 years it was not statistically improved over those who had radiation. Because of the complications, the length of time and expense necessary to use this radiation it was the feeling of these investigators that chemotherapy was the treatment of choice in this group of patients. As a result of this study radiation therapy is not used at most centers in the

Table 7-1. Treatment and Results of Stage I
Cancer of the Ovary

	Recurrence
Surgery Only	5/29 (17%)
Pelvic Radiation	7/23 (30%)
Chemotherapy	2/34 (6%)

United States. There was, however, a renewed interest in this modality as a result of data published from the Princess Margaret Hospital in Toronto.[14] In a prospective randomized study, patients found to have Stage IB and II disease who had at least a total abdominal hysterectomy and bilateral salpingo-oophorectomy were prospectively randomized into three groups: those treated with pelvic and abdominal irradiation, pelvic irradiation alone, and pelvic irradiation plus Chlorambucil. The actual relapse free survival rate for those receiving abdominal and pelvic irradiation at 5 years is 82 percent, for those receiving pelvic irradiation plus chlorambucil, 52 percent and for those who received pelvic irradiation alone 50 percent. Over 40 patients were in the group treated with pelvic and abdominal irradiation and pelvic irradiation plus chlorambucil; however, 5-year survival results are only available for 7 and 8 patients, respectively. These authors do not tell us whether or not these figures are statistically significant. They do state that in a group of patients who had Stage IB, II and "asymptomatic III" who had total abdominal hysterectomy, bilateral salpingo-oophorectomy and were subsequently treated with pelvic plus abdominal irradiation had a significantly better 5-year survival (81 percent) versus those who were treated with pelvic irradiation plus chlorambucil (55 percent). These patients apparently had been closely matched for age, stage, tumor grade and type, completeness of their hysterectomy, bilateral salpingo-oophorectomy and the presence or absence of residual tumor. P value of 0.02 was noted. This study has certainly renewed the interest in radiation therapy as a mode of treatment in early stage ovarian cancer. The authors feel that patients with Stage IA carcinoma of the ovary and those individuals with greater than 2 centimeters of residual disease after surgery should not be treated with radiation therapy. There have been some questions raised concerning this study. These include the surgical staging and the unorthodox designation of symptomatic versus asymptomatic Stage III and the fact that inadequate surgical staging was probably performed in a large number of these patients. It should also be noted that the dosage of chlorambucil used in this study was probably suboptimal and, in fact, amounted to about half of the dose that would be used when the drug is used by itself. The survival in the group of patients considered in this category and treated with radiaton therapy is comparable to those patients treated with chemotherapy or radioisotopes.

THERAPY WITH SMALL RESIDUAL DISEASE REMAINING AFTER SURGERY

Over the last several years those patients with Stage III disease have been divided into two categories, optimal and suboptimal. Data would suggest that those individuals with less than 2 centimeters residual disease have a much better survival than those who have greater than 2 centimeters tumor aggregate left behind after surgery. Although the designation may differ in various protocols, the 2 centimeter designation is probably more commonly accepted for this designation. In this "small residual disease" category, there would be an occasional Stage II patient, but most would be in the Stage III optimal category. Subsequent therapy would be limited to either chemotherapy or radiation therapy. The use of radioisotopes in this group of patients is contraindicated as the penetration for P-32 has a maximum range of 8 mm, but probably of therapeutic importance no more than 1.4 to 3 mm. Therefore, if gross disease is left behind then radioisotope should not be used.

Most experience in this group of patients chemotherapeutically has been again with single agent alkylators. The discussion in the previous section also appears to be valid here. The survival rate using chemotherapy alone of course decreases as the amount of residual disease left behind increases. Recently the use of multiple agent chemotherapy has been advocated in these patients with optimal disease. This is currently being evaluated by the GOG in a two arm protocol using cyclophosphamide and cis-platinum versus cyclophosphamide, Adriamycin and cis-platinum. The results from that study will probably be available in two to three years.

Patients with this amount of residual disease apparently can be treated with radiation therapy with some success. Although results are not as good as in those patients in which no gross disease is left behind after surgery, this therapy may be the best in regards to long-term survival in this highly select group of patients.[14]

THERAPY FOR SUBOPTIMAL DISEASE

Unfortunately, most patients with ovarian cancer at the time that they come to consideration of post-surgical therapy have a significant amount of residual disease. When this situation is encountered chemotherapy appears to be the only therapy available to us that may be of benefit to the patient. Unfortunately all patients do not respond to chemotherapy nor to the same therapeutic agents. This is probably due to the heterogenicity of the malignant cells that make up ovarian cancer. It may be that one clone is highly succeptible to the specific drug, while other cell lines may be highly resistant.

Alkylating Agents

Single agent alkylating agents have been used in ovarian cancer for several decades. Some of the initial reports appeared in the literature in the 1960's and therefore represent the greatest experience of chemotherapy in ovarian cancer. Melphalan (Alkeran), cyclophosphmide (Cytoxan), thiotepa, chlorambucil, and nitrogen mustard make up this group of compounds. Nitrogen mustard, although effective in this cancer, has not routinely been used for several years now because of its considerable toxicity. On the other hand, the other drugs, particularly in the light of toxicity seen with chemotherapeutic agents used today, are relatively mild. Three of these drugs (thiotepa being the exception) can be taken by mouth. Experience from several studies in the literature is presented in regards to alkylating agents in ovarian cancer (Table 7-2).[15] Response rates, complete (CR) plus partial (PR) are similar for all of the drugs; however, the median survival with these agents is relatively limited. One must remember when interpreting data that response rates may be presented in different ways. Although criteria for catagorizing a patient as a responder has become somewhat standardized over the recent past still the length of time that a response is noted may be variable, and this may explain the difference in the results. If only one month of disease regression is required for response obviously there will be more patients

Table 7-2. Alkylating Agents in Ovarian Cancer

Agent (# of patients)	Response	Median Survival
Melphalan (494)	47%	14 months
Cyclophosphamide (126)	49%	13 months
Thiotepa (144)	49%	13 months
Chlorambucil (280)	50%	—

Table 7-3. Non-Alkylating Agents in Ovarian Cancer

Agent (# of patients)	Response
Hexamethylmelamine (53)	42%
Adriamycin (43)	35%
Methotrexate (20)	30%
Cis-platinum (20)	25%
5-Fluorouracil (92)	20%
Vinblastine (10)	20%

categorized as responders than in those studies in which a longer period of time is required for an individual to be counted as a response. Particularly in Phase III studies survival should mirror responses, otherwise the criteria used for response is probably inappropriate. In a large group of patients treated with melphalan at the M.D. Anderson Hospital those individuals categorized as responders lived a considerably longer period of time than those individuals who were nonresponders.[16] Still, of those patients who were responders only 20 percent were alive at 5 years compared with none in the nonresponder category. It would appear that being a responder amounted to an increase of approximately two years' survival time. Still the overall survival for all patients treated in this study with chemotherapy at 5 years was approximately 10 percent.

Other drugs have been evaluated with regard to their response rate in ovarian cancer. These have mainly been evaluated in Phase II studies and as a second line drug after failure usually with an alkylating agent. Several of these drugs, some new, some old, have been listed along with their response rates (Table 7-3).[15] Currently, however, these latter drugs are generally not used as single agent first line therapy.

Combination Chemotherapy

Because of the large number of nonresponders when single agent alkylators were used, beginning over a decade ago, interest was generated in using multiple agent chemotherapy in attempts to increase response and survival in suboptimal carcinoma of the ovary. One of the first attempts was a prospective randomized study using actinomycin-D, 5-fluorouracil and Cytoxan (ACFUCY) versus melphalan by the investigators at M.D. Anderson Hospital.[17] In this prospective randomized study approximately 50 patients were treated with each of these regimens. The response rate (CR + PR) was essentially the same as was the survival at 1 and 2 years. This three drug combination was chosen because each of the drugs appeared to have a different mode of action and also to affect different organ sites in regards to toxicity. The toxicity of this regimen, however, was considerable and greater than melphalan alone. It should be remembered, however, that each individual agent in a drug combination should be effective when used singly in that particular disease. Actinomycin-D has very little if any activity in epithelial ovarian cancer, and 5-fluorouracil has low efficacy. Cytoxan was the only drug in this combination that had considerable activity in this disease.

One of the next combinations studied was that of Adriamycin and Cytoxan, a logical combination since both drugs appeared to be effective as single agents. Several institutions have evaluated this combination with varied results. Parker and associates reported on 41 evaluable women with Stage III/IV ovarian carcinoma who received Adrianycin/Cytoxan every three weeks for five to ten cycles after surgery. Total response rate was 86 percent (CR 46 percent, PR 40 percent). These authors concluded that the absence of pretreatment palpable tumor was a major determinant of drug response, but that further observation was required to demonstrate enhanced survival in this favorable group. Investigators at the Mayo Clinic in evaluating Stage III and IV ovarian cancer patients noted in a prospective randomized study that the addition of Adriamycin to Cytoxan did not increase survival and toxicity was considerably higher in the combination group than with Cytoxan alone.[19]

The Gynecologic Oncology Group in a large Phase III prospective randomized study evaluated Stage III and IV ovarian cancer using melphalan versus Adriamycin + Cytoxan versus melphalan + hexamethylmelamine.[20] The response rate (CR + PR) for Adriamycin + Cytoxan and melphalan + hexamethylmelamine was slightly better than melphalan although not statistically significant. When survival was evaluated, absolutely no difference between the three regimens was noted, with a median survival of slightly more than 1 year in each of the three groups. Again, the toxicity from combination groups was considerably greater than with melphalan alone.

One of the first studies which apparently showed a clear cut benefit of combinaton chemotherapy over a single agent alkylating drug was that reported by Young and associates at the National Cancer Institute.[21] In a prospective randomized study of Stage III and IV ovarian cancer patients were treated either with Alkeran or a combination of hexamethylmelamine, cyclophosphamide, methotrexate and 5-fluorouracil (Hexa-CAF). Those patients treated with Hexa-CAF had a greater response rate (CR + PR) than did melphalan alone (75 percent versus 54 percent, P<0.05). The complete response rate was 33 percent versus 16 percent, which was not statistically significant. Median duration of survival was 29 months for Hexa-CAF versus 17 months for melphalan (p<0.02). When evaluating the data in depth there were a greater number of patients with Grade I and II disease in the melphalan arm compared with those receiving Hexa-CAF, but on the other hand two of seven patients in the group treated with Hexa-CAF had Grade I disease compared with only one of 14 treated with melphalan. (Using the Broder's classification, as these authors did, Grade I is considered by most pathologists as being borderline histologically). When survival was further evaluated it was noted that the only statistically improved survival with the combination was in those patients who had Grade I or II disease. Survival was longer in those patients with Grade III and IV disease and who had been treated with Hexa-

CAF compared with melphalan but it was not statistically significant. The fact that these authors also noted a 54 percent total response with melphalan is somewhat unusual in that most Phase III studies that have recently used melphalan alone as one treatment arm have found no more than 25 to 30 percent total response rate with this single agent. Two subsequent studies using single agent alkylating drug versus Hexa-CAF have found no improvement in response rate or survival of the combination over the single drug. In fact, in one study the objective response rate was significantly better in the patients receiving the alkylating agent versus those receiving Hexa-CAF.[22]

More recently cis-platinum, a heavy metal coordination compound with unique anti-tumor properties, has been used in various combinations. Most of the studies to date have been Phase II or limited Phase III studies. Excellent overall response rates in the range of 70 to 80 percent have been reported by several investigators using a combination of Adriamycin and cis-platinum or Adriamycin, Cytoxan and cis-platinum.[23] The patients treated were individuals with previously untreated Stage III and IV epithelial carcinomas of the ovary. Barker and Wiltshaw from England, in a prospective randomized study of Stage III and IV disease patients with recurrent or residual tumor after radiation therapy, only evaluated the combinaton of low-dose cis-platinum and chlorambucil versus low-dose cis-platinum, chlorambucil and Adriamycin.[24] The response rate and complete remissions were similar in both groups of patients. The addition of Adriamycin did not increase the probability of survival in the complete responders.

The GOG has recently completed a prospective randomized study evaluating Adriamycin and Cytoxan versus Adriamycin, Cytoxan and cis-platinum in suboptimal Stage III and IV ovarian cancer patients. The data is awaiting complete analysis and longer follow-up; however, some preliminary data is available. The response rate to Adriamycin, Cytoxan and cis-platinum appears to be considerably better than those patients treated with Adriamycin, Cytoxan alone. Probably of more significance is the observation that the number of complete responders in the three drug arm is about twice that seen in the patients treated with Adriamycin, Cytoxan alone. The progression free interval between the two regimens is statistically significant with those patients receiving the cis-platinum combination having a longer progression free interval. To date, the survival of those patients with cis-platinum combination appears better but is not statistically significant. Therefore, in those patients receiving a combination with cis-platinum, a larger number of patients appear to be having a response, and a significant number are complete responses. There also appears to be a larger number of patients going to second look laparotomy than was observed when only a single agent alkylator was used. The number of negative second looks also appears to be appreciable, but it is also the unconfirmed observation of this author that there also seems to be an increased recurrence rate in those patients who have had a negative second look and received cis-platinum combination chemotherapy. This, of course, is an extremely important area that must be carefully studied because if survival is not appreciably improved then one must ethically question whether more toxic combinations should be given.

Other drug combinations which appear to be effective in the treatment of advanced ovarian carcinoma include HAD (hexamethylmelamine, Adriamycin and cisplatinum), CHAD (HAD plus cyclophosphamide) and CHAP (cyclophosphamide,

Table 7-4. Chemotherapy in Ovarian Cancer (M.D. Anderson Hospital)

Agent (# of patients)	CR (%)	PR (%)	Median Survival (mos)
Alkeran (104)	19	7	18.6
5-Fluorouracil (21)	19	5	14.3
Hexamethylmelamine (54)	15	17	15
Adriamycin (32)	3	19	16
Hexamethylmelamine +			
Cytoxan (18)	19	10	16.2
Cis-platinum (22)	27	23	21.2
Hexamethylmelamine +			
Adriamycin + Cytoxan (72)	29	3	26.4
Alkeran + Cis-platinum (81)	32	5	29.6

Adriamycin, cis-platinum and hexamethymelamine).[25] To date, only limited studies have been reported but these combinations are apparently being further tested by these investigators.

The group at M.D. Anderson Hospital has recently reported their unique experience testing several different drugs singularly and in combination in a Phase III prospectively randomized study beginning in the early 1970's (as a contract with the National Cancer Institute).[26] In Table 7-4 that study is detailed. Alkeran (melphalan) had been most extensively used at M.D. Anderson Hospital and therefore was the drug to which othr regimens were compared. A set number of patients were studied in each arm, but the number of patients treated with Alkeran was larger because it was used as one of the regimens in several other studies. Results of Alkeran have been combined for convenience since results were essentially the same in all studies. In some combinations (hexamethylmelamine + Cytoxan) the complete response rate was no greater than Alkeran alone and the median survival was less. The more recent combinations of hexamethylmelamine, Adriamycin and Cytoxan, and most recently Alkeran + cis-platinum have shown the highest response rate with the longest survival of any drugs tried. Currently, at the M.D. Anderson Hospital, Alkeran + cis-platinum is the first line chemotherapy regimen in these groups of ovarian cancer patients. From this data the authors were able to identify various risk categories in this suboptimal group of patients. They noted that in a good risk category (Grade I lesions in which tumor left behind after surgery was less than 2 centimeters) the median survival was 34.6 months. In the intermediate risk group (Stage III and disease greater than 2 cms after surgery) the median survival was 24.1 months. In the poor risk category (Stage IV and disease greater than 2 cms post surgery) the median survival was only 12.5 months.

Chemo-Immunotherapy

The use of immunoadjuvants in combination with chemotherapy in ovarian cancer is based on multiple factors. Animal study data, the presence of human ovarian tumor antigens, the immunological capacities of cancer patients, and information regarding chemo-immunotherapy interaction all suggest the possible benefits of this type of therapy in ovarian cancer patients. Several clinical studies have suggested that combined immuno-chemotherapy is of benefit in ovarian cancer. Alberts in 1979 reported the experience of the Southwest Oncology Group (SWOG) using Adriamycin/Cytoxan (AC) with and without nonspecific immuno-therapy with BCG.[27] Patients with Stage III, IV, and recurrent ovarian epithelial cancers were prospectively randomized to receive AC or AC + BCG. Those patients treated with AC + BCG had an overall response rate of 53 percent (12.3 percent CR and 40.4 percent PR). In contrast, those patients who received AC alone had a response rate of 36 percent (CR 1.6 and PR 34.4 percent, p<0.05). The median survival duration of the AC + BCG patients (23.5 months) was statistically better than those who were treated with AC alone (p<0.004). Creasman et al.[28] in 1979 reported a pilot study of the GOG utilizing Corynebacterium (C. Parvum) and melphalan. Forty-four previously untreated Stage III ovarian cancer patients were treated with melphalan and C. Parvum. Patients from current (simultaneous) GOG studies treated with malphalan alone were utilized for comparison. The two groups of patients were similar in regards to histological type and differentiation of tumor. Response rate in the melphalan + C. Parvum group was 53 percent (CR + PR) with only 29 percent (CR + PR) in the melphalan alone group. Progression free interval was longer in the melphalan + C. Parvum group (12 months versus 6 months), and survival was greater in the combined immunochemotherapy group (24 months versus 11.6 months). Currently the GOG is studying cis-platinum, Adriamycin, Cytoxan (PAC) with and without BCG in suboptimal (greater than 1 cm. tumor residual postsurgery) Stage III and IV ovarian cancers. SWOG also is evaluating a PAC combinaton with and without BCG and Adriamycin, Cytoxan plus BCG in Stage III and IV ovarian cancer patients. Preliminary studies suggest the addition of nonspecific immunotherapy may be a benefit in ovarian cancer when given in combination with chemotherapy. Current studies by GOG and SWOG hopefully will answer this important question concerning the efficacy of combined nonspecific immunochemotherapy.

"SECOND LOOK" LAPAROTOMY

The second look laparotomy has become an important part of the total management of a patient with ovarian cancer. The second look laparotomy is a mechanism for evaluating the status of the peritoneal and retroperitoneal spaces in patients with ovarian cancer in which evaluation by other more conventional methods is not definitive. This is particularly apropos for the patient who has no clinical evidence of disease at the completion of prescribed chemotherapy. This is a very detailed, thorough procedure. It should be performed by those individuals who are well aware of the natural history and spread pattern of this malignancy and who have surgical expertise with this cancer. At the time of exploratory laparotomy, peritoneal cytology should be obtained if no free fluid is present within the peritoneal cavity. Many investigators suggest that at least four samples should be obtained. Approximately 100 cc's of saline is instilled into the pelvis, admixed, and then withdrawn for cytological evaluation. Separate like samples are obtained from both lateral abdominal gutters and also from the right diaphragm. This latter sample may be obtained by placing a red rubber catheter against the right diaphragm and the saline injected under force and then allowed to collect posteriorly and then retrieved via the catheter. The entire peritoneal cavity is then evaluated for the presence of gross tumor. If gross tumor is found, attempt is made to resect all of the disease. If none is identified multiple biopsies are obtained, particularly from the area that the tumor was known to have originally been present. All adhesions are sent for microscopic evaluation. If the omentum has not been removed it should be separated at the transverse colon. Our custom is to divide the omentum into at least 10 specimens and send each separately for good histological evaluation of this organ. If the omentum has previously been removed biopsies of any remaining omentum at the transverse colon should be obtained. Pelvic and para-aortic lymph node sampling should then be accomplished if not previously done. Biopsies from areas such as the right diaphragm, lateral abdominal gutters are also advocated by some investigaotrs. The large and small bowel should be run in its entirety with particular attention paid to its mesentery. Any adhesions or questionable areas should be excised if possible for microscopic evaluation. Obviously if any internal pelvic genital organ remains this should be removed in toto. At the completion of this procedure it is not at all unusual to have 40 to 50 separate specimens for histological evaluation. If all of these biopsies including cytology are negative then consideration can be given to stopping chemotherapy—this depends, of course, upon how long the chemotherapy had been given initially. Most investigators suggest that a minimum of 12 to 18 months of chemotherapy is needed before the therapy is stopped.

At the time of the second look laparotomy it is usually considered prudent to become aggressive in regards to removing all of the gross tumor that may be present if possible. This could mean bowel resection, removal of part of the bladder, and large areas of the peritoneum. Removal of vital organs such as partial hepatectomy is not, however, advocated. In some patients who have palpable but stable disease after the completion of the chemotherapy it is felt by some that exploratory surgery should be performed in order to totally "debulk" the patient. If the pattient can be made totally free of gross tumor at this time her survival improves appreciably. Several investigators are now reporting negative "third looks" in patients in whom disease was present at the time of the second look but total debulking was feasible.

Ehrlich has recently reported his experience with the second look laparotomy in those patients who have been treated with combination PAC chemotherapy.[29] About half of his patients did come to a second look laparotomy, and 10 of these 30 patients had a negative second look. In addition, there were four patients who started on the chemotherapy in the "optimal" situation, 5 of 17 (29 percent) had a negative second look. Of those patients with suboptimal disease after their initial surgery only 5 of 39 (13 percent) had a negative second look. The long term survival in these groups of patients having obtained a negative second look after combination chemotherapy is unknown. In those patients who have had a negative second look after single agent alkylating therapy, the vast majority have remained tumor free for prolonged periods of time.

SUMMARY

Although the survival of patients with ovarian cancer has not improved over the last several decades still within the last 10 years a considerable amount of knowledge has been catalogued in regard to this dreaded disease. It is now appreciated that surgery alone (even in what is thought to be early stage disease) is not definitive, with rare exception, and the use of adjunctive therapy in Stage I disease can improve survival from approximatley 60 percent with surgery only to 85 to 90 percent with these other modalities. The identification of the biological activity and spread pattern of this cancer is extremely important and must be thoroughly evaluated at the time of the initial surgical procedure in order to know the exact extent of the disease and therefore give the appropriate treatment postoperatively. The role of surgery not only as far as identifying extent of disease but also as a cytoreductive procedure is now fully appreciated. The initial surgeon must be prepared to carry out this procedure even if ovarian cancer is unexpected preoperatively. Selecting the appropriate therapy postoperatively of course depends upon those findings and what was done at the time of the initial procedure. Unfortunately, the use of chemotherapy empirically, even in combinations, will not result in destruction of residual tumor in all patients. Only time will tell whether the use of in-vitro chemotherapeutic testing procedures currently under evaluation will be of clinical use in the selection of first line chemotherapy. To date, if in-vitro testing notes nonreactivity this is usually the case in the patient but not all patients will respond to the drug which appears in vitro to be active. It does appear to be better than placing all patients on the same protocol. We are now only beginning to understand that heterogenicity of tumors occurs, but have not devised protocols to manage this situation.

The new frontiers that are being opened in the laboratory such as the monoclonal assay may in the future have a direct applicability not only to the diagnosis but in regards to therapy of ovarian cancer. In time, it is hoped that these new mechanisms along with learning how to prevent the disease (such as the recently reported apparent protective effect of the birth control pill against ovarian cancer) will allow us to considerably improve in our efforts to combat this disease.

REFERENCES

1. Tobias JS, Griffiths CT: Management of ovarian carcinoma. N Engl J Med 294:818, 1976.
2. Griffiths CT, Parker LM, Fuller AF: Role of cytoreductive surgical treatment in the management of advanced ovarian cancer. Cancer Treat Rep 63:235, 1979.
3. Kottmeier ED: Annual report on the results of treatment of the uterus, vagina and ovary. 16:14, 1976, Stockholm, Sweden.
4. Aure JC, Hoeg K, Kolstad P: Clinical and histologic studies of ovarian carcinoma. Long term follow up of 990 cases. Obstet Gynecol 37:1, 1971.
5. Creasman WT, Park R, Norris H, et al: Stage I borderline ovarian tumors. Obstet Gynecol 59:93, 1982.
6. Kjorstad KE: Borderline lesions and their therapy. Presented at a Symposium on Ovarian Cancer, Dusseldorf, Germany, June 25, 1982.
7. Rosenshein NR, Leichner PKk, Vogelsang G: Radiocolloids in treatment of ovarian cancer. Obstet Gynecol Survey 34:708, 1979.
8. Currie JL, Bagyne R, Harris C, et al: Radioactive chromic phosphate suspensions: Studies on distribution, dose absorption and effective therapeutic radiation in phantoms, dogs and patients. Gynecol Onc 12:193, 1981.
9. Clarke DCG, Hilaris B, Roussis C, et al: The role of radiation therapy (including isotopes) in the treatment of cancer of the ovary. Progr Clin Cancer 5:227, 1973.

10. Julian CG, Inalsingh A, Barnett LS, et al: Radioactive phosphorus and external radiation as an adjuvant to surgery for ovarian carcinoma. Obstet Gynecol 52:155, 1978.

11. Hreshchyshyn MH, Park RC, Blessing JA, et al: The role of adjunctive therapy in Stage I ovarian cancer. Am J Obstet Gynecol 138:139, 1980.

12. Delclos L, Quinlan EJ: Malignant tumors of the ovary managed with postoperative megavoltage irradiation. Radiology 93:659, 1969.

13. Smith JP,, Rutledge FN, Delclos L: Results of chemotherapy as an adjunct to surgery in patients with localized ovarian cancer. Sem in Onc 2:277, 1975.

14. Dembo AJ, Bush RS, Beale FA, et al: The Princess Margaret Hospital study of ovarian cancer: Stage I, II and symptomatic presentations. Cancer Treat Report 63:249, 1979.

15. Tobias JS, Griffiths CT: Management of ovarian carcinoma. N Engl J Med 294:877, 1976.

16. Smith JP, Rutledge FN: Chemotherapy in the treatment of cancer of the ovary. Am J Obstet Gynecol 107:691, 1970.

17. Smith JP, Rutledge F, Wharton JT: Chemotherapy of ovarian cancer: new approaches to treatment. Cancer 30:1565, 1972.

18. Parker LM, Griffiths CT, et al: Adriamycin/Cyclophosphamide and surgical treatment of advanced ovarian cancer. Proc Am Assoc Cancer Res 19:399, 1978.

19. Edmonson JH, Fleming TR, Decker DG, et al: Different chemotherapeutic sensitivities and host factors affecting prognosis in advanced ovarian carcinoma versus minimal residual disease. Cancer Treat Rep 63:241, 1979.

20. Omura GA, Morrow CP, Blessing JA, et al: A randomized comparison of melphalan versus melphalan plus hexamethylmelamine versus adriamycin plus cyclophosphamide in ovarian carcinoma. Cancer 51:783, 1983.

21. Young RC, Chabner BA, Hubbard SP, et al: Advanced ovarian carcinoma. A prospective clinical trial of melphalan (L-PAM) versus combination chemotherapy. N Engl J Med 299:1261, 1978.

22. Carmo-Pereira J, Costa FO, Henriques E, et al: Advanced ovarian carcinoma: A prospective and randomized clinical trial of cyclophosphamide versus combination cytotoxic chemotherapy (Hexa-CAF). Cancer 48:1947, 1981.

23. Ehrlich CE, Einhorn L, Williams SD, et al: Chemotherapy for Stage III–IV epithelial ovarian cancer with Cis Di Chlorodrammine-platinum (11), adriamycin and cyclophosphamide. A preliminary report. Cancer Treat Report 63:281, 1979.

24. Barker GH, Wiltshaw E: Randomized trial comparing low-dose Cisplatin and chlorambucil with low-dose cis platin, chlorambucil and doxorubicin in advanced ovarian carcinoma. Lancet 4:747, 1981.

25. See whole issue of Cancer Treat Report 63: Feb. 1979.

26. Gershenson DM: Chemotherapy of ovarian malignancies at the M.D. Anderson Hospital. Presented at a Symposium on Ovarian Cancer. Dusseldorf, Germany, June 25, 1982.

27. Alberts DS, Moon TE, Stephens RA, et al: Randomized study of chemoimmunotherapy for advanced ovarian carcinoma. Cancer Treat Report 63:325, 1979.

28. Creasman WT, Gall SA, Blessing JA, et al: Chemo-immunotherapy in management of primary Stage III ovarian cancer. Cancer Treat Report 63:319, 1979.

29. Ehrlich CE: Personal communication.

8 | Chemotherapy of Advanced Ovarian Carcinoma

Thomas B. Hakes

The chemotherapy of ovarian carcinoma has undergone a number of changes in the past several years. Standard treatment of advanced ovarian carcinoma in the 1960's and early 1970's usually included 1 to 2 years of therapy with an oral alkylating agent sometimes followed by a second look laparotomy. Initial response rates with alkylating agents were in the range of 35 to 65 percent with an average of perhaps 45 percent. At the end of 2 years 5 to 15 percent were continuing responders. Long term responders, i.e., greater than five years, and patients with negative second look laparotomies constituted approximately 10 percent of an intial group of patients with stage III and IV disease.[1] While these results were not encouraging the small group of long term survivors was always of interest. These were often patients who had gross disease left behind at surgery and yet had no disease found at second look surgery. Certainly we have not throught of "cure" in other common adenocarcinomas such as colon, lung, breast, pancreas when gross disease is left behind.

In the late 1960's and early 1970's a number of new drugs such as 5-fluorouracil, methotrexate, vinblastine, and actinomycin D were tried in ovarian carcinoma.[2,3] While showing activity in ovarian carcinoma they were clearly not as active as the alkylating agents. These drugs were often used in combination with alkylating agents following the successful lead of MOPP therapy in Hodgkin's disease[4] and the Cooper regimen in breast carcinoma.[5] In randomized studies comparing alkylating agents to combination regimens the response rates were improved with combination chemotherapy but survival times remained the same.[6]

In the middle 1970's a number of drugs were introduced whose activity in ovarian carcinoma approximated that of the alkylating agents, specifically these were doxorubicin (adriamycin), hexamethylmelamine, and cisplatin. Combinations including these drugs and alkylating agents have routinely resulted in response rates of 60 to 85 percent.[6] The question awaiting answer at the moment is whether survival will be improved over that seen with traditional alkylating agent therapy. Early results from trials comparing these new combinations to alkylating agents show substantially higher response rates and response durations but the data on survival is not yet available.[7,8,9] Actually the question posed by most of these new studies is: "Is combination therapy superior to sequential therapy?", since most patients failing the alkylating agent arm of such studies receive a cisplatin containing combination.[10] While most investigators are awaiting the results of these ongoing randomized studies popular opinion already regards these new combinations as superior and they are generally used as standard therapy.

Hopes for improved survival in ovarian carcinoma center on the search for new drugs or treatment modalities. There have not been any particularly promising new drugs for ovarian carcinoma since cisplatin was introduced several years ago. In fact the success of present combination chemotherapy assures that most patients eligible for new drug trials will be very heavily pretreated. This virtually assures a low response rate for any new drug no matter how active in untreated ovarian cancer. Thus there is interest in new "in vitro" testing methods to identify active new drugs[11] as discussed elsewhere in this book. Hormones have always played a minor role in the treatment of ovarian cancer, but the finding that many ovarian carcinomas are estrogen receptor positive[12] has renewed interest in this area. Other developments discussed elsewhere in this volume include intraperitoneal chemotherapy, intraperitoneal radioactive colloids, and monoclonal antibodies.

A word of caution regarding the evaluation of studies mentioned in this review. Comments will refer to treatment of stage III/IV epithelial ovarian carcinoma unless otherwise noted. Responses to treatment may be defined surgically or clinically. The surgical response is defined at second look laparotomy and is certainly the most accurate and objective measure of response. The criteria for surgical responses are the same as those of clinical responses. Clinical responses are defined as follows: complete response is the disappearance of all measureable disease for a minimum of 1 to 3 months; partial response is a 50 to 99 percent reduction in the size of measurable disease as defined by the two greatest diameters; and no response is no change or progressive growth of disease. The terms stable disease and minor response will not be mentioned in this review as they are too ambiguous. For practical purposes we are interested in complete response rates because partial responders do not survive much longer than non-responders with ovarian carcinoma (Fig. 8-1).[13,14] Therefore in evaluating any study we will be particularly interested in the complete response rates. Older studies, particularly with the alkylating agents, often fail to define response criteria. In the past, ascites and pleural effusions were often regarded as measureable, a practice that is not presently accepted due to the difficulty in evaluating effusions. In addition, older single drug studies were done on untreated patients, while most newer drugs have been evaluated in patients who have already failed alkylating agents. These differing response criteria and patient populations are the reasons for the sometimes widely divergent response rates quoted for various drugs.

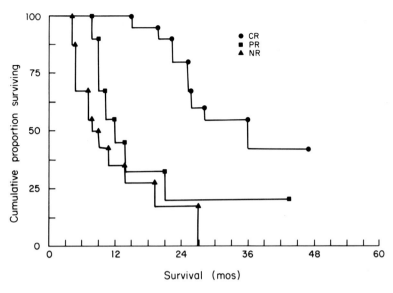

Fig. 8-1.   Survival versus clinical response for 88 patients treated with Cytoxan, Adriamycin and cisplatin for stage III–IV ovarian carcinoma.[14]

ALKYLATING AGENTS

Among the earliest alkylating agents used in ovarian carcinoma were triethylene thiophosphoramide (thio-tepa),[15] chlorambucil,[16,17] L-phenylalanine mustard (melphalan),[1] and cyclophosphamide.[18] The collected response rates for the various alkylating agents are shown in Table 8-1.

Response rates for alkylating agents average about 45 percent with complete responses in the range of 5 to 20 percent. Many of these studies were done in the 1960's when response criteria were not well defined. Effusions were often accepted as measureable disease.[15] Normally these studies were done with patients who had received no prior chemotherapy as opposed to studies with newer drugs where most patients have received prior chemotherapy. Thus due to liberal response criteria and no prior treatment, studies with alkylating agents may appear much superior to newer agents such as cisplatin, adriamycin, and hexamethylmelamine. However, as will be discussed later and as is demonstrated in Table 8-2 the newer agents are as active or more active than the alkylating agents.

Median survival among patients with advanced ovarian carcinoma treated with alkylating agents range from 10 to 16 months in the studies summarized in Table 8-1. As mentioned previously partial responses were of little use. Luciani et al.[19] showed that survival of partial responders to thio-tepa was not significantly longer than nonresponders. However, complete responders lived significantly longer.

The alkylating agents appear cross resistant in ovarian cancer. Response rates to a second alkylating agent are quite low.[18,20,21] A recent trial using "double alkyla-

Table 8-1. Single Agent Chemotherapy in Stage III/IV Ovarian Carcinoma

Drug	Number Treated	Response Rate (%)	Reference
Melphalan[1]	541	47	3
Cyclophosphamide	335	43	3
Chlorambucil	388	51	3
Thio-tepa[2]	337	48	3
Nitrogen mustard	99	31	6
Prednimustine[3]	36	28	65
CCNU[4]	74	14	6
BCNU[5]	34	2	6
Methyl CCNU[6]	26	0	6
Yoshi 864	33	0	27
5-Fluorouracil	92	20	3
Mtx[7] (conventional dose)	25	20	6
Mtx (leucovorin rescue)	27	20	6
Vincristine	22	0	3
Vinblastine	10	20	3
VP 16-213[8]	57	5	37,38,39
VM 26[9]	16	0	41
	20	40	40
Doxorubicin (adriamycin)	224	14	6
	63	36	44,45,46
4'-Epi-doxorubicin	16	6	86
Hexamethylmelamine	142	25	6
	53	36	29,46
Cisplatin	237	31	6
Actinomycin D			
6-Mercaptopurine	19	5	87
m-AMSA[10]	58	7	88,89,90
Piperazinidine	26	0	91
Dianhydrogalacititol	39	15	92
Spirogermanium	46	4	93,94,95
Progestins	60	38	3
	146	5	58,59,60,61
Diethylstilbesterol	14	36	62
Tamoxifen	16	25	63,64

1 = L-phenylalanine mustard, 2 = Triethylene thiophosphoramide, 3 = Leo 13, a chlorambucil-steroid ester, 4 = 1-(2-chloroethyl)-3-cyclohexyl-1-nitrosourea, 5 = 1,3-bis (2-chloroethyl)-1-nitrosourea, 6 = 1-(2-chloroethyl)-3-(4-methyl cyclohexyl)-nitrosourea, 7 = methotrexate, 8 = 4'-demethyl-1-0-(4,6-0-(ethylidene)-B-D-glucopyranosyl)-epipodophyllotoxin, 9 = 4'-demethyl-1-0-(4,6-0-(2-thenylidene) = B-D-glucopyranosyl)-epipodophyllotoxin, 10 = 4'-(9-acridinylamino) methanesulfon-m-anisidine

tor'' therapy with thio-tepa and chlorambucil after initial failure of an alkylating agent containing combination regimen, showed no responses in the 18 patients treated.[21]

There is little evidence that oral, intravenous, continuous, intermittent, or high dose drug schedules are superior one over the other. High dose cyclophosphamide enjoyed a period of popularity when Buckner et al.[22] noted responses in 8 of 9 patients treated with cyclophosphamide (120 mg/m^2). However, a small randomized study comparing oral melphalan to a high dose cyclophosphamide regimen (Table 8-2) showed no difference in response rate or survival.[23] However, the toxicity of the high dose regimen was substantially greater with marked leukopenia, several episodes of sepsis, and one toxic death. Though this study is quite small it is frequently cited as evidence

Table 8-2. Single Agent Trials in Untreated Patients with Stage III/IV Ovarian Carcinoma

Drug	Number Treated	Response Rate (%)	Complete Responses (%)	Reference
Thio-tepa vs	12	66		31
Methotrexate (daily po)	10	0		
Methotrexate/Thio-tepa	8	50		
Melphalan vs	50	30	22	29
Hexamethylmelamine	22	46	32	
5-fluorouracil	24	17	17	
Melphalan vs	14	64	14	23
Cyclophosphamide (80 mg/k)	10	60	20	
Melphalan vs	20	25	10	44
Adriamycin	19	42	5	
Melphalan vs	31	25	11	46
Adriamycin	32	27	12	
Hexamethylmelamine	31	29	13	
Hexamethylmelamine +				
Cyclophosphamide	32	40	34	
Adriamycin vs	12	50	25	45
Melphalan + Adriamycin	14	29	21	
Cisplatin (1 mg/k/week)	12	83	33	70
Cyclophosphamide vs	11	45		28
BCNU	11	9		

that intensive alkylating agent regimens are not superior to conventional dose regimens.

It was during the 1960's that the thought of second look laparotomies arose. Rutledge lists several reasons to justify reexploration: "(1) the patient may have had a sufficient amount of the drug; (2) the tumor may become more localized and possibly resectable for the first time; (3) the benefit from the drug may be exhausted and it is time to switch to another drug; (4) the mass may now be suitable for irradiation; and (5) the mass that has served as a guide to the drug action is suspected not to be cancer as presumed, but is possibly composed of benign agglutinated organs rather than a neoplastic mass."[24] Certainly the thought of limiting the duration of alkylating agent therapy was given impetus by the finding of an increased incidence of acute myelocytic leukemia with long term alkylating agent therapy.[25,26] However, it was also during the same time that treatment periods of 12 to 24 months were accepted as standard for alkylating agents in advanced ovarian carcinoma. Smith et al. (Table 8-3) suggested, in a retrospective review of patients with negative second look laparotomies after alkylating agent therapy, that survival was substantially better among

Table 8-3. Survival by Number of Cycles of Melphalan Before "Second Look" Operation

Chemotherapy Cycles	(%) 2-Year Survival	(%) 5-Year Survival
1–4	38	13
5–9	64	30
10+	85	65

patients receiving 10 or more monthly courses of treatment. Among patients with a negative second look laparotomy done after 1 to 4 courses of alkylating agent the 5-year survival rate was 13 percent compared to 65 percent for those receving 10 or more courses.[1]

Among a group of 800 patients treated with melphalan at MD Anderson Hospital in the 1960's 12 percent came to second look laparotomy and 6 percent had a negative second look laparotomy and were long-term survivors.[24] Thus we see a small group of patients possibly cured by alkylating agent therapy. However, the small size of the group demonstrates that this treatment was clearly inadequate.

Yoshi 864, a new busulfan analog active against experimental tumors resistant to mechlorethamine, gave no responses in 33 patients with ovarian carcinoma who had received prior chemotherapy.[27]

The nitrosoureas are traditionally included among the alkylating agents. They do not appear to be active in ovarian carcinoma (Table 8-1). A small randomized study of 1,3-bis-(2-chloroethyl)-3-(4-methyl cyclohexyl)-nitrosourea (BCNU) versus cyclophosphamide showed progression of disease in 10 of 11 patients treated with BCNU as opposed to only 5 of 11 treated with cyclophosphamide.[28] There is little interest in this group of agents at the moment for the treatment of ovarian carcinoma.

ANTIMETABOLITES, VINCAS, AND ACTINOMYCIN D

5-Fluorouracil (5-FU) has shown consistent but minor activity in ovarian carcinoma (Table 8-1). Response rates in untreated patients range from 15 to 20 percent.[3] In a randomized study of untreated patients with advanced ovarian carcinoma treatment with melphalan, hexamethylmelamine or 5-FU gave response rates of 30, 46 and 17 percent respectively (Table 8-2).[29] 5-FU is rarely used as a single agent today, but is a frequent component in combination chemotherapy regimens, particularly in the older non-cisplatin regimens[13,30] or salvage regimens after failure of cisplatin.

Methotrexate as a single agent in advanced ovarian carcinoma has a response rate in the range of 15 to 20 percent. In a small randomized study of untreated patients comparing thio-tepa to oral methotrexate to combination thio-tepa/methotrexate response rates of 66, 0 and 50 percent respectively were noted (Table 8-2).[31] This study suggests little or no activity for oral methotrexate in ovarian carcinoma. Small groups of patients have been treated with conventional dose intravenous methotrexate and the response rates average 25 percent.[6] High dose methotrexate has been used in patients who failed treatment with alkylating agents, and response rates of 11 to 13 percent have been noted.[32,33] Barlow and Piver have suggested a synergistic effect for the combination of cyclophosphamide and high dose methotrexate. In a group of prior treated patients they found a response rate of 11 percent for high dose methotrexate alone as opposed to 43 percent for the cyclophosphamide/high dose methotrexate combination.[32] Methotrexate has been most frequently used in conventional intravenous doses as a component of non-cisplatin combination regimens such as HexaCMF[13] or CMF.[34]

Vincristine has shown no activity in ovarian carcinoma (Table 8-1)[3] though the studies are small and all patients treated had prior chemotherapy.

Vinblastine demonstrated a 20 percent response rate in 10 prior treated patients with ovarian carcinoma. This drug has not been widely used in the past. However, recent studies with human tumor stem cell assays suggest vinblastine may be quite active in ovarian carcinoma.[35] In a recent study by Budman et al.[36] in advanced ovarian carcinoma a combination of cisplatin, vinblastine, cyclophosphamide, and hexamethylmelamine appeared equivalent to CHAP by historical comparison.

The epipodophyllotoxins VM 26 and VP 16-213 have been tested in ovarian cancer (Table 8-1). Several independent trials show little activity for VP 16 as a second line drug.[37,38,39] Radice et al. in reviewing several broad phase II studies of VM 26 suggested a 40 percent response rate as a second line drug in ovarian carcinoma.[40] However, the only disease specific study in ovarian carcinoma shows no responses among the 16 patients treated.[41]

There is little or no published data on actinomycin D as a single agent in ovarian carcinoma.[3] In spite of this the drug has been frequently used in combination.[1,42,43] Table 8-3 lists three studies comparing single alkylating agents to combinations containing actinomycin D. Two studies show no increase in response rate with actinomycin D.[1,43] The third study shows an increased response rate with the three drug combination of actinomycin D, 5-fluorouracil, and cyclophosphamide but no improvement in survival.[42] Thus there is very little data to suggest that actinomycin D has any activity in ovarian carcinoma.

ADRIAMYCIN

Adriamycin (doxorubicin) came into widespread clinical use in the early 1970's. A recent review notes a 14 percent response rate in a compilation of 224 patients (Table 8-1).[6] Such figures, however, suffer the shortcomings of drug trials conducted among heavily pretreated patients. If we look at studies in patients where adriamycin was used as a first line drug response rates of 27 to 50 percent are noted (Table 8-1 and 8-2).[44,45,46] The average response rate among 63 patients with no prior treatment was 36 percent (Table 8-1). Thus adriamycin would appear to be an effective drug in ovarian carcinoma with activity comparable to the alkylating agents.

HEXAMETHYLMELAMINE

Weiss noted a 32 percent response rate with hexamethylmelamine in patients with ovarian carcinoma who had received no prior chemotherapy and a 19 percent response rate among those with prior chemotherapy.[47] Another recent review notes a response rate of 25 percent overall (Table 8-1).[6] In two additional studies among 53 patients with no prior treatment the average response rate was 53 percent (Tables 8-1 and 8-2).[29,46] Thus hexamethylmelamine also appears to be an active drug in ovarian carcinoma with activity comparable to or superior to the alkylating agents.

CISPLATIN

Cisplatin is considered one of the most active drugs in ovarian carcinomas. There are virtually no studies of cisplatin as a single agent in untreated patients. In a compilation of 237 patients with prior treatment a 31 percent response rate is quoted.[6] Cisplatin has been given in a multiplicity of schedules in attempts to ameliorate toxicity or increase its effectiveness. Probably the most widely used schedule is 50 mg/m² given intravenously over a period of 15 minutes to a few hours. Doses of 100 to 120 mg/m² are purported to be more effective. There is evidence for this in breast[48] and testicular cancers. Wiltshaw et al.[49] in treating 82 patients with ovarian carcinoma who had prior alkylating agent therapy noted a response rate of 33 percent for patients treated with cisplatin 30 mg/m² as opposed to 52 percent for cisplatin 100 mg/m². Piver et al. noted a response rate of 5 percent in 20 patients treated with cisplatin 100 mg/m² every 3 weeks as third line therapy.[50] However, the same group noted a 70 percent response rate in 10 patients treated with cisplatin 100 mg/m² every week as third line therapy and a 83 percent response rate when used as first line treatment.[51] Bruckner et al.[52] noted responses in 4 of 20 patients treated with cisplatin 120 mg/m² who had previously failed cisplatin at 50 mg/m². A study by Ehrlich et al.[53] compared a combination of cyclophosphamide, adriamycin, and cisplatin 20 mg/m² times 5 days to the same combination with cisplatin lowered to 50 mg/m². Both combinations induced responses in approximately 80 percent of patients with complete responses in 44 and 40 percent respectively. To date there is no difference in survival between the two groups. Thus at least in combination we see no difference between the 50 and 100 mg/m² doses. The schedule of 20 mg/m² times 5 days was developed in an attempt to reduce nausea and nephrotoxicity, but this was not particularly successful.[54] Cisplatin at present is the mainstay in most combination chemotherapy regimens for advanced ovarian carcinoma.

MISCELLANEOUS SINGLE AGENTS

6-Mercaptopurine, m-AMSA, dianhydrogalactitol, 4'-epi-doxorubicin, and spirogermanium have shown minimal activity in ovarian carcinoma (Table 8-1). Piperazinidine showed no activity (Table 8-1). However, as previously mentioned, most new drug trials today are done in heavily pretreated patients, and it is difficult to know what these negative results mean. Even cisplatin, probably the most active drug in ovarian carcinoma, has only a 5 percent response rate when used as third line chemotherapy in ovarian carcinoma.[51]

HORMONES

In 1976 Tobias and Griffiths summarized the studies relating to progestational agents in ovarian cancer.[3] The cumulative response rate for 60 patients taken from several studies was 38 percent. They noted that these studies suffered from small numbers and questionable definitions of response.

Recently it has been noted that many ovarian carcinomas contain receptors for estrogen and progesterone.[12,55,56,57] In these studies, encompassing 60 to 70 patients, approximately 50 percent of the tumors were estrogen receptor positive with values ranging from 0 to 300 fm/mg (femntomoles per milligram of protein). The positive values averaged 74 fm/mg with a median of 60 fm/mg. No correlations were made with hormone responses in ovarian carcinoma. It is suggested that patients with estrogen receptor positive carcinomas may have a better prognosis.[55] Only 15 percent of the carcinomas were positive for progesterone receptor protein with values ranging from 0 to 60 fm/mg. Positive values averaged 23 fm/mg with a median of 11 fm/mg. Again no correlations were available for hormone responses in ovarian carcinoma. Thus it appears that a major percentage of ovarian carcinomas contain estrogen receptor protein and a substantially smaller portion progesterone receptor protein.

As noted above early studies of progestational agents in ovarian carcinoma suggested a 38 percent response rate. However, a compilation of recent studies shows only a 5 percent response rate.[58,59,60,61] These patients were probably more heavily pretreated than those in the prior series, but the criteria for responses were also more objective. There is a suggestion that high dose intramuscular progestins may be superior to the oral route of administration. Margioni et al.[61] found a 15 percent response rate in 30 patients treated with high dose intramuscular medroxyprogesterone as opposed to no responses among 30 patients treated with a high dose oral regimen.

There is a single report of diethylstilbesterol use in advanced ovarian carcinoma.[62] Fourteen patients, most of whom had prior radiation or alkylating agent therapy, were treated. Five responses were noted, three of which were disappearance of ascites.

Myers et al.[64] reported three out of three partial responses to antiestrogen (tamoxifen, nafoxidine) therapy in patients with ovarian carcinoma resistant to standard chemotherapy. Schwartz et al.[64] noted one response among 13 patients treated with tamoxifen as third line therapy.

Prednimustine a chlorambucil ester of prednisolone induced 28 percent remissions in a group of 36 patients with ovarian carcinoma.[65] Among 21 patients with no prior therapy the response rate was 38 percent as opposed to 13 percent in the 15 patients who had received prior melphalan. It was hoped this compound might have a special affinity for estrogen receptor positive cells in ovarian carcinomas. However, in the above study the response rate and hematologic toxicity were comparable to that seen with conventional alkylating agents.

COMBINATION CHEMOTHERAPY

The discussion of combination chemotherapy in ovarian carcinoma has been split into two sections, non-cisplatin combinations and cisplatin combinations. Combinations without cisplatin have shown response rates in the range of 30 to 60 percent (Table 8-4) whereas cisplatin combinations routinely give response rates of 60 to 85 percent (Table 8.5). On this basis these combinations appear fundamentally different. However, the newer cisplatin combinations are more toxic, and the question remains whether survival has been improved along with these higher response rates.

Table 8-4. Combination Chemotherapy in Ovarian Carcinoma: Non-Cisplatin Combinations in Patients Without Prior Treatment

Drugs*	# Pts.	CR+PR (%)	CR (%)	Median* Surv. (mo)	Reference
Melphalan vs	50	42	20	12	1
ActD + 5-FU + Ctx	47	45	30	10	
Melphalan vs	22	45	40		42
ActD + 5-FU + Ctx	22	63	18		
Melphalan vs	96	29	17	9	43
Melphalan + 5-FU	77	27	16	13	
Melphalan + 5-FU + ActD	85	32	17	13	
ActD + 5-FU + Ctx	45	26	9	8	
Melphalan vs	114	26	17	11	96
Ctx + 5-FU + Mtx	110	41	19	9	
Melphalan + 5-FU + Mtx(HD) vs	119	47	19	12	97
Sequential melphalan +					
5-FU + Mtx(HD)	121	60	24	12	
Melphalan vs	70	11	6		98
Thio-tepa + Mtx	72	15	6		
Ctx + Adria + 5-FU	71	30	10		
Thio-tepa + Mtx alternating with					
Ctx + Adria + 5-FU	62	21	3		
Ctx + Adria	41	86	46		99
Melphalan vs	23	30	3	14	100
Ctx + Adria	24	71	8	14	
Ctx vs	35	31		12	101
Ctx + Adria	36	36		12	
Melphalan vs	72	29	7	11	102
Melphalan + Adria	70	54	21	17 +	
Melphalan vs	64	38	13	ND	103
Melphalan + HMM	97	52	27	ND	
Ctx + Adria	35	49	23	ND	
Adria + Ctx vs	20	59	35	17	104
HMM + Ctx	23	50	30	14	
Melphalan vs	37	54	16	17	13
Ctx + Mtx + 5-FU + HMM	40	75	33	29	

*Abbreviations- ActD (actinomycin D); 5-FU (5-fluorouracil); Ctx (cyclophosphamide); Mtx (methotrexate); Mtx(HD) (high dose methotrexate with citrovorum rescue); Thio-tepa (triethylene thiophosphoramide); Adria (doxorubicin); HMM (hexamethylmelamine); ND (no significant difference).

COMBINATIONS WITHOUT CISPLATIN

A large number of combination regimens are listed in Table 8-4. There are a number of similarities among these studies. Most response rates fall in the range of 30 to 45 percent with 15 to 20 percent complete responses and median survival times of 10 to 15 months. With the addition of adriamycin or hexamethylmelamine to the combinations response rates of 50 to 60 percent are commonly seen with 25 to 35 percent complete responses. Most of these studies show increased response rates for combinations as opposed to single alkylating agent therapy but no improvement in survival. The sole exception to this is the National Cancer Institute sponsored study comparing melphalan therapy to a combination of cyclophosphamide, methotrexate, 5-fluorouracil and hexamethylmelamine (HexaCMF) where the median survival was 17 versus 29 months respectively (Table 8-4, p = .02).[13]

Table 8-5. Combination Chemotherapy in Ovarian Carcinoma: Cisplatin Combinations in Patients with no Prior Chemotherapy

Drug*	Patients	CR + PR (%)	CR (%)	Median* Surv. (mo)	Reference
Clb + CPDD + Adria vs	24	66	41		49
Clb + CPDD	34	59	32		
Clb	16	25	0		
Ctx + CPDD	21				9
Ctx	21				
Ctx + Adria + CPDD vs	22	59	22	ND	8,69
Ctx + Mtx + 5-FU + HMM	24	37	8	ND	
Melphalan	21	43	10	ND	
Ctx + HMM + Adria + CPDD vs	123	63	41	19	7,70
Melphalan	123	44	20	17	
CPDD + Adria + Ctx (PAC V) vs	25	88	44	23	53,105
CPDD + Adria + Ctx (PAC I)	31	75	40	23	
CPDD + Adria vs	18	72		20	66
CPDD	18	20		20	
Thio-tepa + Mtx	17	20		10	
CPDD + Adria + Ctx + HMM vs	36	80	40	19 +	66,67
CPDD + Adria	18	70	30	19 +	
Ctx + Adria + CPDD vs		71	43		106
Ctx + Adria + HMM		62	31		
Ctx + Adria + CPDD vs	91	71	44		68
Ctx + Adria	101	46	20		

*Abbreviations- CPDD (cisplatin); others as per table 8-4.

Along with increased response rates came increased toxicity. Oral alkylating agents such as melphalan and chlorambucil had few side effects beyond leukopenia and thrombocytopenia. The combination chemotherapy regimens introduced nausea, vomiting, alopecia, mucositis, diarrhea, and cystitis. With the addition of hexamethylmelamine came peripheral neuropathy and with adrimaycin came cardiomyopathy. Thus it was disappointing that most randomized studies showed no increased survival with combination chemotherapy.

CISPLATIN COMBINATION CHEMOTHERAPY

Cisplatin combination chemotherapy routinely gives clinical response rates of 60 to 85 percent with 35 to 45 percent complete responses and median survivals of 19 to 25 months (Table 8-5). Two,[49,66,67] three,[8,49,53,68] and four[7,67] drug combinations with cisplatin seem to give similar response rates (Table 8-5). Cytoxan and cisplatin (CP), adriamycin and cisplatin (AP), cytoxan, adriamycin and cisplatin (CAP) and cytoxan, hexamethylmelamine, adriamycin and cisplatin (CHAP) are the cisplatin combinations commonly used today. The addition of cisplatin to these combinations has increased not only response rates but also toxicity. Cisplatin commonly causes nephropathy, peripheral neuropathy, anemia, and high-frequency hearing loss. Thus there are a number of trials comparing cisplatin combination chemotherapy to single alkylating agent therapy (Table 8-5).[7,9,69] To date these studies show increased response rates for cisplatin combination chemotherapy but no improvement in survival.

However, in most of these trials the patients who fail alkylating agent therapy go on to treatment with a cisplatin combination. For example, in the Eastern Cooperative Oncology Group study comparing CHAP to melphalan those who fail melphalan are treated with hexamethylmelamine/adriamycin/cisplatin. This combination gives a 27 to 33 percent response rate in patients failing an alkylating agent.[70,71] Thus the question in most of these randomized comparisons of single alkylating agent to cisplatin combination chemotherapy is one of sequential versus combination treatment. But, two pieces of information suggest the superiority of cisplatin combinations. First, as noted in Table 8-5 median survivals are in the range of 20 to 25 months as opposed to 10 to 15 months seen for single alkylating agents and older combination chemotherapy regimens (Tables 8-4 and 8-5). Second, the complete response rates with cisplatin combinations are in the range of 35 to 45 percent as compared to 5 to 20 percent for alkylating agents (Tables 8-4 and 8-5) and as shown in Figure 8-1 and noted in other studies[13] patients with complete responses to chemotherapy live significantly longer.

PROGNOSTIC FACTORS

Cytologic grade and residual tumor volume affect survival and chemotherapy responses in ovarian carcinoma.[72,73] Griffiths[73] noted that survival time in stage III-IV ovarian carcinoma was related to the size of the largest residual tumor masses. Those patients whose tumor was less than 1.5 cm in diameter had considerably better survival times. Decker et al.[72] correlated survival with cytologic tumor grade. Those patients with well-differentiated low grade tumors survived significantly longer than

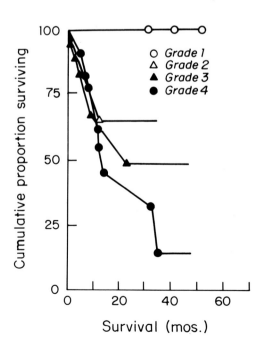

Fig. 8-2. Survival versus cytologic tumor grade for 47 patients treated with hexamethylmelamine, cyclophosphamide, methotrexate and 5-fluorouracil for stage III–IV ovarian carcinoma. (Reprinted with permission from Young RC, Chabner BA, Hubbard SP, et al: Advanced ovarian adenocarcinoma—A prospective clinical trial of nelphalan versus combination chemotherapy. N Engl J Med 299:161, 1978.)

those with poorly differentiated high grade tumors. This correlation was independent of histologic type. Both these studies were done in the era of single alkylating agent chemotherapy. A more recent study correlated survival and cytologic grade in patients treated with hexamethylmelamine/cytoxan/methotrexate/5-fluorouracil (HexaCAF) (Fig. 8-2).[74] Patients with low cytologic grade carcinomas survived longer. Two recent studies with cisplatin based chemotherapy regimens suggest that volume of residual disease is still an important prognostic factor.[53,75] In both studies the chance of a surgically documented complete response was considerably greater when the diameter of the largest residual tumor mass was less than 3 centimeters. In one study,[75] 20 of 24 patients with residual tumor masses less than 3 centimeters had a complete response to CHAP chemotherapy as documented by surgery.

Cytologic grade and residual tumor mass were correlated with survival in a group of 88 patients with stage III-IV ovarian carcinoma treated at Memorial Hospital with 12 monthly cycles of CAP followed by second look laparotomy.[14] Residual tumor mass was, as noted before, an important prognostic indicator of survival. This is demonstrated in Figure 8-3 where survival is plotted as a function of the largest tumor mass left behind at initial surgery. Survival is significantly better (logrank test, p = .0001) for patients with smaller residual tumor masses. This correlation is also present (Fig. 8-4) when we consider total residual tumor volume (sum of the volume of all residual tumor masses). A volume of 14 cm^3 is equivalent to a mass 3 cm in diameter, 66 cm^3 to 5 cm and 268 cm^3 to an 8 diameter mass. Again survival is better among those with less residual tumor (logrank test, p = .0001). Correlation of survival with cytologic grade is less clear (Fig. 8-5). Survival is not significantly different among patients with various cytologic grades (logrank test, p = .93). This is in

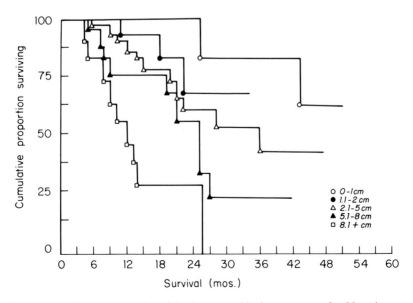

Fig. 8-3. Survival versus diameter of the largest residual tumor mass for 88 patients treated with Cytoxan, Adriamycin and cisplatin for stage III–IV ovarian carcinoma.[14]

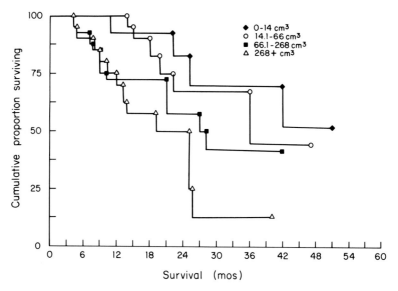

Fig. 8-4. Survival versus total residual tumor volume for 88 patients treated with Cytoxan, Adriamycin and cisplatin for stage III–IV ovarian carcinoma.[14]

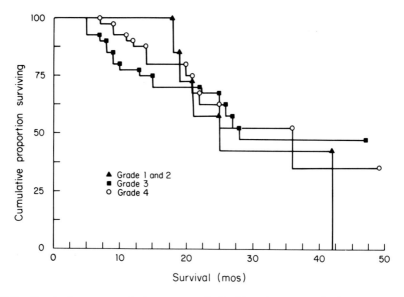

Fig. 8-5. Survival versus cytologic tumor grade for 88 patients treated with Cytoxan, Adriamycin and cisplatin for stage III–IV ovarian carcinoma.[14]

contrast to the clear correlation shown in earlier studies by others (Fig. 8-2).[74] We might take our data as showing no correlation between cytologic grade and survival in ovarian carcinoma, or alternatively we might interpret it as showing an improved prognosis for patients with high grade carcinomas treated with CAP. Indeed this is suggested by the fact that the median survival for the 88 patients in this study is 25 months, quite good compared to prior studies with noncisplatin chemotherapy regimens (Table 8-4).

OVARIAN GERM CELL MALIGNANCIES

Germ cell malignancies of the ovary (dysgerminoma, endodermal sinus tumor, embryonal carcinoma, immature teratoma and mixed germ cell tumors) have a different spectrum of chemotherapeutic sensitivities than epithelial ovarian carcinomas. Minimal single agent data exists for ovarian germ cell malignances. Alkylating agents have activity.[1] On the basis of combination chemotherapy studies the following agents probably have activity: alkylating agents, actinomycin D, vinblastine, bleomycin, and cisplatin.[76] The standard regimens until recently were vincristine, actinomycin D and cyclophosphamide (VAC) or methotrexate, actinomycin D and chlorambucil (MAC).[78] It is difficult to discuss response rates in these studies utilizing the VAC and MAC regimens owing to the variety of stages and histologic subtypes treated. However, excellent survivals are reported using these regimens in both the adjuvant and advanced disease settings. Most patients with ovarian germ cell malignancies are treated with chemotherapy even if the tumor is completely resected owing to their tendency to recur.[76] Exceptions might be a small, completely resected grade I ovarian teratoma, or a dysgerminoma. Most dysgerminomas are successfully treated with surgery and radiation therapy. More recently combinations of vinblastine, actinomycin D, bleomycin and cisplatin (VABP)[76] and cisplatin, vinblastine and bleomycin (PVB)[79] have been reported to give response rates of 77 and 90 percent respectively. The VABP study included several patients with prior treatment (radiation, VAC, MAC), while the PVB study included only untreated patients. Thus there are at least four chemotherapy combinations reported to have a high order of activity in ovarian germ cell malignancies: VAC, MAC, VABP, and PVB. There are no direct comparisons of these regimens. VABP is active in patients who have failed VAC or MAC.[76] Cisplatin which is very active in ovarian epithelial carcinomas and testicular germ cell malignancies is used in higher doses of 100 to 120 mg/m^2 in the PVB and VABP regimens. There is no experience with the lower cisplatin doses of 50 to 60 mg/m^2 so often used in epithelial ovarian carcinomas. There is evidence however in testicular germ cell malignancies to suggest that cisplatin doses of 100 mg/m^2 are more effective than 50 mg/m^2.[80]

Our present strategy in ovarian germ cell malignancies is surgical debulking, three courses of VABP over three months, a second look laparotomy if the patient has no evidence of disease and one additional cycle of VABP post-operatively. If the patient has residual disease the therapy is tailored to the circumstances. Bulky residual disease, liver, and bone marrow involvement, poor performance status and prior systemic therapy are poor prognostic factors.[76] Bulky residual disease is a particularly bad prognostic factor as in epithelial ovarian carcinoma and thus aggressive surgical debulking is warranted.

FUTURE DIRECTIONS

The trend in treatment of stage III-IV epithelial ovarian carcinoma is towards more intense treatment for shorter periods of time. Oral alkylating agents were given for 18 to 24 months, cisplatin based combination chemotherapy is commonly given for 12 months and now there are several studies which suggest that 5 to 6 months of treatment with cisplatin combination chemotherapy may give equivalent results.[75,81] Treatment intensity has been increased by adding more drugs to chemotherapy combinations such as the four drug CHAP regimen[70] or by pushing individual drugs harder as in a weekly cisplatin regiment.[51] Bruckner et al.[82] have combined both approaches with an intensification schedule for a combination of CHAP given to produce leukopenia in the range of 1000 to 1500 cells cm^3. An alternating regimen of CAP with HexaCMF is being evaluated.[83] Low dose whole abdominal plus pelvic radiation therapy has been combined with a regimen of cisplatin and hexamethylmelamine in patients with bulky residual ovarian carcinoma.[84] After a six-month induction with CHAP patients are given two courses of radiation therapy, 1050 rads over 6 to 7 weeks, with concurrent chemotherapy.

New drugs remain a possibility though there are no apparent candidates at the moment.

Perhaps as many as 25 percent of complete responders documented at surgery are relapsing in the 1 to 2 years following cessation of chemotherapy.[14,53,75] Most of these relapses are in the peritoneal cavity. Thus the possibility of some sort of intraperitoneal consolidation therapy is of interest. Such an approach is under evaluation at the National Cancer Institute with intraperitoneal 5-fluorouracil following systemic therapy with cyclophosphamide, hexamethylmelamine, cisplatin and 5-fluorouracil.[85]

Since residual tumor volume remains such an important prognostic variable the possibility of preoperative chemotherapy is an attractive possibility. The thought being that more complete surgical debulking might be possible after two or three courses of ciaplatin based combination chemotherapy. The major impediment to such an approach is the frequent necessity for a full laparotomy to establish the diagnosis of ovarian carcinoma.

Monoclonal antibodies and in vitro drug assays which are promising approaches are discussed elsewhere in this volume.

REFERENCES

1. Smith JP, Rutledge F, Wharton JT: Chemotherapy of ovarian cancer. Cancer 30:1565, 1972.
2. DeVita VT, Wasserman TH, Young RC, et al: Perspectives on research in gynecologic oncology. Cancer 38:509, 1976.
3. Tobias JS, Griffiths CT: Management of ovarian carcinoma. N Eng J Med 294:818, 877, 1976

4. Devita VT, Serpick AA, Carbone PP: Combination chemotherapy in the treatment of advanced Hodgkin's disease. Ann Intern Med 73:881, 1970.

5. Cooper RJ: Combination chemotherapy in hormone resistant breast cancer. Proc Am Assoc Cancer Res 10:15, 1969.

6. Katz ME, Schwartz PE, Kapp DS, et al: Epithelial carcinoma of the ovary: Current strategies. Ann Intern Med 95:98, 1981.

7. Vogl SE, Pagano M, Kaplan B: Cyclophosphamide, hexamethylmelamine, adriamycin, and diamminedichloroplatinum vs melphalan for advanced ovarian cancer-A randomized prospective trial of the eastern cooperative oncology group. Proc Am Soc Clin Oncol 22:473, 1981.

8. Sturgeon JFG, Fine S, Bean HA, et al: A randomized trial of melphalan alone versus combination chemotherapy in advanced ovarian cancer. Proc Am Soc Clin Oncol 21:422, 1980.

9. Decker DG, Fleming TR, Malkasian GD, et al: A treatment program for stage III and IV ovarian cancer-Cyclophosphamide versus cyclophosphamide and cis-platinum. Obstet Gynecol 60:481, 1982.

10. Vogl SE, Kaplan BH, Greenwald E: Prognostic factors for platinum-based combination chemotherapy of advanced ovarian cancer. Proc. Am Soc Clin Oncol 21:429, 1980.

11. Salmon SE, Hamburger AW, Soehnlen B, et al: Quantitation of differential sensitivity of human-tumor stem cells to anticancer drugs. N Engl J Med 298:1321, 1978.

12. Holt JA, Caputo TA, Kelly KM, et al: Estrogen and progestin binding in cytosols of ovarian adenocarcinomas. Obstet Gynecol 53:50, 1979.

13. Young RC, Chabner BA, Hubbard SP, et al: Advanced ovarian adenocarcinoma-A prospective clinical trial of melphalan versus combination chemotherapy. New Engl J Med 299:1261, 1978.

14. Hakes TB: Memorial Hospital, unpublished data.

15. Blinick G, Kabakow B, Wallach RC, et al: Treatment of advanced inoperable ovarian carcinoma with thio-tepa. Am J Obstet Gynecol 96:425, 1966.

16. Lebherz T, Huston JW, Austin JA, et al: Sustained palliation in ovarian carcinoma. Obstet Gynecol 25:475, 1965.

17. Masterson JG, Nelson JH: The role of chemotherapy in the treatment of gynecologic malignancy. Am J Obstet Gynecol 93:1102, 1965.

18. Beck RE, Boyes DA: Treatment of 126 cases of advanced ovarian carcinoma with cyclophosphamide. Can Med Assoc J 98:539, 1968.

19. Luciani L, de Palo GM, Conti U, et al: Carconomi ovarici in fase avanzata trattati con thio-tepa. Tumori 59:259, 1973.

20. Stanhope CR, Smith JP, Rutledge F: Second trial drugs in ovarian cancer. Gynecol Oncol, 5:52, 1977.

21. Ozols RF, Howser DM, Young RC: Double alkylator therapy (thio-tepa plus chlorambucil) for previously treated advanced ovarian cancer. Cancer Treat Rep 65:731, 1981.

22. Buckner CD, Brigs R, Clift RA, et al: Intermittent high-dose cyclophosphamide (NSC-26271) treatment of stage III ovarian carcinoma. Cancer Chemother Rep 58:697, 1974.

23. Young RC, Canellos GP, Chabner BA, et al: Chemotherapy of advanced ovarian carcinoma: a prospective randomized comparison of phenylalanine mustard and high dose cyclophosphamide. Gynecol Oncol 2:489, 1974.

24. Rutledge F: Treatment of epithelial cancer of the ovary. In Rutledge F, Boronow RC, Wharton JT (eds): Gynecologic Oncology. New York, John Wiley and Sons, 1976.

25. Reimer RR, Hoover R, Fraumeni JF, et al: Acute leukemia in patients receiving chlorambucil as long term therapy of ovarian cancer. New Engl J Med 297:177, 1977.

26. Lerner HJ: Acute myelogenous leukemia in patients receiving chlorambucil as long term

adjuvant chemotherapy for stage II breast cancer. Cancer Treat Rep 62:1135, 1978.

27. Slavik M, Muss H, Blessing JA, et al: Phase II clinical study of Yoshi 864 in epithelial ovarian carcinoma: A Gynecologic Oncology Group study. Cancer Treat Rep 66:1775, 1982.

28. Jorgensen EO, Malakasian GD, Webb G: Pilot study evaluating 1, 3-bis-(2-chloroethyl)-1-nitrosourea in the treatment of advanced ovarian carcinoma. Am J Obstet Gynecol 116:769, 1973.

29. Smith JP, Rutledge FM: Random study of hexamethylmelamine, 5 fluorouracil and melphalan in the treatment of advanced carconoma of the ovary. Natl Cancer Inst Monogr 42:169, 1975.

30. Izbicki RM, Baker LH, Samson MK, et al: 5-FU infusion and cyclophosphamide in treatment of advanced ovarian cancer. Cancer Treat Rep 61:1573, 1977.

31. Greenspan EM, Bruckner HW: Comparison of regression induction with triethlyene thiophosphoramide or methotrexate in bulky stage IIIb ovarian carcinoma Natl Cancer Inst Monogr 42:173, 1975.

32. Barlow JJ, Piver MS: Methotrexate with citrovorum factor rescue, alone and in combination with cyclophosphamide, in ovarian carcinoma. Cancer Treat Rep 60:527, 1976.

33. Parker LM, Griffiths CT, Yankee RA, et al: High-dose methotrexate with leucovorin rescue in ovarian cancer: a phase II study. Cancer Treat Rep 63:275, 1979.

34. Brodovsky HS, Temkin N, Sears ML: Melphalan versus cyclophosphamide, methotrexate and 5 fluorouracil in women with ovary cancer. Proc Am Soc Clin Oncol 18:308, 1977.

35. Salmon SE, Meyskens FL, Alberts DS, et al: New Drugs in ovarian cancer and malignant melanoma: in Vitro phase II screening with the human tumor stem cell assay. Cancer Treat Rep 65:1, 1981.

36. Budman D: Personal communication.

37. Slayton R, Creasman WT, Petty W, et al: Phase II trial of VP-16-213 in the treatment of advanced squamous cell carcinoma of the cervix and adenocarcinoma of the ovary: a Gynecologic Oncology Group study. Cancer Treat Rep 63:2089, 1979.

38. Edmonson JH, Decker DG, Malkasian GD, et al: Phase II evaluation of VP-16-213 (NSC 141540) in patients with advanced ovarian carconoma resistant to alkylating agents. Gynecol Oncol 6:7, 1978.

39. Maskers AP, Armand JP, Lacave AJ, et al: Phase II clinical trial of VP-16-213 in ovarian cancer. Cancer Treat Rep 65:329, 1981.

40. Radice PA, Bunn PA, Ihde DC: Therapeutic trials with VP16-213 and VM26: Active agents in small cell lung cancer, non-Hodgkins lymphoma and other malignancies. Cancer Treat Rep 63:1231, 1979.

41. Samson MK, Baker LH, Talley RW, et al: VM26 (NSC-122819) a clinical study in advanced cancer of the lung and ovary. Eur J Cancer 14:1359, 1978.

42. Barlow JJ, Piver MS: Single agent vs combination chemotherapy in the treatment of ovarian cancer. Obstet Gynecol 49:609, 1977.

43. Park RC, Blum J, DiSaia PJ, et al: Treatment of women with disseminated or recurrent advanced ovarian cancer with melphalan alone, in combination with 5-fluorouracil and dactinomycin, or with the combination of cytoxan, 5-fluorouracil and dactinomycin. Cancer 45:2529, 1980.

44. dePalo GM, DeLena M, Luciani L, et al: Melphalan versus adriamycin in the treatment of advanced carcinoma of the ovary. Surg Gynecol Obstet 141:899, 1975.

45. dePalo GM, DeLena M, Bonadonna G: Adriamycin versus adriamycin plus melphalan in advanced ovarian carcinoma. Cancer Treat Rep 61:355, 1977.

46. Smith JP: Chemotherapy in gynecologic cancer. Surg Clin North Am 581:201, 1978.

47. Weiss RB: The role of hexamethylmelamine in advanced ovarian carcinoma treatment. Gynecol Oncol 12:141, 1981.

48. Forastiere AA, Hakes TB, Wittes JT, et al: Cisplatin in the treatment of metastatic breast carcinoma-A prospective randomized trial of two dosage schedules. Am J Clin Oncol 5:243, 1982.

49. Wiltshaw E, Subramarian S, Barker GH, et al: Cancer of the ovary: A summary of experience with cis-dichlorodiammineplatinum(II) at the Royal Marsden Hospital. Cancer Treat Rep 63:1545, 1979.

50. Piver MS, Barlow JJ, Lele SB, et al: cis-Dichlorodiammineplatinum(II) as third-line chemotherapy in advanced ovarian adenocarcinoma. Cancer Treat Rep 62:559, 1978.

51. Piver MS, Lele S, Barlow J: Weekly cis-diamminedichloroplatinum(II): Active third-line chemotherapy in ovarian carcinoma-A preliminary report. Cancer Treat Rep 64:1379, 1980.

52. Bruckner HW, Wallach R, Cohen CJ, et al: High-dose platinum for the treatment of refractory ovarian cancer. Gynecol Oncol 12:64, 1981.

53. Ehrlich CE, Einhorn LH, Roth L, et al: Response, ''second look'' status and survival in stage III-IV epithelial ovarian cancer treated with cis-dichlorodiammineplatinum(II), adraimycin and cyclophosphamide. Proc A Soc Clin Oncol 21:423, 1980.

54. Dentino M, Luft F, Yum MN, et al: Long term effect of cis-diamminedichloride platinum on renal function and structure in man. Cancer 41:1274, 1978.

55. Creasman WT, Sasso RA, Weed JC, et al: Ovarian carcinoma: Histologic and clinical correlation of cytoplasmic estrogen and progesterone binding. Gynecol Oncol 12:319, 1981.

56. Hahnel R, Kelsall GRH, Martin JD, et al: Estrogen and progesterone receptors in tumors of the human ovary. Gynecol Oncol 13:145, 1982.

57. Crickard K, Baker DT, Wittliff JL: Association of steroid hormones with intracellular binding components in normal and neoplastic ovaries of women. Am Assoc Cancer Res 18:239, 1977.

58. Aabo K, Pedersen AG, Hald I, et al: High-dose medroxyprogesterone acetate in advanced chemotherapy-resistant ovarian carcinoma: A phase II study. Cancer Treat Rep 66:407, 1982.

59. Malkasian GD, Decker DG, Jorgensen EO, et al: Medroxyprogesterone acetate for the treatment of metastatic and recurrent ovarian carcinoma. Cancer Treat Rep 61:913, 1977.

60. Trope C, Johnsson JE, Sigurdsson K, et al: High-dose medroxyprogesterone acetate for the treatment of advanced ovarian carcinoma. Cancer Treat Rep 66:1441, 1982.

61. Mangioni C, Franceschi S, LaVecchia C, et al: High-dose medroxyprogesterone acetate in advanced epithelial ovarian cancer resistant to first or second-line chemotherapy. Gynecol Oncol 12:314, 1981.

62. Long RT, Evans AM: Diethylstilbestrol as chemotherapeutic agent for ovarian carcinoma. Misouri Med 60:1125, 1963.

63. Myers AM, Moore GE, Major FJ: Advanced ovarian carcinoma: Response to antiestrogen therapy. Cancer 48:2368, 1981.

64. Schwartz PE, Keating G, MacLusky N, et al: Tamoxifen therapy for advanced ovarian cancer. Am Soc Clin Oncol 21:430, 1980.

65. Johnson JE, Trope C, Mattsson W, et al: Phase II study of Leo 13 (prednimustine) in advanced ovarian carcinoma. Cancer Treat Rep 63:421, 1979.

66. Holland JF, Bruckner HW, Cohen CJ, et al: Cis-platinum therapy of ovarian cancer. In Prestayko AW, Crooke ST (eds): Cisplatin: Current Status and New Developments. New York, Academic Press, 1980.

67. Bruckner HW, Cohen CJ, Wallach WJ, et al: Prospective controlled randomized trial comparing combination chemotherapy of advanced ovarian carcinoma with adriamycin and

cis-platinum + / − cyclophosphamide and hexamethylmelamine. Proc Am Soc Clin Oncol 20:414, 1979.

68. Omura GA, Ehrlich CE, Blessing JA: A randomized trial of cyclophosphamide plus adriamycin with or without cis-platinum. Proc Am Soc Clin Oncol 1:104, 1982.

69. Sturgeon JFG, Fine S, Gospodarowicz MK, et al: A randomized trial of melphalan alone versus combination chemotherapy in advanced ovarian cancer. Proc. Am Soc Clin Oncol 1:108, 1982.

70. Vogl SE, Kaplan B, Pagano M: Diamminedichoroplatinum based combination chemotherapy is superior to melphalan for advanced ovarian cancer when age is greater than 50 and tumor diameter greater than 2 cm. Proc Am Soc Clin Oncol 1:119, 1982.

71. Bernath A, Andrews T, Curry S, et al: HAP (hexamethylmelamine, adriamycin, cisplatinum) vs CAP (cyclophosphamide, adriamycin, cisplatinum) in aikylating agent resistant advanced ovarian carcinoma. Proc Am Soc Clin Oncol 1:470, 1982.

72. Decker DG, Malkasian GD, Taylor WF: Prognostic importance of histologic grading in ovarian carcinoma. Natl Cancer Inst Monogr 42:9, 1975.

73. Griffiths CT: Surgical resection of tumor bulk in the primary treatment of ovarian cancer. Natl Cancer Inst Monogr 42:101, 1975.

74. Ozols RF, Garvin AJ, Costa J, et al: Advanced ovarian cancer—a correlation of histologic grade with response to therapy and survival. Cancer 45:572, 1980.

75. Greco FA, Burnett LS, Wolff SN, et al: Limited residual advanced ovarian cancer—a cureable neoplasm? Proc Am Soc Clin Oncol 1:106, 1982.

76. Bradoff JE, Hakes TB, Ochoa M, et al: Germ cell malignancies of the ovary-treatment with vinblastine, actinomycin D, bleomycin and cisplatin containing chemotherapy combinations. Cancer 50:1070, 1982.

77. Slayton R, Hreshchyshyn M, Shingleton H, et al: Treatment of malignant ovarian germ cell tumors: Response to vincristine, dactinomycin and Cytoxan. Cancer 42:390, 1978.

78. Creasman W, Fether B, Hammond C, et al: Germ cell malignancies of the ovary. Obstet Gynecol 53:226, 1979.

79. Williams S, Slayton R, Silverberg S, et al: Response of malignant ovarian germ cell tumors to cis-platinum, vinblastine and bleomycin. Proc Am Soc Clin Oncol 22:463, 1981.

80. Samson MK, Stephens RL, Klugo RC: Positive dose-response of high versus low dose cis-platinum, vinblastine and bleomycin in disseminated germ cell neoplasms of the testis. Proc Am Soc Clin Oncol 1:470, 1982.

81. Stiff P, Boblick J, Lanzotti V, et al: Aggressive combination chemotherapy followed by early second look laparotomy for patients with advanced ovarian carcinoma. Proc Am Soc Clin Oncol 1:111, 1982.

82. Bruckner HW, Cohen CJ, Deppe G, et al: Ovarian cancer: schedule modification and dosage intensification of cyclophosphamide, hexamethylmelamine, adriamycin and cisplatin regimen (CHAP II). Proc Am Soc Clin Oncol 1:107, 1982.

83. Young JA, Kroener JF, Lucas WE, et al: Cisplatin, adriamycin, and cyclophosphamide alternating with hexamethylmelamine, cyclophosphamide, methotrexate and 5-fluorouracil for advanced ovary cancer. Proc Am Soc Clin Oncol 1:115, 1982.

84. Vogl SE, Seltzer V, Greenwald E, et al: Safe concurrent whole abdominal radiation, Diamminedichloroplatinum and hexamethylmelamine as consolidation therapy for bulky advanced ovarian cancer. Proc Am Assoc Cancer Res 23:155, 1982.

85. Young RC, Houser DM, Myers CE, et al: Combination chemotherapy (Chex-UP) with intraperitoneal maintenance in advanced ovarian adenocarcinoma. Proc Am Soc Clin Oncol 22:465, 1981.

86. Trope C: A phase II study of 4'-epi-doxorubicin in advanced ovarian carcinoma. Proc Am Soc Clin Oncol 1:121, 1982.

87. Moore GE, Bross IDJ, Ausman R, et al: Effect of 6-mercaptopurine (NSC-755) in 290 patients with advanced cancer: Eastern Clinical Drug Program. Cancer Chemother Rep 52:655, 1968.

88. Dombernowsky P, Hansen HH: m-AMSA in advanced ovarian carcinoma-a phase II study. Proc Am Soc Clin Oncol 21:426, 1980.

89. Schneider RJ, Woodcock TM, Howerd J, et al: Phase II trial of AMSA in previously treated patients with stage III and IV ovarian cancer. Cancer Treat Rep 66:1589, 1982.

90. Kearsley JH, Page J, Levi JA: Phase II study of AMSA in patients with advanced ovarian cancer. Cancer Treat Rep 66:1242, 1982.

91. Delgado G, Thigpen T, Dolan T, et al: Phase II trial of piperazinidine in treatment of advanced ovarian adenocarcinoma. Proc Am Soc Clin Oncol 19:332, 1978.

92. Blom J, Blessing J, Maldineo J, et al: Dianhydrogalactitol in the treatment of advanced gynecologic malignancies. Proc Am Soc Clin Oncol 21:416, 1980.

93. Trope C, Mattsson W, Gynning I, et al: Phase II study of spirogermanium in advanced ovarian malignancy. Cancer Treat Rep 65:119, 1981.

94. Weiselberg L, Budman DR, Schulman P, et al: Phase II trial of spirogermanium in advanced epithelial carcinoma of the ovary. Cancer Treat Rep 66:1675, 1982.

95. Brenner D, Forastiere A, Rosenschein N, et al. A phase II study of spirogermanium in patients with advanced carcinomas of the ovary and cervix. Proc Am Soc Clin Oncol 1:115, 1982.

96. Brodovsky HS, Temkin N, Sears M: Melphalan versus cyclophosphamide, methotrexate and 5-fluorouracil in women with ovarian cancer. Proc Am Soc Clin Oncol 18:308, 1977.

97. Klaassen DJ, Boyes DA, Gerulath A, et al: Preliminary report of a clinical trial of the treatment of patients with advanced stage III and IV ovarian cancer with melphalan, 5-fluorouracil, and methotrexate in combination and sequentially: A study of the Clinical Trials Group of the National Cancer Institute of Canada. Cancer Treat Rep 63:289, 1979.

98. Bruckner HW, Pagano M, Falkson G, et al: Controlled prospective trial of combination chemotherapy with cyclophosphamide, adriamycin and 5-fluorouracil for the treatment of advanced ovarian cancer: a preliminary report. Cancer Treat Rep 63:297, 1979.

99. Griffiths CT, Yankee RA, Knapp RC, et al: Adriamycin/cyclophosphamide and surgical treatment of advanced ovarian cancer. Am Soc Clin Oncol 19:399, 1978.

100. Turbow MM, Jones H, Yu VK, et al: Chemotherapy of ovarian carcinoma: a comparison of melphalan vs adriamycin-cyclophosphamide. Proc Am Soc Clin Oncol 21:196, 1980.

101. Edmonson JH, Fleming TR, Decker DG, et al: Different chemotherapeutic sensitivities and host factors affecting prognosis in advanced ovarian carcinoma versus minimal residual disease. Cancer Treat Rep 63:241, 1979.

102. Trope C: A prospective and randomized trial comparison of melphalan vs adriamcyin-melphalan in advanced ovarian carcinoma. Proc Am Soc Clin Oncol 22:469, 1981.

103. Omura GA, Blessing JA, Morrow CP, et al: Follow-up on a randomized trial of melphalan vs melphalan plus hexamethylmelamine vs adriamycin plus cyclophosphamide in advanced ovarian adenocarcinoma. Proc Am Soc Clin Oncol 22:470, 1981.

104. Schwarz PE, Lawrence R, Katz M: Combination chemotherapy for advanced ovarian cancer: A prospective randomized trial comparing hexamethylmelamine and cyclophosphamide to doxorubicin and cyclophosphamide. Cancer Treat Rep 65:137, 1981.

105. Ehrlich CE, Einhorn L, Williams SD, et al: Chemotherapy for stage III–IV epithelial ovarian cancer with cis-dichlorodiammineplatinum(II), adriamycin, and cyclophosphamide: a preliminary report. Cancer Treat Rep 63:281, 1979.

106. Mangioni C, Bolis G, Bortolozzi G, et al: Cis-dichlorodiammineplatinum, adriamycin cyclophosphamide vs hexamethylmelamine, adriamycin, cyclophosphamide in advanced ovarian cancer. Proc Am Assoc Cancer Res 21:149, 1980.

9 | New Investigational Techniques in Ovarian Cancer

Robert F. Ozols
Charles E. Myers
Robert C. Young

The treatment of ovarian cancer is entering a new era in which empirically derived therapies will be replaced by more rational and disease-specific approaches. The new investigational modalities of treatment are based upon an increased understanding of the biology of ovarian cancer as well as upon experimental and theoretical advances in radiation oncology and in the pharmacology of antineoplastic drugs. The need for more effective therapy of ovarian cancer is readily apparent from the survival results of standard therapy presented in the previous chapter and can be summarized in Table 9-1. The standard practice of using combination chemotherapy following surgery in patients with stage III–IV disease has resulted in only an 11 percent pathologically confirmed complete response rate in patients who have residual masses greater than 3.0 cm following surgery. In contrast, patients who have small volume disease (<3.0 cm masses) following surgery have a 69 percent complete response rate to combination chemotherapy. Since the vast majority of ovarian cancer patients present with stage III–IV disease and since most patients have bulky disease following the initial surgery, only a minority of ovarian cancer patients will achieve a complete response to therapy and it is only in these patients that survival is improved.[1]

In this chapter we will review the advances in our understanding of the biology of ovarian cancer and describe some new investigational therapies which hold promise for improving upon the generally unsatisfactory results of standard therapy. Finally, we will summarize the standard approaches to the treatment of patients with

Table 9-1. Effect of Residual Disease on Response to Chemotherapy

Chemotherapy Regimen		Disease Status Prior to Chemotherapy (Number, Percent)		Percent Pathologic Complete Remissions	
	Reference	Non-Bulky	Bulky	Non-Bulky	Bulky
Hexa-CAF	(1)	8 (20%)	32 (80%)	100% (8/8)	16% (5/32)
ChexUP	(2)	14 (27%)	37 (73%)	36% (5/14)	14% (5/37)
H-CAP	(3)	21 (42%)	29 (58%)	86% (18/21)	11% (3/29)
A-C	(4)	12 (33%)	24 (67%)	92% (11/12)	4% (1/24)
PAC	(5)	17 (30%)	39 (70%)	30% (5/17)	13% (5/39)
	MEAN	31% (20–42%)	69% (58–80%)	69% (30–100%)	11% (4–16%)

ovarian cancer and discuss the potential role of the investigational modalities in each stage of this disease.

ETIOLOGY, PATTERNS OF METASTASES AND BIOLOGY OF OVARIAN CANCER

The common epithelial ovarian carcinomas arise from the surface "germinal" epithelial cells which are not the source of germ cells as originally proposed but are actually modified mesothelium of mesodermal origin. The surface epithelium is also closely related embryologically to the paramesonephric or Mullerian system. This accounts for the development of serous, endometroid, and mucinous carcinomas as the transformed malignant surface epithelial cell recapitulates the respective Mullerian epithelia, i.e., tubal, endometerium, and endocervical. The less common clear cell carcinoma of the ovary most likely represents a variant of endometroid carcinomas and therefore also is of Mullerian epithelial origin. Thus all the common epithelial tumors potentially may be responsive to biological control mechanisms which influence the development of Mullerian ducts. For example, Mullerian inhibition substance (MIS) obtained from fetal calf testes can inhibit the growth of ovarian carcinoma cells in experimental systems.[6–9] Potential therapeutic applications of MIS will be discussed in a later section.

The etiology of ovarian cancer remains to be precisely established. The epidemiologic profile of the women with an increased risk (single, relative infertility) as well as the increased incidence of ovarian cancer surrounding menopause suggest that a change in the hormonal milieu of the surface epithelium may be important in the development of ovarian tumors.[10] The establishment of tissue culture cell lines of rat surface germinal epithelia[11] has provided a model system for the investigation of hormonal effects[12] and should allow for the direct evaluation of other factors potentially involved in the neoplastic transformation of the surface epithelium. Further support for the role of hormones in the etiology of ovarian cancer is provided by the observation that patients with breast cancer have twice the risk of developing ovarian cancer. In addition there is some evidence that endocrine therapy (see below) may be of benefit in certain patients with ovarian cancer. Direct experimental evidence for the role of hormones in either the development of ovarian cancer or in the regulation of malignant ovarian cancer cell growth is currently not available. However, the finding [10,13,14] that common epithelial tumors frequently have estrogen receptors (30 to 50 percent) and androgen receptors (80 percent) suggests that some steroid hormone influences may exist in epithelial ovarian malignancies. The recent characterization in our laboratory of a human ovarian cancer cell line which has cytoplasmic estrogen and androgen receptors will allow for the direct investigation of hormonal effects upon the proliferation of receptor positive malignant ovarian cancer cells. [15]

Once the malignant transformation has occurred in the surface epithelium, neoplastic cells from the ovary can insidiously spread by several mechanisms. Contiguous growth of the tumor mass can result in involvement of any structure within the pelvis which is in close proximity to the ovary, e.g., pelvic side walls, uterus, bladder, colon. More distant spread occurs as the result of lymphatic drainage primarily to the paraaortic lymph nodes and secondarily to the iliac nodes. Perhaps the most important mechanism of metastases of ovarian cancer is via peritoneal seeding. Free floating malignant cells are frequently observed in peritoneal washings even in the absence of malignant ascites. [16] Once malignant ascites does develop (due to lymphatic and diaphragmatic obstruction from tumor cells) the entire peritoneum is at risk for the development of plaque-like surface tumor deposits which frequently are initially asymptomatic and undetectable by non-invasive diagnostic studies. The unsuspected spread of tumor cells has recently been clinically documented by the Ovarian Cancer Study Group. [17] Systematic restaging was prospectively performed in 100 patients referred with early (stage Ia–IIb) ovarian cancer. Ninety-two percent of the patients were felt to be disease free after the initial laparotomy. Upon referral, the patients underwent exhaustive restaging procedures including a second laparotomy in 68 patients. Thirty-one percent of the patients were found to have a more advanced stage and the majority of these (77 percent) had stage III disease. Sites of unsuspected disease included: pelvic peritoneum, peritoneal washings and ascites, paraaortic lymph nodes and the diaphragm. This study has important therapeutic implications both for the application of standard therapy as well as for the design of new investigational modalities of treatment. [18]

INVESTIGATIONAL THERAPIES

Intraperitoneal Chemotherapy

From the pattern of metastases described in the previous section, it is apparent that the determining factor for the successful treatment of ovarian cancer is the eradication of all intra-abdominal disease. Combination chemotherapy regimens produce clinical complete responses (CCR) in approximately 40 percent of the patients. [1-5,19] However, pathologic complete responses (PCR) as determined by a negative "second look" laparotomy are achieved in only 11 percent of patients who have bulky disease at the initiation of chemotherapy (Table 9-1). It is in this clinical setting of residual small volume disease where intraperitoneal chemotherapy has its greatest potential impact.

Intraperitoneal chemotherapy is not a new technique in the management of patients with ovarian cancer. The injection of antineoplastic agents directly into the peritoneal cavity has been used in the past to aid in the control of malignant ascites. In contrast to the previous use of intraperitoneal chemotherapy as a palliative measure, the current methods of intraperitoneal chemotherapy have the potential to directly improve the end results of treatment. The major differences between previous methods of intraperitoneal chemotherapy and current techniques[20–27] are (1) the use of a semi-permanent Tenckhoff dialysis catheter and (2) the delivery of the antineoplastic agents in a large volume (2 liters of dialysate) instead of in 50 to 100 ml of saline. The use of a large volume of dialysate for drug administration is based, in part, upon theoretical pharmacokinetic modeling studies. Dedrick et al.[28] have predicted that a maximum pharmacologic advantage for intraperitoneal chemotherapy will be achieved by the repetitive administration of a drug in a large volume to allow for uniform distribution of drug throughout the peritoneal cavity. The pharmacologic advantage (the ratio of peak intraperitoneal levels to peak blood level) is based upon the difference in peritoneal clearance and clearance from the circulation. The slower the peritoneal clearance of a drug the greater the potential pharmacologic advantage. The peritoneal clearance is a function of the molecular weight and the hydrophilic properties of the drug. High molecular weight compounds with a low lipid solubility have a slow peritoneal clearance leading to an increased pharmacologic advantage.[20,23] Two other properties are necessary for a drug to be useful in the intraperitoneal treatment of ovarian cancer: (1) the concentrations achievable in the peritoneal cavity must be cytotoxic to ovarian cancer cells and (2) the cytotoxic drug concentration should produce an acceptable degree of peritoneal irritation.

The technical considerations in the use of the Tenckhoff catheter for the administration of intraperitoneal chemotherapy have recently been described in detail.[27] The catheter, a flexible silastic tube with a Dacron cuff, was originally used in the mangement of patients with chronic renal failure. The catheter is surgically implanted through the anterior abdominal wall with the Dacron cuff eliciting a fibrotic reaction in the subcutaneous fat resulting in a barrier to infectious organisms. In the NCI series, 68/78 catheter insertions were performed under local anesthesia. The remaining catheters were placed during laparotomies which were performed for staging or re-staging purposes. Major complications of catheter placement were unusual (Table 9-2): 3/78 (5 percent) of catheter placements resulted in intestinal perforations. Minor bleeding into the peritoneal cavity following catheter insertion occurred in the majority of patients which cleared with the initial exchanges of dialysate. Similarly, pain at the insertion site usually resolved within the first 4 to 6 hours postoperatively. The most significant threat to prolonged catheter usage is infection. However, in the NCI series only 3/78 (3.8 percent) catheter insertions were associated with intra-abdominal infections. The overall incidence of catheter related peritonitis in this group of patients in whom the catheters were maintained independently was 10 percent per catheter year. The intra-abdominal sepsis responded in all patients to intravenous and intra-pertitoneal administration of antibiotics. There were three other instances of exit site infections which required removal of two of the catheters. The catheters functioned satisfactorily in the majority of patients. Occasionally there developed outflow or inflow obstruction but this responded to repositioning of the catheter in most instances. The use of 2

Table 9-2. Complications of Tenckhoff Catheters in 78 Patients[27]

Aspect of Catheter Maintenance	Complication Rate
1. Catheter implantation	—3/78 (4%) intestinal perforation —Transient mild bleeding and pain occurred in the majority of patients
2. Septic complications	—3/78 (4%) intra-abdominal sepsis —3/78 (4%) exit site infections
3. Catheter function	—14/78 (18%) of catheters required repositioning to overcome transient obstruction to inflow or outflow

liters of dialysate produced uniform distribution of drug throughout the peritoneal cavity as demonstrated by computerized tomographic studies with intraperitoneal Hypaque.[29]

It must be emphasized that the low catheter complication rate in our series was due, in part, to (1) the same experienced surgeon performing the vast majority of the catheter insertions and (2) the use of CT scans and abdominal ultrasounds to identify patients who, because of either adhesions or size and location of metastases, would have an unacceptable risk for catheter implantation. Furthermore, it is possible that technical refinements could be made in the catheter to facilitate the dialysis, particularly to improve upon the outflow rate.

Phase I and II Trials of Intraperitoneal Chemotherapy in Ovarian Cancer

Table 9-3 summarizes the results of three Phase I trials of intraperitoneal chemotherapy in ovarian cancer performed at the NCI. The initial drug evaluated was methotrexate.[20,25] This preliminary study demonstrated that a pharmacologic advantage could be achieved with intermittent intraperitoneal dialysis. However, the high incidence of local toxicity and the fact that clinical responses were not observed in the NCI study with intraperitoneal methotrexate led to the evaluation of more active agents. Howell et al.[30] used a different technique with 2 separate catheters which allowed continuous infusion of methotrexate for up to 120 hours. In this pilot study 2 minor responses to intraperitoneal methotrexate were observed in ovarian cancer patients.

Intraperitoneal 5-fluorouracil was initially evaluated in a Phase I trial[21] and recently a Phase II trial has been completed.[24] In the Phase I trial, myelosuppression and mucositis were the dose-limiting toxicities. The Phase I trial demonstrated a marked pharmacologic advantage for intraperitoneal 5-fluorouracil with the mean 4 hour peritoneal concentration being 298 times greater than the simultaneously measured plasma level. The dose limiting toxicity in the Phase I trial was myelosuppression and mucositis. Fourteen patients with refractory ovarian cancer were treated in the Phase II trial with a total of 69 cycles of intraperitoneal 5-FU. Twelve of the patients had

Table 9-3. Phase I Trials of Intraperitoneal Chemotherapy in Ovarian Cancer at the NCI

PHARMACOLOGIC PARAMETERS

Drug	Schedule	Pharmacologic Advantage (Ratio of peak intraperitoneal level to peak plasma level)
Methotrexate	50 uM: 8 x 4 hr exchanges q 2 wk	18–36
5-Fluorouracil	4 mM: 8 x 4 hr exchanges q 2 wk	298
Adriamycin	36 uM: 4 hr dwell every 2 wks	474

TOXICITY

Drug	Dose Limiting Toxicity	Other Toxicities
Methotrexate	Peritonitis	Myelosuppression
5-Fluorouracil	Myelosuppression Mucositis	Abdominal Pain
Adriamycin	Peritonitis	Mild Nausea and Vomiting Myelosuppression (mild)

received prior therapy with intravenous 5-FU. While the response rate to intraperitoneal 5-FU was only 7 percent, in 7/8 (88 percent) patients with small volume disease there was no evidence for disease progression while on therapy with intraperitoneal 5-fluorouracil. In contrast, in 4/6 (67 percent) of patients with bulky intraabdominal disease there was progression intraperitoneally while on therapy. The major toxicity was abdominal pain which was experienced to varying degrees by all patients while on therapy. Other toxicities included: myelosuppression (14 percent of patients had WBC counts less than 1500/mm^3), mucositis (7 percent), and nausea and vomiting (93 percent of patients had mild-moderate discomfort).

The results of a Phase I trial of intraperitoneal adriamycin have also been recently reported.[22] Adriamycin is an active agent in the treatment of ovarian cancer with a 40 percent response rate in previously untreated patients.[31] It is however without significant activity in patients who have failed non adriamycin-containing regimens.[32,33] In a series of studies with a murine model of ovarian cancer it was demonstrated that intraperitoneally administered adriamycin was curative to 70 percent of tumor bearing mice whereas an equitoxic intraveous dose had no effect on survival.[34,35] The survival advantage of intraperitoneal adriamycin was due to increased intra-abdominal levels of adriamycin and a subsequent suppression of DNA synthesis in tumor cells. Using the specific fluorescence of adriamycin it was also demonstrated that intraperitoneally administered drug could readily diffuse into the outermost 4 to 6 cell layers of intra-abdominal tumor masses.[35] Further experimental rationale for intraperitoneal adriamycin was provided by direct cloning studies using malignant ascites or malignant peritoneal washings.[36,37] Three distinct patterns of in vitro cytotoxicity were demonstrated with human ovarian cancer cells. The most sensitive cells were from previously untreated patients, and the most resistant cells were from patients who had relapsed after therapy with adriamycin-containing combination chemotherapy regimens. The in vitro resistance to adriamycin in these cells could not be overcome by exposure to concentrations of adriamycin potentially achievable by intraperitoneal therapy. Cells from patients who had failed a non adriamycin-containing regimen had a dose-dependent sensitivity to adriamycin. Significant cytotoxicity was observed only after exposure to concentrations of adriamycin which while not achievable by intravenous administration could be achieved by intraperitoneal therapy. These in vitro studies were consistent with the low response rate of intravenous adriamycin in relapsed patients and suggested that higher concentrations of adriamycin, such as achievable by intraperitoneal administration, would potentially be useful in some patients with ovarian cancer.

The intraperitoneal administration of adriamycin was evaluated in 10 patients who were refractory to systemic chemotherapy. None of the patients, however, had received prior therapy with intravenous adriamycin. Adriamycin was administered for a 4 hour dwell every 2 weeks with concentrations ranging from 9 to 54 μM. The dose limiting toxicity of intraperitoneal adriamycin was a dose dependent sterile peritonitis. Severe abdominal pain associated with the development of a sterile inflammatory ascites and asymptomatic adhesions occurred at concentrations greater than 36 μM. In this Phase I trial there were 3 objective responses and 2 other patients had a transient marked reduction in ascites formation while on therapy. The objective responses were observed only in patients who had non-bulky (<2 cm masses) disease. The clinical activity of intraperitoneal adriamycin was likely the result of an antitumor effect, and not a sclerotic effect, since the reduction of ascites in two patients was accompanied with a decrease in the number of malignant cells. In addition, malignant cells collected from the peritoneal cavity immediately after intraperitoneal therapy with adriamycin no longer had a proliferative capacity as demonstrated by their inability to form tumor colonies in soft agar.

Adriamycin concentrations were measured by HPLC chromatography.[22,38] The maximum pharmacologic advantage was 474 which was higher than achieved with either 5-fluorouracil or methotrexate (Table 9-3). The peak plasma levels after a 60 mg/2L intraperitoneal dose were 10 times lower than after a 60 mg intravenous dose. The intraperitoneal levels of adriamycin achieved had previously been demonstrated to be cytotoxic to human ovarian cancer cells obtained from patients who were refractory to non-adriamycin containing regimen.

A pilot study of intraperitoneal cis-platinum in refractory ovarian cancer patients has also been recently reported by Howell et al.[26] In contrast to the NCI experience with methotrexate, 5-fluorouracil or adriamycin, the intraperitoneal administration of platinum was not reported to produce any local toxicity. The cis-platinum was administered at a dose of 90 mg/m^2 with a 4 hour dwell time. Concurrent intravenous sodium thiosulfate was administered in some patients to neutralized systemic toxicity.[34] The area under the curve (AUC) for the peritoneal cavity/plasma was 12. The administration of thiosulfate reduced the nephrotoxicity presumably by forming a covalent bond with cis-platinum resulting in a stable non-reactive compound. However, it was felt by the authors that the concentration of cis-platinum in the peritoneal cavity was sufficiently greater than that in the plasma to prevent thiosulfate from interfering with the antitumor effects of cis-platinum in the peritoneal cavity. One of seven relapsed ovarian cancer patients had an objective response to intraperitoneal cis-platinum.

Table 9-4 summarizes the clinical situations where intraperitoneal chemotherapy

Table 9-4. Intraperitoneal Chemotherapy in Ovarian Cancer

I. Clinical situations where intraperitoneal therapy not likely to be of benefit
  A. Patients with bulky disease
  B. Patients who have become clinically resistant to a drug will probably not respond to the same drug administered intraperitoneally.
II. Clinical situations where intraperitoneal therapy is potentially useful
  A. Local Disease
    1. In patients with early stage disease who are at a high risk for relapse after surgery [poorly differentiated stage Ia, Ic, and stage II].
  B. Advanced Stage III
    1. As maintenance therapy for patients who achieve a complete response to induction therapy.
    2. In patients who have small volume residual disease after induction therapy.
    3. Combined with systemic therapy as part of induction therapy.

should be evaluated in patients with ovarian cancer. From the results of (1) the Phase I–II clinical trials, (2) the dose response relationship of ovarian cancer cells from relapsed patients, and (3) from experimental studies of drug penetration into solid tumors, it is not likely that intraperitoneal therapy with most drugs will be beneficial in ovarian cancer patients who have (a) bulky disease and (b) who have become refractory to the same drug when administered either p.o. or intravenously. In contrast, intraperitoneal therapy may be of benefit in patients with non-bulky disease where tumors are responsive to the higher doses of drug achievable by intraperitoneal administration. Perhaps the greatest potential for intraperitoneal therapy is in that group of patients who have had a good but only partial response to induction chemotherapy and have residual non-bulky disease. The use of intraperitoneal therapy with either 5-fluorouracil or adriamycin (depending upon the nature of the primary induction regimen) in this clinical setting is currently under evaluation at the National Cancer Institute as well as by the Gynecologic Oncology Group.

Another potential role for intraperitoneal chemotherapy is in patients who have achieved a complete response to chemotherapy. It has previously been demonstrated[1] that this group of patients remain at risk for relapse. Patients who achieve a complete response to induction therapy at the NCI are randomized to receive either no maintanence or 6 cycles of intraperitoneal chemotherapy.[2] At present, the role of intraperitoneal chemotherapy in preventing relapses has not been established in part due to the small number of patients with bulky disease who have achieved a complete response with combination chemotherapy (Table 9-1).

Other clinical situations where intraperitoneal therapy needs further evaluation include adjuvant therapy in high risk patients with early stage disease and combined with systemic treatment as part of the induction therapy for patients with stage III disease. In addition, the Tenckhoff catheter allows for administration of other agents, such as the chemotherapy and radiation sensitizing agent misonidiazole (to be discussed below) as well as a means by which to collect malignant cells. Potentially this can be used to aid in the selection of chemotherapy (see below) as well as an additional way to follow the response to therapy by assessing the number of tumor cells which remain after therapy.

The optimum drug for intraperitoneal therapy also remains to be determined. As previously discussed it should be a cytotoxic drug that produces a marked pharmacologic advantage while not resulting in prohibitive local toxicity. The development of sterile peritonitis has been a major problem in most studies with intraperitoneal therapy in ovarian cancer. It is possible that in vitro tests of dose response relationships in ovarian cancer cells can be coupled with the development of new drugs and analogues of available active drugs to help select a drug which not only is cytotoxic to ovarian cancer but also does not produce an inflammatory effect in the peritoneum. A potential candidate for such a drug is aclacinomycin. This anthracycline analog has been demonstrated in vitro to be as cytotoxic to ovarian cancer cells as the parent compound adriamycin.[40] Since this drug can be administered orally[31] and has not been associated with any soft tissue injury when extravasated during intravenous therapy, it may not be as irritating to the peritoneum as is adriamycin.

High Dose Chemotherapy

An alternate approach to the attainment of high concentrations of antineoplastic drugs, other than by their direct intraperitoneal instillation, has been with high dose intravenous administration. Initial studies with high dose (9 mg/kg) cyclophosphamide failed to demonstrate a clinically useful dose-response relationship.[41] However, recent clinical and experimental studies have suggested that high dose intravenous cis-platinum may be useful even in the treatment of patients who have stopped responding to standard dose cis-platinum.

The rationale for high dose platinum is summarized in Table 9-5. A clinically useful dose-response in ovarian cancer patients has been previously established.[42] Ovarian cancer patients who have relapsed after therapy with platinum at 50 mg/m^2 have a 20 percent response rate to higher doses of platinum, 120 mg/m^2. Experimental evidence for a dose response has also been provided by in vitro studies of platinum cytotoxicity in human ovarian cancer cell lines.[43] The steepest part of the dose response occurred at platinum concentrations of 0.5 to 2.0 ug/ml, which approximate the peak achievable plasma levels after standard dose platinum administration. A one hour exposure at 0.5 ug/ml resulted in 75 percent colony survival whereas a one hour exposure at 2.0 ug/ml produced <10 percent colony survival. Recent experimental studies in animals that the administration of platinum in hypertonic saline[44] markedly decreases the toxicity of platinum led to the use of 3 percent hypertonic saline as the

Table 9-5. Rationale for High Dose Cis-Platinum in Ovarian Cancer

I. Clinical Evidence for a Dose-Response to Platinum
  A. Ovarian cancer patients who have relapsed after treatment with cis-platinum at 50 mg/m^2 have a 20% response rate to cis-platinum at 120 mg/m^2.
II. Experimental Evidence for a Dose-Response
  A. Human ovarian cancer cell lines have a steep dose-response to cis-platinum.
III. Experimental Evidence that Renal Toxicity of Cis-Platinum Can be Reduced by Pharmacologic Manipulation
  A. Administration of cis-platinum in hypertonic saline
  B. Use of thiosulfate to neutralize toxicity
IV. Clinical Evidence that High-Dose Platinum Can be Safely Administered
  A. High dose platinum 40 mg/m^2 x 5 administered in hypertonic saline in testicular cancer patients without any increased renal toxicity.

vehicle for a high dose (40 mg/m^2 × 5) cis-platinum study in patients with poor prognosis testicular cancer.[45] In this study there were no instances of renal toxicity associated with high dose cis-platinum. The mechanism of the apparent protective effect of hypertonic saline is unknown. It may relate to the aquation equilibria of cis-platinum. The presence of a high chloride concentration may decrease the formation of diamino dihydroxy platinum which is presumably the toxic metabolite of cis-platinum. An alternate pharmacologic manipulation which may decrease cis-platinum toxicity is the concurrent administration of thiosulfate.[26]

On the basis of these observations a clinical Phase II trial of high dose cis-platinum (40 mg/m^2 × 5) is currently in progress at the Medicine Branch, NCI. Refractory ovarian cancer patients, all of whom have received prior cis-platinum, are treated with high dose cis-platinum which is administered in 250 ml of 3 percent saline. The patients are also vigorously hydrated prior to cis-platinum administration. The preliminary results of this study indicate that some patients who have relapsed on standard dose cis-platinum will respond to high dose cis-platinum. Furthermore, the dose limiting toxicity in these patients may be myelosuppression and not nephrotoxicity. In particular, platelet nadirs below 10,000/mm^3 were frequently observed with high dose platinum in these heavily treated refractory ovarian cancer patients. Transient nephrotoxicity has also been noted during treatment although the creatinine clearances have returned to pre-treatment values. The hypertonic saline does not protect from ototoxicity or peripheral neuropathy. The actual response rate in this group of patients for high dose cis-platinum remains to be defined. The demonstration that it can be administered without any increased nephrotoxicity and the presence of clinical activity in relapsed patients indicates that high dose platinum be evaluated in previously untreated patients.

Immunotherapy

Any role of immunotherapy in ovarian cancer has not been firmly established. The rationale for immunotherapy in this disease is based upon (1) the presence of a variety of human ovarian cancer tumor-associated antigens, (2) the demonstration that patients with ovarian cancer have a defect in B-cell function while T-cell function remains normal,[46] (3) the observation that ovarian cancer patients have a decrease in the number of natural killer (NK) cells,[47–49] and (4) experimental studies with immunotherapy in a murine model of ovarian cancer. In this transplantable tumor which has a pattern of metastases similar to patients with ovarian cancer, the intraperitoneal administration of corynebacterium parvum and heterologous tumor antisera produces a prolongation of survival.[50–51]

There have been several uncontrolled studies of immunotherapy in patients with ovarian cancer.[52,53] The types of immunotherapy used have included: BCG, c. parvum, irradiated allogeneic cryopreserved tumor cells, neurominidase treated tumor cells, and heterologous immune antiserum. The immunotherapy in these trials was administered subcutaneously, intravenously or intraperitoneally, and it was usually combined with other modalities of therapy making it impossible to define the contribution of the immunotherapy toward the overall treatment results.

There has been one trial, however, that does suggest a role for immunotherapy in ovarian cancer. Advanced stage patients were randomized in a Southeast Oncology Group study to receive no immunotherapy or BCG by scarification.[54] All patients received adriamycin + cyclophosphamide chemotherapy. The overall response rate in the chemotherapy + immunotherapy group was 53 percent compared to 36 percent for those receiving chemotherapy alone. The latter group also had a lower complete response rate (2 percent vs. 12 percent) and a shorter survival (13.1 months vs. 23.5 months) compared to the group receiving immunotherapy. This provocative study is being repeated by the Gynecology Oncology Group in an effort to confirm or deny the beneficial role of nonspecific immunotherapy with BCG. The patients in this study will be stratified for all known prognostic features including extent of disease and histologic grade.

There are several investigational immunotherapeutic approaches which are specific for ovarian cancer and which may hold a greater therapeutic promise than does non-specific immunotherapy. As previously discussed, the epithelial human ovarian cancers histologically resemble tissues derived from the Mullerian duct. Mullerian inhibiting substance (MIS) is a fetal testicular product which induces regression of the Mullerian duct in male embryos. Using a partially purified fraction of MIS isolated from newborn calve testes, Donohue et al.[6,7] have demonstrated that MIS is cytotoxic to a human serous cystadenocarcinoma cell line in vitro and also inhibits the growth of the cell line in nude mice.[8] MIS is at least partially specific for ovarian cancer since there was no inhibition of a growth in a colon cancer cell line.[6-8] MIS is a complex glycoprotein which has been purified 7000-fold.[9] Therapeutic trials of MIS will require new technology to prepare sufficient quantities of MIS since the current method of isolation from calf testes can only provide sufficient material for laboratory investigations.

Monoclonal antibodies against ovarian cancer antigens have also recently been prepared.[55,56] If these antibodies can be demonstrated to be specific for ovarian cancer then they may prove to be useful not only for therapy (either as cytotoxic antibodies or as antibodies complexed with toxins) but also for diagnostic studies.

Another potential immunotherapy for ovarian cancer would be the specific stimulation of endogenous cells capable of inhibiting tumor growth. Mantovani[48] has demonstrated that ascites from ovarian cancer patients contains a low number of NK cells. In an effort to stimulate NK activity Mantovani treated 8 patients with intraperitoneal C. parvum. Solid tumor masses were not affected by the intraperitoneal C. parvum although ascites was controlled in the majority of patients. An augmentation of intraperitoneal NK activity however was not demonstrated in this study.

Hormone Therapy

Hormonal treatment of ovarian cancer remains an unproven therapy.[52,53] It appears that progestins have a low level of clinical activity in unselected patients with epithelial ovarian cancer. Mangoni[57] treated 75 patients with either oral or intramuscular medroxyprogesterone acetate. While there were no responses in patients receiving oral MPA, there was a 15 percent response rate in patients receiving the i.m. drug suggesting that the higher systemic levels of MPA achieved by i.m. administration may be important in increasing the response rate. Endometroid tumors appeared to be more sensitive than other histologic types. However, the results of the Eastern Cooperative Oncology Group with MPA in heavily treated ovarian cancer patients suggest that the increased blood levels of MPA which occur after the i.m. route of administration are not the major factor for response to hormonal therapy. In the ECOG study i.m. MPA was administered to 19 heavily pretreated ovarian cancer patients and in contrast to the previous trial there were no responses observed.[50] Histologic subtypes were not reported in this study.

Numerous studies have confirmed the presence of cytoplasmic steroid receptors in epithelial ovarian carcinomas.[10] Approximately 50 to 67 percent of common epithelial ovarian cancers have cytoplasmic estrogen receptors. A more recent study has demonstrated that nearly all epithelial ovarian tumors have cytoplasmic androgen binding proteins.[14] The binding site concentrations (range 4 to 88 fmol/mg cytosol protein) and dissociation constants (K_d range 0.5 to 5.9 nmol/1) are characteristic of a cytoplasmic androgen receptor. However, there are no reported clinical studies of androgens or antiandrogens in ovarian cancer patients. There also have been no studies correlating the presence of receptors with additive hormonal therapy in ovarian cancer. The high incidence of estrogen receptors in ovarian tumors and the low (<10 percent) response rate in unselected ovarian cancer patients clearly indicates that response to additive hormonal therapy in ovarian cancer does not have as significant a correlation as exists in breast cancer patients.

There have been 2 reports which have suggested that antiestrogen therapy with Tamoxifen may be of some benefit to selected patients with ovarian cancer. Myers et al.[59] reported a complete remission with Tamoxifen in a refractory ovarian cancer patient lasting 18+ months. This patient's tumor contained both an estrogen and progesterone receptor. Schwarz et al.[60] reported on 13 patients who received Tamoxifen. One patient had a partial response and 4 patients had prolonged stable disease periods. All these patients had estrogen receptor levels that were borderline (15 to 29 fmol/mg protein) or high (58 to 162 fmol/mg protein).

In summary, all hormonal therapy in ovarian cancer remains strictly investigational. It is hoped that laboratory studies with an estrogen receptor positive human ovarian cancer cell line[15] and clinical studies correlating hormonal response with the presence of specific cytoplasmic steroid receptors will help establish the definitive role of hormonal therapy in ovarian cancer patients. In addition, it is possible that while hormones may not have a direct cytotoxic effect on ovarian cancer cells, they may have growth regulatory effects which could potentially be exploited to increase the cytotoxicity of cycle specific anticancer drugs.

Multimodality Treatment of Advanced Ovarian Cancer

The extent of residual disease after the initial laparotomy and prior to chemotherapy has been a major predictive factor for long term survival. In the M. D. Anderson series,[61] stage III patients with residual tumor masses all being less than 1.0 cm had a 5-year survival of 41 percent compared to only 9 percent for patients with tumor masses greater than 3.0 cm. Further support for the influence of tumor volume upon the ability to achieve a complete remission and thereby improve survival can be obtained from Table 9-1. The mean complete remission rate was only 11 percent for patients with bulky disease and 69 percent in patients with small volume disease. In addition, Griffith[62] has demonstrated that aggressive debulking surgery may improve survival in some patients with bulky ovarian cancer. These observations have led to the acceptance of debulking surgery as an integral part in the combined modality approach to the management of advanced ovarian cancer. However, as can be seen in Table 9-1, even at major cancer centers, most of which have aggressive gynecologic surgery, the vast majority (70 percent) of patients will still have bulky disease prior to the initiation of chemotherapy. Furthermore, the true value of debulking surgery in those 20 to 30 percent of advanced stage patients who can be successfully debulked to less than 2.0 cm disease can only be established in a prospective randomized trial.

The routine use of postoperative pelvic radiotherapy has not resulted in an improvement in survival for the vast majority of patients with stage III ovarian cancer.[63] Newer, more extensive radiotherapy techniques[64-66] in which the entire abdomen (including the diaphragm, liver and kidneys) is radiated are based upon careful staging studies (see above) which have demonstrated that the entire peritoneal surface is at risk for micrometastatic disease. The Princess Margaret Group has demonstrated that whole abdominal radiotherapy in asymptomatic patients with small volume stage III disease was superior to pelvic irradiation + chlorambucil.[64,65] The observations that (1) most patients with ovarian cancer cannot be surgically debulked, (2) radiotherapy appears to be an effective modality for small volume disease, and (3) the vast majority of stage III patients respond to therapy but most patients are left with residual disease have formed the basis of investigational studies of combined modality approaches to ovarian cancer. Fuks et al.[67] have used chemotherapy as the modality to achieve the initial debulking with the aim of increasing the number of patients who will be subsequently amenable to cytoreductive surgery and thereby likely to benefit from post-operative radiotherapy. After the initial chemotherapy and surgery to reduce all tumor masses to less than 2.0 cm, the patients are then treated with total abdominal radiotherapy administered via a series of AP/PA opposed fields. The whole peritoneal cavity is treated to a dose of 3000 rad in 20 fractions in 4 weeks, the pelvis receives 5100 rad in 33 fractions over 6 to 7 weeks, and the paraaortic lymph nodes and medial parts of the diaphragm receive 4200 rad in 28 fractions in 5 to 6 weeks. Finally, the total dose to the liver is 2250 rad and to the kidneys 2000 rad. In their initial series, 7 of 15 patients (11 of whom had bulky disease) have completed the proscribed course of chemotherapy-surgery-radiotherapy. Six of seven of these patients have remained disease-free 1 to 10 months after completion of radiotherapy.

The Johns Hopkins Group[68] has added immunotherapy together with aggressive surgery, chemotherapy, and irradiation in an investigative combined modality approach to stage III–IV ovarian cancer. Patients who have small volume disease after the initial debulking surgery receive intraperitoneal colloidal ^{32}P, followed by whole abdominal irradiation, and a year of melphalan. In addition, one half of these patients are randomized to receive intraperitoneal human ovarian antitumor serum (HOATS). Patients with residual macrometastatic disease following the initial surgery receive chemotherapy with hexamethylmelamine + cyclophosphamide and either adriamycin or cis-platinum on alternating cycles. These patients are also randomized to receive HOATS or no added immunotherapy. The toxicity of the whole abdominal radio-

Table 9-6. Rational for Combined Modality Approach (CHIPS) in Ovarian Cancer

I. Alternating non-cross resistant regimens
II. Radiation therapy with chemotherapy
III. Hypoxic cell sensitizers
  A. Intraperitoneal misonidazole
  B. Intravenous cis-platinum
IV. Implanted Tenckhoff catheter
  A. Increased intraperitoneal levels of misonidazole with decreased peak plasma levels leading to potentially decreased rate of neurotoxicity.
  B. Allows for collection of malignant cells to evaluate response to therapy.

therapy included mild/moderate nausea and vomiting and one instance of a bowel obstruction. Of the 13 patients who received HOATS, 6 developed a skin rash and 2 of these also had serum sickness. The results of this study have been presented in preliminary form. In patients with small volume disease the cumulative survival at 2½ years was 70 percent. In patients with bulky stage III or IV disease, the 1-year survival was 50 percent. The impact of the different therapeutic modalities upon end results in this study cannot be determined. The results in bulky stage III and IV patients (50 percent 1-year survival) are similar to previous reports for combination chemotherapy alone.

The Clinical Oncology Program, NCI, has recently instituted a radically different combined modality approach to the treatment of patients with stage III–IV ovarian cancer. In this study cycles of chemotherapy (cyclophosphamide + hexamethylmelamine) are alternated with cycles of combined modality therapy (total abdominal irradiation, intravenous cis-platinum and intraperitoneal misonidazole as a radiation sensitizer). The rationale for CHIPS study (C-cyclophosphamide, H-hexamethylmelamine, I-irradiation, S-sensitizer) is summarized in Table 9-6. Non cross-resistant modalities are used to threotically minimize the selection of drug resistant variants. Total abdominal radiation is included as one type of non cross-resistant therapy and is given every other month for a 5-day period at a daily dose of 200 rad by a split field approach. The total dose to the abdomen using this fractionation is 3000 rad. In addition, bulky masses receive a CT directed boost dose of irradiation. During each 5 day segment of radiation, the patients also receive 20 mg/m^2 of cis-platinum intravenously as well as 4 grams of misonidazole intraperitoneally. This appears to optimize the concentration of sensitizers within intraperitoneal tumors while decreasing the peripheral neuropathy associated with high dose intravenous misonidazole. The insertion of the Techkhoff catheter prior to therapy also allows for the collection of malignant cells for experimental studies as well as an additional means to follow therapy via cytologic examination of peritoneal washings. Since few patients have, as of this date, completed the prescribed therapy, the efficacy of this treatment remains to be established. However, preliminary analysis of toxicity results indicate that acceptable levels of myelosuppression are the major toxicity of this combined modality approach.

In Vitro Drug Sensitivity Testing

In 1978, Hamburger and Salmon[69,70] described an in vitro assay for determining the sensitivity of a wide variety of solid tumors to chemotherapeutic agents. The initial correlations between in vitro sensitivity/resistance[71] and clinical response led to a proliferation of laboratories performing in vitro tests and to the near acceptance of the human tumor stem cell assay (HTSCA) as a routine method for the individualization of chemotherapy. In many ways epithelial ovarian cancer is the prototype solid tumor for in vitro selection of chemotherapy: (1) the presence of malignant ascites and peritoneal washings frequently provide a ready source of tumor cells and invasive procedures are not required, (2) malignant effusions are easier to process than solid tumors which must be enzymatically dissociated to prepare the cell suspension required for drug testing, (3) there are a variety of drugs which have a response rate of 20 to 40 percent in previously untreated ovarian cancer patients, and (4) the response rate in relapsed patients is less than 10 percent.[33]

The initial report by Alberts et al.[72] demonstrated a 99 percent accuracy rate in predicting clinical resistance and a 62 percent accuracy rate in predicting a clinical response to therapy. The median duration of response in this trial was only 4 months. This same group recently[73] reported an update of this trial. In 22 patients treated on the basis of in vitro test results the overall response rate was 73 percent and the median survival was 12.6 months. In contrast, in 15 patients treated empirically, since only drug resistance was detected in vitro, the response rate was 20 percent and the median duration of survival was 4.5 months. Similar results were obtained by Natale and Kushner.[74] In 28 in vitro/in vivo correlations, the assay had a predictive accuracy of 77 percent for clinical sensitivity and 93 percent for resistance.

In contrast to these initial reports, subsequent larger studies with solid tumors pointed out some serious shortcomings of the HTSCA. Von Hoff[75] reported that sufficient tumor colony growth for in vitro testing (>30 colonies per plate) was obtained in only 199/800 (25 percent) of tumor specimens. Our experience with 156 malignant effusions[76] or malignant washings from ovarian cancer patients have been similar to those reported by Von Hoff.[75] Only 40 percent of the specimens produced sufficient colony growth for in vitro testing and in only 20 percent of these was an active drug identified. Thus in specimens from 100 relapsed ovarian cancer patients who have received prior therapy with a 3 to 4 drug combination chemotherapy regimen, only 8 to 10 instances of in vitro sensitivity can be expected and only 5 to 6 patients will likely respond to HTSCA directed therapy. Since the median duration of these responses will only be 4 to 6 months, it is clear that HTSCA therapy is not likely to be of benefit in the treatment of the vast majority of relapsed ovarian cancer patients. This of course is not due solely to the technical limitations of this assay but reflects the lack of available active agents for relapsed ovarian cancer patients.[33]

Some technical limitations of the HTSCA have recently been identified and include (1) difficulty in preparation of single cell suspensions, (2) lack of optimum growth conditions for specific tumor types and (3) growth of colonies from clusters of cells instead of from single clonogenic cells. In addition, it remains to be established that the assay is predictive for a specific drug(s) or merely is identifying those patients who are more generally responsive to chemotherapy. These technical limitations, coupled with the absence of sufficient numbers of active drugs for relapsed ovarian cancer patients together with the short duration of response in relapsed patients, make the HTSCA an experimental tool and not a clinically proven means for selection of chemotherapy in the standard practice of gynecologic oncology. There is no justification for withholding standard therapy merely on the basis of HTSCA results nor should patients undergo invasive procedures, e.g. laparotomy, solely to obtain tissues for stem cell analysis.

In contrast to the limitations of the HTSCA in the individualization of a patient's chemotherapy, the HTSCA has generated useful information regarding the patterns of cross-resistance in ovarian cancer.[37,77] It has also been useful as a model system in which to study dose-response relationships, in particular, how they relate to new therapeutic modalities such as intraperitoneal chemotherapy (discussed above) and high dose platinum. While the HTSCA allows for the assessment of patterns of drug resistance and the nature of the dose-response relationship, it is of limited utility in the study of the actual molecular mechanisms of resistance since the size of the colonies precludes most biochemical analyses. The HTSCA studies are therefore complemented by ongoing biochemical studies in established cell lines[15] which may help solve the vexing problem of drug resistance in ovarian cancer.

The HTSCA also has potential in the identification of new active agents for the treatment of ovarian cancer. In vitro "Phase II" trials may be a more rapid way to screen a variety of potential new agents.[78] The NCI is sponsoring an ongoing trial in which the HTSCA is being evaluated as a screening mechanism for new drugs. As part of this study, tumors from previously untreated patients including ovarian cancer are screened blindly against known active agents. The results of this study will provide the most definitive information to date regarding the validity of the assay as a means for identifying clinically useful anticancer drugs.

Table 9-7. Potential Role for Investigational Therapies in Ovarian Cancer

---

I. Stage I (Ia–Ib with well and moderately well differentiated tumors)
  A. Current Practice
    1. A beneficial role for any form of adjuvant therapy has not been established. The OCSG-GOG has an ongoing protocol of post-operative melphalan vs. no adjuvant therapy.
  B. Investigational therapy
    1. If the OCSG-GOG study demonstrates a need for adjuvant therapy, then the optimum type of therapy will need to be established.
II. Stage II and Poor Prognosis Stage I
  A. Current Practice
    1. The optimum standard modality has not been determined: single agent or combination chemotherapy, intraperitoneal ^{32}P, whole abdominal radiation.
  B. Investigational Therapies
    1. Intraperitoneal chemotherapy or immunotherapy, monoclonal antibodies, simultaneous intravenous and intraperitoneal chemotherapy, combined chemotherapy (i.p. or i.v.) and immunotherapy, HTSCA directed chemotherapy.
III. Small Volume Stage III
  A. Current Practice
    1. Combination chemotherapy or whole abdominal radiotherapy
  B. Investigational Therapies
    1. Same as for Stage II
IV. Bulky Stage III and Stage IV
  A. Current Practice
    1. Combination Chemotherapy
  B. Investigational Therapies
    1. Combined modality treatment [optimum timing of debulking surgery chemotherapy and radiation therapy], combined i.v. and i.p. chemotherapy, combination chemotherapy and immunotherapy, HTSCA directed therapy, and high dose chemotherapy (± autologous bone marrow support).

CONCLUSION

Table 9-7 compares the potential role of investigational therapeutic modalities to standard therapy in the management of patients with all stages of ovarian cancer. The cornerstone of present, and future, management of ovarian cancer is a careful and comprehensive laparotomy in which all sites of disease are documented. The following discussion of potential therapies assumes that definitive surgical staging has been performed.

Stage I

The need for postoperative adjuvant therapy in patients with stage Ia-Ib with well or moderately well-differentiated tumors remains to be established. The Ovarian Cancer Study Group together with the Gynocology Oncology Group are randomizing these patients to either observation or melphalan.[18] If this trial demonstrates that adjuvant therapy is beneficial then future studies will be required to determine the optimum adjuvant modality. It may be, however, that the survival of definitively staged stage I patients is so good that no adjuvant therapy is required. If definitive staging has not been performed, then it is likely that some form of adjuvant therapy will be useful (see below) since many of these patients will have unsuspected stage II–III disease.[17]

Stage II

The optimum postoperative treatment for stage II patients and poor prognosis stage I patients has not been determined. Therapeutic modalities currently under investigation include: single agent or combination chemotherapy; total abdominal irradiation, and intraperitoneal colloidal[32] P. If none of these modalities is demonstrated to be satisfactory, then those investigational procedures which have an experimental and theoretical basis to be of potential value in small volume residual disease will require evaluation, including: intraperitoneal chemotherapy or immunotherapy, HTSCA directed chemotherapy, simultaneous intravenous and intraperitoneal chemotherapy, and combined modality approaches.

Stage III—Small Volume Disease

It is clear that both combination chemotherapy and whole abdominal irradiation are effective therapeutic modalities for patients with small volume disseminated stage III disease. A direct comparison of the two modalities has not however been reported. In both previously untreated small volume stage III patients and in initially bulky patients who are left with small volume residual disease after induction therapy, the same investigational modalities as listed for stage II disease require evaluation.

Bulky Stage III and Stage IV

It is this group of patients in whom current treatment approaches are inadequate. Unfortunately, this group of patients also comprises the vast majority of patients with ovarian cancer. The standard approach to therapy with combination chemotherapy following the initial laparotomy has led to a PCR rate of only 11 percent. Accordingly it is appropriate that investigational therapies be evaluated in previously untreated patients with bulky disease since the standard approach is likely to produce long term survival in a small minority of patients. There are two major therapeutic goals in patients with bulky disease: (1) decrease the bulk of the disease and (2) eliminate the small volume disease which frequently is left after standard induction therapy. In an effort to control the bulk disease the major modalities are surgery and chemotherapy. The optimum sequence and timing for these two modalities remains to be established. In addition, new approaches to the induction chemotherapy such as high dose chemotherapy using the most active agents (cisplatinum and cyclophosphamide) perhaps even with autologous marrow support, or selection of active combinations using the HTSCA deserve immediate evaluation. Once the bulk disease is eliminated and patients are left with small volume disease, the same modalities previously discussed for stage III small volume disease may prove beneficial in inducing a complete remission. Again, the feasibility of immunotherapy will have to be established prior to studies aimed at optimizing the sequence and combination of this modality with other potentially active forms of treatment, including radiotherapy and intraperitoneal chemotherapy. The overall responsiveness of ovarian cancer and the development of a variety of new therapeutic modalities provides optimism that major therapeutic advances will be forthcoming in the not too distant future.

REFERENCES

1. Young RC, Chabner BA, Hubbard SP, et al: Advanced ovarian adenocarcinoma. A prospective randomized trial of melphalan (L-PAM) versus combination chemotherapy. N Eng J Med 299:1261, 1978.
2. Young TC, Howser DM, Myers CE, et al: Combination chemotherapy (CHex-UP) with intraperitoneal maintenance in advanced ovarian adenocarcinoma. Proc Amer Soc Clin Oncol 22:465, 1981.
3. Greco FA, Julian CG, Richardson RL, et al: Advanced ovarian cancer: brief intensive combination chemotherapy and second-look operation. Obstet Gynecol 58:199, 1981.
4. Parker LM, Griffiths CT, Yankee RA, et al: Combination chemotherapy with adriamycin cyclophosphamide for advanced ovarian adenocarcinoma. Cancer 46:669, 1980.
5. Ehrlich CE, Einhorn LH, Stehnman FB, et al: Response, "second look" status and survival in stage III–IV epithelial ovarian cancer treated with cis-platinum, adriamycin and cyclophosphamide. Proc Amer Soc Clin Oncol 21:423, 1980.
6. Donahoe PK, Swan DA, Hayashi A, et al: Mullerian duct regression in the embryo correlated with cytotoxic activity against human ovarian cancer. Science 205:913, 1979.
7. Fuller AF, Guy SR, Budzik GP, et al: Mullerian inhibition factor inhibits colony growth of a human ovarian carcinoma cell line. J Clin Endocrinol Metab 54:1051, 1982.
8. Donohoe P, Fuller AF, Scully RE, et al: Mullerian inhibiting substance inhibits growth of a human ovarian cancer in nude mice. Ann Surg 194:477, 1981.
9. Budzik G, Swann DA, Hayashi A, et al: Enhanced purification of Mullerian inhibiting substance by lectin affinity chromatography. Cell 2:909–915, 1980.
10. Hamilton TC, Davies P: Hormonal relationships in ovarian cancer. Rev and Rel Cancer, 1983 (in press).
11. Hamilton TC, Henderson WJ, Eaton C: Isolation and growth of the rat germinal epithe-

lium. In Richards RJ, Rajan KT (eds): Tissue Culture in Medical Research. Oxford, Pergamon Press, 1980, pp. 237–244.

12. Hamilton TC, Davies P, Griffiths K: Oestrogen receptor-like binding in the surface germinal epithelium of the rat ovary. J Endocr 95:377, 1982.

13. Holt JA, Little CR, Lorinez MA, et al: Estrogen receptor and peroxidase activity in epithelial ovarian carcinomas. J Nat Cancer Inst 67:307, 1981.

14. Hamilton TC, Davies P, Griffiths K: Androgen and oestrogen binding in cytosols of human ovarian tumors. J Endocr 90:412, 1980.

15. Hamilton TC, Foster BJ, Grotzinger KR, et al: Development of drug sensitive and resistant human ovarian cancer cell lines: A model system for investigating new drugs and mechanisms of resistance. Proc Amer Assoc Cancer Res, 1983 (in press).

16. Ozols RF, Fisher RI, Anderson J, et al: Peritoneoscopy in the management of ovarian cancer. Am J Obstet Gynecol 140:611, 1981.

17. Young RC, Wharton JT, Decker DB, et al: Staging laparotomy in early ovarian cancer. Proc Am Soc Clin Oncol 20:399, 1979.

18. Young RC, Walton L, Decker D, et al: Early stage ovarian cancer: Results of randomized trials after comprehensive initial staging. Proc Amer Soc Clin Oncol, 1983 (in press).

19. Vogl SE, Berenzweig M, Kaplan BH, et al: The CHAD and HAD regimens in advanced ovarian adenocarcinoma: Combination chemotherapy for ovarian carcinoma with cyclophosphamide, adriamycin and cis-dichlorodiammineplatinum (II). Cancer Treat Rep 62:1021, 1979.

20. Jones RB, Myers CE, Guarino AM, et al: High volume intraperitoneal chemotherapy ("belly bath") for ovarian cancer. Cancer Chemotherapy Pharmacol 1:161, 1978.

21. Speyer JL, Collins JW, Dedrick RL, et al: Phase I and pharmacologic studies of 5-fluorouracil administered intraperitoneally. Cancer Res 40:567, 1980.

22. Ozols RF, Young RC, Speyer JL, et al: Phase I and pharmacologic studies of adriamycin administered intraperitoneally to patients with ovarian cancer. Cancer Res 42:4265, 1982.

23. Speyer JL, Myers CE: The use of peritoneal dialysis in delivery of chemotherapy in intraperitoneal malignancies. In Mathe G, Muggia F (eds): Recent Results in Cancer Research. New York, Springer-Verlag, 1980, pp. 274–279.

24. Ozols RF, Speyer JL, Jenkins J: Phase II trial of 5-fluorouracil administered intraperitoneally to patients with refractory ovarian cancer. 1983 (in press).

25. Jones RB, Collins JM, Myers CE, et al: High volume intraperitoneal chemotherapy with methotrexate in patients with cancer. Cancer Res 41:55, 1981.

26. Howell SB, Pfeifle CE, Wung WE, et al: Intraperitoneal cisplatin with systemic thiosulfate protection. Ann Int Med 1982, (in press).

27. Jenkins JJ, Sugarbaker PH, Gianola FJ, et al: Technical considerations in the use of intraperitoneal chemotherapy administered by Tenckhoff catheter. Surgery 154:858, 1982.

28. Dedrick RL, Myers CE, Bugnay PM, et al: Pharmacokinetic rationale for peritoneal drug administration in treatment of ovarian cancer. Cancer Treat Rep 62:1, 1978.

29. Dunnick NR, Jones RB, Doppman JL, et al: Intraperitoneal contrast infusion for assessment of intraperitoneal metastases and fluid dynamics. Am J Roentgenol 133:221, 1979.

30. Howell SB, Chu BCF, Wung WA, et al: Long duration intracavitary infusion of methotrexate with systemic leucovorin protection in patients with malignant effusions. J Clin Invest 67:1161, 1981.

31. Young RC, Ozols RF, Myers CE: The anthracycline antineoplastic drugs. N Engl J Med 305:139, 1981.

32. Hubbard SM, Barkes P, Young RC: Adriamycin therapy for advanced ovarian carcinoma recurrent after chemotherapy. Cancer Treat Rep 62:1375, 1978.

33. Stanhope RC, Smith JP, Rutledge F: Second trial drugs in ovarian cancer. Cynecol Oncol 5:52, 1977.

34. Ozols RF, Grotzinger KR, Fisher RI, et al: Kinetic characterization and response to chemotherapy in a transplantable murine cancer. Cancer Res 39:3202, 1979.
35. Ozols RF, Locker GY, Doroshow JH, et al: Pharmacokinetics of adriamycin and tissue penetration in murine ovarian cancer. Cancer Res 39:3209, 1979.
36. Ozols RF, Willson JKV, Grotzinger KR, et al: Cloning of human ovarian cancer cells in soft agar from malignant effusions and peritoneal washings. Cancer Res 40:2743, 1980.
37. Ozols RF, Willson JKV, Weltz MD, et al: Inhibition of human ovarian cancer colony formation by adriamycin and its major metabolites. Cancer Res 40:4109, 1980.
38. Israel M, Pegg WJ, Wilkinson PM, et al: Liquid chromatographic analysis of adriamycin and metabolites in biological fluids. J Liq Chromatogr 1:795, 1978.
39. Howell SB, Taetle R: The effect of sodium thiosulfate on cis-dichloro-diammineplatinum (II) nephrotoxicity and antitumor activity in L1210 leukemia. Cancer Treat Rep 64:611, 1980.
40. Ozols RF, Myers CE, Young RC: The potential role of anthracyclines in the intraperitoneal chemotherapy of ovarian cancer. Excerpta Medica, 1983 (in press).
41. Young RC, Canellos GP, Chabner BA, et al: Chemotherapy of advanced ovarian carcinoma. A prospective randomized comparison of phenylalanine mustard and high dose cyclophosphamide. Gynecol Oncol 2:489, 1974.
42. Bruckner HW, Wallach R, Cohen CJ, et al: High dose platinum for the treatment of refractory ovarian cancer. Gynecol Oncol 12:64, 1981.
43. Ozols RF, Hamilton TC, Young RC, et al: Unpublished data.
44. Litterst CL: Alterations in the toxicity of cis-dichlorodiammineplatinum (II) and in tissue localization of platinum as a function of NaCl concentration in the vehicle of administration. Toxicol and Appl Pharmacol 61:97, 1981.
45. Ozols RF, Javadpour N, Deisseroth AB, et al: Treatment of poor prognosis non germinomatous testicular cancer with an effective high dose platinum regimen. Cancer, (in press).
46. Mandell GL, Fisher RI, Bostick F, et al: Ovarian Cancer: A solid tumor with evidence of normal cellular immune function but abnormal B cell function. Amer J Med 66:621, 1979.
47. Mantovani A, Polentaratti N, Gritti P, et al: K-Cell activity in ovarian cancer patients given chemotherapy. Eur J Cancer 15:797, 1979.
48. Mantovani A, Allavena P, Sessa C, et al: Natural killer activity lymphoid cells isolated from human ascitic ovarian tumors. Int J Cancer 25:573, 1980.
49. Mantovani A, Sessa C, Peri G, et al: Intraperitoneal administration of corynebacterium parvum in patients with ascitic ovarian tumors resistant to chemotherapy: Effects of cytotoxicity on tumor-associated macrophages and NK cells. Int J Cancer 27:437, 1981.
50. Knapp RC, Berkowitz DS: Cornyebacterium parvum as an immunotherapeutic agent in an ovarian cancer model. Am J Obstet Gynecol 128:782, 1977.
51. Order SE, Donahue U, Knapp R: Immunotherapy of ovarian carcinoma. An experimental model. Cancer 32:573, 1973.
52. Young RC: Gynecologic malignancies. In Pinedo R (ed): Chemotherapy Annual. 1981, pp 321–350.
53. Hogan WM, Young RC: Gynecologic malignancy. In Pinedo R (ed): Chemotherapy Annual. 1982, pp 309–338.
54. Alberts DS, Moon TE, Stephens RA, et al: Randomized study of chemoimmunotherapy for advanced ovarian carcinoma: A preliminary study of a Southwest Oncology Group study. Cancer Treat Rap 63:325, 1979.
55. Bast RC, Feeney M, Lazarus H, et al: Reactivity of a monoclonal antibody with human ovarian carcinoma. J Clin Invest 68:1331, 1981.
56. Bhattacharya M, Chatterjee SK, Barlow JJ, et al: Monoclonal antibodies recognizing tu-

mor associated antigen of human mucinous cystadenocarcinomas. Cancer Res 47:1650, 1982.

57. Mangioni C, Francheschi S, LaVecchia CB, et al: High-dose medroxy progesterone acetate (MPA) in advanced epithelial ovarian cancer resistant to first or second-line chemotherapy. Gynecol Oncol 12:314, 1981.

58. Slayton RE, Pagano M, Creech RH: Progestin therapy for advanced ovarian cancer: A Phase II Eastern Cooperative Oncology Group Trial. Cancer Treat Rep 65:895, 1981.

59. Myers AM, Moore GE, Major FJ: Advanced ovarian carcinoma: Response to antiestrogen therapy. Cancer 48:2368, 1981.

60. Schwartz PE, Keating G, MacLusky N, et al: Tamoxifen therapy for advanced ovarian cancer. Obstet Gynecol 59:583, 1982.

61. Smith JP, Day TA: Review of ovarian cancer at the University of Texas Systems Cancer Center, M.D. Anderson Hospital and Tumor Institute. Am J Obstet Gynecol 135:989, 1979.

62. Griffiths CT, Parker LM, Fuller AF: Role of cytoreductive surgical treatment in the management of advanced ovarian cancer. Cancer Treat Rep 63:235, 1979.

63. Fuks Z: External radiotherapy of ovarian carcinoma: Standard approaches and new frontiers. Sem Oncol 2:253, 1975.

64. Dembo AJ, Bush RA, Beale FA, et al: Ovarian Carcinoma: Improved survival following abdominopelvic irradiation in patient with a completed pelvic operation. Am J Obstet Gynecol 134:793, 1979.

65. Dembo AJ, Bush RS, Beale FA, et al: The Princess Margaret Hospital study of ovarian cancer: Stages I, II, and asympomatic III presentation. Cancer Treat Rep 63:249, 1979.

66. Glatstein E, Fuks Z, Bagshaw MA: Diaphragmatic treatment in ovarian carcinoma: A new radiotherapeutic technique. Int J Radiation Oncology Biol Phys 2:357, 1977.

67. Fuks Z, Rizel S, Anteby S, et al: The multimodal approach to the treatment of Stage III ovarian carcinoma. Int J Radiation Oncology Biol Phys 8:903, 1982.

68. Torres JLP, Bross DS, Hernandez E, et al: Multimodality treatment of patients with advanced ovarian carcinoma. Int J Radiation Oncology Biol Phys 8:1671, 1982.

69. Hamburger AW, Salmon SE: Primary bioassay of human tumor stem cells. Science (Wash. DC) 197:461, 1977.

70. Hamburger AW, Salmon SE: Primary bioassay of human myeloma stem cells. J Clin Invest 60:846, 1977.

71. Salmon SE, Hamburger AW, Soehnlen B, et al: Quantitation of differential sensitivity of human tumor stem cells to anticancer drugs. N Engl J Med 298:1321, 1978.

72. Alberts DS, Chen HSG, Soehnlem B, et al: In vitro clonogenic assay for predicting response of ovarian cancer to chemotherapy. Lancet 2:340, 1980.

73. Alberts DS, Chen HSG, Young L, et al: Improved survival for relapsing ovarian Cancer (OV CA) patients (pts) using the human tumor stem cell assay (HTSCA) to select chemotherapy (CRX). Proc Amer Soc Clin Oncol 22:462, 1981.

74. Natale RB, Kushner B: Applications of the human tumor cloning assay to ovarian cancer. Proc Amer Assoc Cancer Res 22:156, 1981.

75. Von Hoff DD, Casper J, Bradley E, et al: Association between human tumor colony-forming assay results and response of an individual patient's tumor to chemotherapy. Amer J Med 70:1027, 1981.

76. Ozols RF, Hogan WM, Young RC: Unpublished data.

77. Alberts DS, Chen HSG, Salmon SE, et al: Chemotherapy of ovarian cancer directed by the human tumor stem cell assay. Cancer Chemother Pharmacol 6:279, 1981.

78. Salmon SE, Meyskens FL, Alberts DS, et al: New drugs in ovarian cancer and malignant melanoma: In vitro Phase II screening with the human tumor stem cell assay. Cancer Treat Rep 65:1, 1981.

10 Epidemiology of Endometrial Cancer: A Review of Hormonal and Non-Hormonal Risk Factors

Noel S. Weiss

The endometrium is the lining of the body (corpus) of the uterus, and is the tissue in which most malignant tumors of this organ originate. In the past, tumors of the endometrium have not been unduly common, and they have been (and remain) tumors in which the case fatality is low. Nonetheless, sharp changes in incidence during recent years in the United States have brought endometrial carcinoma under close scrutiny by both the professional and lay community. One of the benefits of this scrutiny is an improved understanding of why endometrial carcinoma occurs.

This chapter reprinted in part with permission from Reviews in Cancer Epidemiology, edited by AM Lilienfeld, Vol. II, pp. 47–60, Copyright 1983 by Elsevier Science Publishing Co., Inc.

DEMOGRAPHIC CORRELATES OF THE OCCURRENCE
OF ENDOMETRIAL CARCINOMA

Time

In the United States, the last decade has seen large, rapid changes in the incidence of endometrial cancer. After a number of years of relative stability, the incidence in the early 1970's began to rise in most areas.[1] The increase in incidence was experienced primarily by women in the postmenopausal years, and was generally greater in the western than in the eastern part of the country (Table 10-1). The increase shown in the table is actually a modest *underestimate* of the true one that occurred.[2] The rate of hysterectomy (95 percent of which is performed for reasons other than cancer) rose rapidly during the same period, but the denominators of the cancer rates presented have not been corrected for this change.

Table 10-1. Annual Incidence[a] of Invasive Carcinoma of the Uterine Corpus, by Age: Connecticut and Alameda County (California), 1960–75

Time Period	Connecticut Age (years) 30–49	Connecticut Age (years) 50–69	Alameda County[b] Age (years) 30–49	Alameda County[b] Age (years) 50–69
1960–64	15.4	66.5	11.0	70.6
1965–69	13.7	67.9	15.7	109.8
1970–71	11.6	77.1	17.0	135.6
1972–73	16.7	84.4	23.2	195.4
1974–75	14.7	99.4	17.8	168.9
1976–77	12.6	87.9	13.4	200.3
1978–79	11.8	80.0	6.7	138.8

(Data from Marrett LD, Elwood JM, Meigs JW, et al: Recent Trends in the Incidence and Mortality of Cancer of the Uterine Corpus in Connecticut. Gynecol Oncol 6:183, 1978, and Uterine Cancer Incidence. Vol. V #1, State of California, Department of Health, 1978; and personal communications.)
[a] Rate per 100,000 adjusted, within the broad age groups shown, to a uniform standard (10-year age groups for Connecticut, 5-year age groups for Alameda County).
[b] Whites only.

Table 10-2. Annual Incidence of Endometrial Cancer[a] in Women 35–74 Years Old[3]

Range of Ages of Women, Yr	TNCS,[b] 1969–71	San Francisco– Oakland, 1969–71	CSS,[c] 1975, Excluding Carcinoma in Situ	CSS,[c] 1975, Post Histologic Review
			Annual Incidence of Endometrial Cancer According to:	
35–44	8.6	9.0	9.3	9.3
45–54	42.6	54.7	86.3	71.9
55–64	79.2	122.5	238.3	177.0
65–74	79.5	103.7	147.2	141.9
Total[d]	47.3	65.2	108.2	88.5

[a] Rate per 100,000 women.
[b] Third National Cancer Survey.
[c] Cancer Surveillance System of Western Washington.
[d] Adjusted to the age distribution of the 1970 U.S. population 35–74 years old.

Table 10-3. Annual Incidence[a] of Invasive Cancer of the Uterine Corpus Plus Uterine Cancer not Further Specified as to Site; Denmark, 1958–72

	Age (years)	
	30–49	50–69
1958–62	7.6	53.5
1963–67	6.8	53.3
1968–72	8.0	51.4

(Data from Clemmesen J: Statistical Studies in Malignant Neoplasms. V Munksgard, Copenhagen 1977, with permission.)

[a]Rate per 100,000 population, adjusted (within the broad age groups shown) to a uniform standard (5-year age groups).

Some of the elevation in incidence may be due to changes in the criteria used by pathologists for the diagnosis of endometrial carcinoma, and some is probably due to the increased incidence of estrogen-induced endometrial hyperplasia, a lesion whose morphology has many features in common with that of endometrial cancer and is sometimes labelled as such. Nonetheless, histologic reviews of cases diagnosed during the years of peak incidence, the mid-1970's, performed by pathologists using conservative criteria for the presence of cancer, found the incidence to be unequivocally raised over that of earlier years (Table 10-2).[3,4]

In the late 1970's in the United States the incidence of endometrial carcinoma declined (Table 10-1). In contrast to these rapid changes, the incidence during the past several decades *outside* of North America only increased slightly or not at all (Table 10-3).

All the trends cited above run parallel to patterns of postmenopausal estrogen use. Though introduced into medical practice in the 1920's, estrogens were not widely taken by postmenopausal women in this country until the 1960's. Even then, consumption was greater in the western U.S. than in other regions,[5] and outside of North America it remained sporadic.[6] Beginning in 1976, coincident with the documentation of the association between estrogens and endometrial cancer, there began a steady decline in the use of estrogens by American women.[7]

Nationality

Even prior to the estrogen-stimulated increase in the incidence of corpus cancer, rates among United States' Caucasians were greater than those among European women (Table 10-4).[8] The incidence among black and Asian women in the United States also has been considerably above that of their counterparts in Africa and Asia. In Hawaii, Chinese and Japanese women have higher rates of corpus cancer than Caucasians in Europe. The high rate among Asian women in Hawaii was present in the early 1960's as well,[9] arguing that factors other than exogenous estrogens have been responsible for it.

Table 10-4. Incidence of Cancer of the Uterine Corpus in Selected Populations[a]

Continent	Country	Area	Race	"Truncated" Incidence[b]
Africa	Nigeria	Ibadan	All	4.2
South America	Brazil	Recife	All	4.1
	Columbia	Cali	All	11.3
North America	USA	Detroit	White	44.1
			Black	20.8
		New Mexico	Spanish	17.9
			Other white	39.0
			Indian	11.4
Asia	India	Bombay	All	3.1
	Israel	All	Jews	22.9
			Non-Jews	3.1
	Japan	Miyagi	All	3.2
Europe	Norway	All	All	23.2
	U.K.	Oxford	All	20.7
	Yugoslavia	Slovenia	All	21.2
Oceania	USA	Hawaii	White	71.4
			Japanese	40.7
			Chinese	49.0
			Hawaiian	63.8
	New Zealand	All	Maori	58.1
			Non-Maori	22.8

(Data from Waterhouse J, Muir C, Correa P, Powell J (eds): Cancer Incidence in Five Continents, Vol. III. Lyon, IARC Scientific Publications No. 15, 1976, with permission.)

[a] Depending on population, rates apply to a part of the period 1969–72.

[b] Annual rate per 100,000 population ages 35–64 standardized to the age distribution of the world standard population.

Age

The relation of the incidence of endometrial cancer to age depends, in part, on the degree of exposure of the postmenopausal female population to estrogens. When estrogen use is uncommon, the rates rise rapidly in late reproductive life, peak in the 50's and 60's, and plateau or slightly decline in later life (Fig. 10-1). In populations in which estrogen use is widespread among women in their 50's and 60's, the peak in incidence at these ages is accentuated.

Race

Maoris in New Zealand experience a rate of corpus cancer more than twice that of non-Maoris (Table 10-4); the incidence among the latter is comparable to that of European whites. The high rate among Maoris is *not* due to an unusually high incidence of corpus cancer that is non-endometrial in nature (F. Foster: Personal communication). Hawaiian women also have a relatively high incidence of corpus cancer (Table 10-4), so it may be that some feature of their shared Polynesian background is responsible.

In other parts of the world the incidence of corpus cancer among Caucasians exceeds that among women of other races (Table 10-4). However, the white/black difference in the United States depends on age (Fig. 10-1), as it is not present in

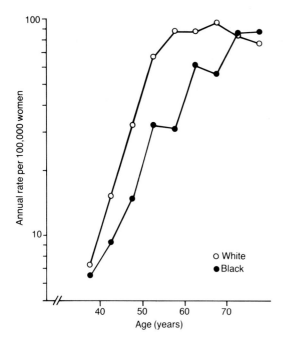

Fig. 10-1. Incidence of Cancer of the Uterine Corpus, by Age and Race: U.S. Third National Cancer Survey, 1969–71. (From The Third National Cancer Survey: Incidence Data. National Cancer Institute Monograph 41, March 1975—Third National Cancer Survey, with permission.)

women before the age of 40 nor beyond age 70. The similarity of rates at older ages is due at least in part to the inclusion of non-endometrial tumors (whose incidence rises rapidly with age and is higher in blacks than in whites) in the published data.

RISK FACTORS

Hormonal

Endogenous Estrogens. Cellular proliferation is a prerequisite for carcinogenesis.[10] Since estrogens are the primary stimulants of endometrial proliferation, it follows that their presence may be a necessary condition for the development of at least some endometrial carcinomas. The data available support such a role for estrogens:

1. In the presence of estrogen-secreting ovarian tumors, the prevalence of endometrial carcinoma at the time of oophorectomy ranges from 6 to 11 percent.[11–13] Even allowing for possible biases in the selection of cases and in the use of liberal criteria for the presence of uterine cancer, it is likely that the observed frequency of this second primary tumor is considerably greater than that expected.

2. Elevated levels of estrogens can arise from an excessive production of other hormones that can be converted to estrogens. For example, women who have polycystic ovaries and amenorrhea or oligomenorrhea (the polycystic ovary syndrome) secrete abnormally large quantities of androstenedione. This is aromatized peripherally, resulting in persistent estrone levels characteristic of the peak of the normal ovulatory

cycle.[14] An unusually high proportion of young women with endometrial cancer[15] and endometrial hyperplasia[16] have polycystic ovaries.

Several groups of women with the polycystic ovary syndrome have been followed with no cases of endometrial cancer found[17,18] but, as the expected incidence in these young women was exceedingly low, the presence of an increased *relative* risk could not be ruled out.

3.   Even when hormones such as androstenedione are produced in normal quantities, overly-high rates of conversion can produce elevated estrogen levels. For example, there is a 15- to 20-fold difference between very light and very heavy women in the speed with which they convert androstenedione into estrone[19] (the conversion is believed to occur primarily in adipose tissue, and represents the primary source of estrogens in postmenopausal women), and as a consequence serum estrogen levels of heavy women are far higher.[20] A consistent finding in studies of endometrial cancer is that cases are more likely to be overweight than controls;[21–27] the relative risk associated with being overweight has been estimated to be 2 to 20, depending in part on the criterion used to define it.

4.   The presence of menstrual cycles attests to the presence of estrogens, and women who continue to have cycles till relatively late ages, e.g. their 50's, are subsequently at greater risk of endometrial cancer than are other women.[22–27] Studies of this relationship need to avoid the potential bias of having uterine bleeding due to the presence of a tumor being mistaken for continuing menstrual activity. One study that did, by restricting the analysis to cases diagnosed at age 60 or greater, estimated that women whose menopause occurred at or after age 52 were at 2.4 times the risk of endometrial cancer of women whose menopause occurred before age 49.[23]

5.   Finally, the rate of androstenedione-to-estrone conversion, and the levels of plasma estrogens themselves, are higher in women with endometrial cancer than in controls.[20,28,29] While most of the difference can be accounted for by a difference in body weight between the two groups, the fact that the in vitro conversion rate in adipose tissue[30] of cases is higher than that in controls argues that other factors may be responsible as well.

Lack of Endogenous Progestogens.   Progesterone is the only endogenous progestogen of biologic importance. The surge of progesterone secretion that begins just prior to ovulation each month in the premenopausal woman causes endometrial proliferation to cease and shedding to take place. These are events that would be expected to discourage the development of cancer. Epidemiologic evidence is compatible with a protective effect of progesterone:

Premenopausal women.   Endometrial cancer is rare in premenopausal women. Its peak incidence occurs during the first or second decade after the menopause (Fig. 10-1), a time of life in which estrogen production continues (through peripheral conversion of adrenal androgens) but in which there is no cyclic progesterone available.

Polycystic ovary syndrome.   Women with the polycystic ovary syndrome, at increased risk of endometrial cancer (see above), are characterized not only by excessive production of estrogens (from androgens) but by the absence of cyclic progesterone secretion.[31]

Number of children.   A woman's probability of developing endometrial cancer is inversely related to the number of children she has borne.[22–26,32] While this observation has a number of possible explanations, there is at least a suggestion from other data that impaired fertility due to inadequate progesterone secretion could be responsible:

1. In women with endometrial cancer but no estrogen exposure, a history of long-standing menstrual irregularity is common.[33] Menstrual irregularity is often due to estrogen secretion that is not balanced by secretion of progesterone.

2. In contrast to the incidence of breast cancer, the incidence of endometrial cancer is unaffected by the age at which the first birth has occurred.[22-24] Thus a competing explanation for the association of endometrial cancer with low parity—that hormonal events acting at a specific susceptible period early in reproductive life are playing a role—is unlikely to be a valid one.

Exogenous Estrogens. For several decades, estrogens have been taken by women after the menopause, and early on it was appreciated that they develop adenomatous hyperplasia of the uterus more commonly than do other women.[34] Though the magnitude of this association has not been quantified well, its credibility is strengthened by the fact that some of these lesions regress completely when estrogens are discontinued.[35] Adenomatous hyperplasia itself probably represents an early stage in the development of carcinoma, as it frequently coexists with endometrial cancer in estrogen users and has been observed to precede the appearance of carcinoma.[36,37] Indeed, the histologic criteria for distinguishing the more advanced hyperplasias from early endometrial carcinoma are ambiguous (the morphologic characteristics of the ''minimal'' endometrial lesion whose growth is no longer under control are not known), and differences among pathologists exist in their use. Thus, differences among studies in the degree to which they find estrogens to be associated with endometrial cancer (see below) can partly be attributed to this classification problem.

A listing of published studies that have examined menopausal estrogen use in relation to endometrial cancer incidence is shown in Table 10-5. Excluded from the list are those whose design led to a falsely low measure of the magnitude of the association: (1) studies that failed to exclude women who had undergone hysterectomy from the control group, and (2) studies that included as controls women with estrogen-induced conditions, e.g. postmenopausal vaginal bleeding.

All but one of the 16 studies shown found that a greater proportion of women with endometrial cancer had taken estrogens than had controls. In addition, every one that examined the question found that the case-control difference increased with increasing duration of use. In general, the estimates of relative risk associated with long duration of use, e.g., >5 years obtained by the studies were in greater agreement than those for all durations combined.

Apart from duration of use, an estrogen user's excess risk of endometrial cancer depends upon various factors.

Time since first use. All studies showing a positive association agree that the estrogen user's risk of endometrial cancer exceeds that of the nonuser by the fifth year of use or earlier. The time at which the excess risk is *first* present is not clear: Some find it within the first year of use,[38,45] others not until the fifth year,[39,42] the rest in between.

Time since last use. All five studies that have examined this question observed

Table 10-5. Summary of Published Articles Relating Use of Menopausal Estrogens to the Incidence of Endometrial Cancer

First Author	Reference	Area of Residence or Hospitalization	Years of Diagnosis	#	% Estrogen Users	Relative Risk[a]	Time Since 1st Use	Time Since Last Use	Type of Estrogen	Dose	Cycling
				Cases			Information on Excess Risk Related to Patterns of Use				
Antunes	38	Balitmore, MD	1973–77	344	19	4.9	+	–	+	+	+
Gray	39	Louisville, KY	1947–76	205	22	3.0	+	–	+	+	–
Hoogerlund	40	Madison, WI	1960–74	587	18	2.3	+	–	+	–	–
Hulka	41	Chapel Hill, NC	1970–76	186	33	1.4	+	+	+	+	+
Jelovsek	42	Durham, NC	1940–75	431	12	2.4	+	–	–	–	–
Jick	43	Seattle, WA	1975–77	67	90	11.3	+	–	+	+	–
Kelsey	55	New Haven, CT	1977–79	148	32	3.0	+	–	+	–	–
MacDonald	44	Olmsted County, MN	1945–74	106	23	2.3	–	–	+	+	+
Mack	45	Southern California	1971–75	63	83	8.0	+	+	+	+	+
Salmi	46	Turku, Finland	1970–76	282	33	0.6	–	–	+	–	–
Shapiro	47	13 North American hospitals	1976–79	149	40	3.9	+	+	+	–	+
Smith	48	Seattle, WA	1960–72	317	48	7.5	–	–	–	–	–
Spengler	26	Toronto, Canada	1977	88	45	3.2	+	–	–	+	–
Stavraky	27	London, Canada	1976–78	206	47	4.8	+	+	–	+	+
Weiss	49	Seattle-Tacoma, WA	1975–76	322	78	7.0	+	+	+	+	+
Ziel	50,51	Los Angeles, CA	1970–74	94	57	7.6	+	–	+	–	–

[a]Risk of endometrial cancer among estrogen users relative to risk of 1.0 in nonusers. Definition of "use" varies by study, ranging from "any" to use for ≥ 1 year.

a fall in the excess risk once estrogen use ceased. In one of them there remained no residual excess risk once two drug-free years had elapsed,[41] but in the other four[27,45,47,49] some excess persisted. In none of the studies was the number of women who had discontinued estrogens large enough to arrive at a very precise answer to this question.

Type of estrogen. Every study listed found the use of conjugated estrogens to be associated with an increased risk of endometrial cancer. The one study that failed to find any excess risk associated with estrogen use[46] was conducted in Finland, where conjugated estrogens are rare among those hormones that are prescribed. Of the U.S. studies that examined the effect of other estrogens, e.g. stilbestrol or ethinyl estradiol, neither of which was in common use, eight of eleven observed a similar positive relationship for them.

Dose. In the range commonly prescribed, 0.3 mg to 1.25 mg per day of conjugated estrogens (or equivalent amount of other estrogens), the risk of endometrial cancer is elevated for all doses and appears to rise with increasing dose.

Periodic Interruption of Use. Many women who take estrogens are instructed to discontinue them for 1 week each month. Of the seven studies that compared this method to that of continuous exposure, two found risks highest from continuous use, two from cyclic use, and three found no difference. The fact that the incidence of endometrial hyperplasia is no different in groups of women on the two regimens[52] also argues that there is little to distinguish them in terms of subsequent cancer risk.

Though the most common reason for prescribing noncontraceptive estrogen preparations is the amelioration of symptoms of the menopause, estrogen use by other groups of women has permitted some evaluation of its long-term effects. Young women with gonadal agenesis who received stilbestrol (a synthetic, nonsteroidal estrogen) for prolonged periods had an unusually high incidence of endometrial cancer.[53] (Though there have been no studies of cancer incidence among untreated women with this condition, there is no biologic reason to suspect gonadal dysgenesis *per se* as an etiologic factor.) In a group of patients with breast cancer who had received estrogenic hormones (primarily stilbestrol) for treatment of their disease, the subsequent incidence of endometrial cancer was about twice that expected on the basis of rates in other breast cancer patients.[54]

The results of the studies of endometrial cancer in relation to use of noncontraceptive estrogens, taken together with: (1) the correlation of time trends in the incidence of endometrial cancer and estrogen use in the U.S.; (2) the growth-stimulating effect of exogenous estrogens on endometrial tissue that can lead to the development of pre-malignant lesions; and (3) the role that endogenous estrogens are known to play in the etiology of this cancer, argue strongly that exogenous estrogens are a cause of endometrial cancer. Endometrial neoplasms that arise from the action of these hormones do so relatively quickly, often in less than 5 years. In many women, this adverse effect of estrogens is "reversible," in that stopping the drug reduces the size of the excess risk within a year or two. Thus, it appears that exogenous estrogens act at a relatively late stage in the development of endometrial cancer, most likely through the stimulation of growth of cells with malignant potential.

Endometrial tumors that develop in estrogen users tend to be less invasive and more highly differentiated than the tumors of non-users.[38,41,42,44,49,59] This is reflected in a more favorable survival experience among estrogen-using cases.[56-59] There are reasons to believe that all of the following are responsible for this phenomenon:[60]

1. Some cases of estrogen-related adenomatous hyperplasia are falsely labelled as early endometrial cancer (see above).
2. On the average, endometrial cancer is detected earlier in estrogen users than in nonusers.
3. Endometrial tumors that arise in the presence of high estrogen levels tend to be biologically less aggressive than other endometrial tumors.

Lack of Exogenous Progestogens. When estrogen therapy is accompanied by periodic supplementation with a progestogen, the incidence of hyperplastic changes in the endometrium is greatly reduced.[61,62] It might be expected that the incidence of endometrial carcinoma would be reduced as well, and data from several studies suggest this is the case, whether that therapy is given for symptoms of the menopause[63,64] or for gonadal agenesis.[65] Women who are exposed to progestogens through their use of "combined" oral contraceptives have about one-half the incidence of endometrial cancer as do nonusers (Table 10-6),[55,66-69] despite the fact that these preparations contain an estrogen as well. The one oral contraceptive whose use led to an increased risk of

Table 10-6. Use of Combined Oral Contraceptives[a] Among Women with Endometrial Cancer and Among Controls

Use of Combined Oral Contraceptives	Patients With Cancer	Controls	Relative Risk[b]	95 Percent Confidence Limits
Yes[c]	17	76	0.5	0.1–1.0
No	93	173	1.0	—

(From Weiss NS, Sayvetz TA: Incidence of endometrial cancer in relation to the use of oral contraceptives. N Engl Med 302:551, 1980, with permission.)
[a] Subjects who had used sequential oral contraceptives for one or more years are excluded.
[b] Standardized for age and use of menopausal estrogens.
[c] Use for one or more years.

Table 10-7. Use of Sequential Oral Contraceptives Among Women with Endometrial Cancer and Among Controls

Use of Sequential Oral Contraceptives	Patients With Cancer	Controls	Relative Risk[a]	95 Percent Confidence Limits
Yes[b]	7	19	2.2	0.6–7.3
Oracon	6	8	7.3	1.4–38.8
Other	1	11	0.3	0.0–2.9
No	110	376	1.0	—

(From Weiss NS, Sayvetz TA: Incidence of endometrial cancer in relation to the use of oral contraceptives. N Engl J Med 302:551, 1980, with permission.)
[a] Standardized for age (35 to 39, 40 to 49, 50 to 54 years), use of combined contraceptives (less than a year vs. a year or more), and use of menopausal estrogens (less than a year vs. a year or more).
[b] Use for one or more years.

endometrial cancer (Table 10-7),[66,70] Oracon, was a sequential preparation that employed dimethisterone, a quite weak progestogen. (Oracon also contained a relatively large dose of ethinyl estradiol, a potent estrogen.)

How much progestogen is needed to obviate the increased risk of endometrial cancer in women who are taking postmenopausal estrogens? Because of the concern over the adverse effect of progestogens on the occurrence of cardiovascular disease, the answer to this question is more than academic. It appears that at least 10 days per month of progestogen is required, as the incidence of endometrial hyperplasia remains high if the hormone is used for shorter durations.[71,72] However, because relatively low doses of progestogen, e.g., 150 μg/day of D/L-norgestrel, 1 mg/day of norethindrone, have nearly the same effect as higher doses in: (1) reducing DNA synthesis and nuclear estradiol reception concentrations in endometrial cells; and (2) preventing the endometrial ultrastructural changes that occur with estrogen use,[73] these lower doses are appropriate to use at present.

Risk Factors not Known to be Hormonal

Abnormal Glucose Tolerance and Diabetes Mellitus. Though the relationship between diabetes and endometrial cancer has been commonly investigated and long-cited, there remains some doubt as to its nature and magnitude. Many studies have documented the frequency of abnormal glucose tolerance in cases but not in controls, and those studies that examined controls as well tended not to take into account confounding variables, e.g. body weight. In any event, the relevance of a woman's glucose tolerance after the diagnosis of cancer to that prior to the inception of cancer is uncertain. A case-control study which attempted to take account of these problems[23] *did* find an elevated frequency of antecedent diabetes among endometrial cancer patients, but three others observed no such relationship.[26,27,69] Finally, two studies that monitored the occurrence of cancer among cohorts of diabetics found neither the incidence of nor the mortality from endometrial cancer to be elevated.[74,75] However, both studies lacked statistical power to detect a relatively small excess. In summary, though abnormal glucose tolerance might predispose a woman to the development of endometrial cancer, the question is by no means settled.

Elevated Arterial Pressure. The study of the role of high blood pressure in the etiology of endometrial cancer is plagued by the same kinds of difficulties present for elevated blood sugar: inaccuracies in the retrospective assessment of hypertension, lack of standardized blood pressure measurements in routine clinical records, and the presence of important confounding variables which require control. At the present time it is unclear whether any relationship exists. Two studies that controlled for age and weight estimated the endometrial cancer risk in hypertensive women to be 50 to 100 percent greater than that among normotensives.[23,24] A third study also found a higher proportion of cases than controls to have high blood pressure, but there was an excess of women among the cases with low blood pressure as well.[22] Three additional studies found no association at all.[26,27,69]

Gall Bladder Disease. After taking exposure to exogenous estrogens into account, two studies[24,45] found a greater proportion of women with prior gall bladder disease among endometrial cancer cases than among controls. It is possible that this association is due to the association of endogenous estrogens to both conditions.

Radiation Exposure.   It is difficult to make any strong statement regarding the effect of radiation on the occurrence of endometrial cancer, for the results of a number of studies are in conflict; some favor a strong association,[76,77] others none at all.[78,79] Even in the studies that demonstrated a relationship, the possible confounding influence of the condition which led to therapeutic radiation was not evaluated.

Cigarette Smoking.   In the one study that examined the relationship,[24] a history of cigarette smoking was estimated to reduce the incidence of endometrial cancer by more than 50 percent. This benefit was present in both estrogen users and nonusers. The only measure of the amount of cigarette smoke to which the women were exposed was a fairly crude one (maximum number of cigarettes smoked per day), and no relationship of reduced risk to this measure was observed.

Cigarette smoking has an effect similar to that of estrogen lack on other body systems: Cigarette smokers have a greater prevalence of osteoporosis[80] and tend to experience menopause at an earlier age[81–85] than do nonsmokers. Thus, it is at least plausible that cigarette smoking could act to reduce the incidence of endometrial cancer through an anti-estrogen effect.

Genetic Factors.   In a study conducted in a population in which estrogen use was uncommon, there was little if any tendency for endometrial cancer to occur in families more often than would have been expected by chance.[22] It is not known whether one or more genetic factors act synergistically with exogenous estrogens to produce endometrial cancer.

FUTURE DIRECTIONS

It seems likely that the action of estrogens on the endometrium, whether the hormones are endogenously- or exogenously-derived, encourages the development of carcinoma. It seems equally likely that the action of progestogens, derived from whatever source, is the opposite. Knowledge of these effects will allow, through the judicious use (or nonuse) of these hormones, the prevention of many cases of endometrial cancer. Nonetheless, there will continue to be many women who produce relatively great amounts of estrogen and/or small amounts of progesterone. Many others will continue to use "unopposed" noncontraceptive estrogen preparations, because of concern with short-term and potential long-term adverse effects of supplemental progestogens. Thus, probably the most important thrust of future research into the etiology of endometrial cancer will be the identification of characteristics and exposures that interact with these gonadal hormones to produce or prevent the disease. Such characteristics and exposures as hypertension, low parity, obesity, etc., do not appear to interact with exogenous hormones in an important way, for the added risk of endometrial cancer attributable to estrogen use is similar whether or not these are present.[24] Nonetheless, to the extent that modifying factors can be identified, the knowledge of their presence in an individual woman can make her decision to use estrogens (and/or progestogens) a more informed one.

REFERENCES

1. Weiss NS, Szekely DR, Austin DF: Increasing incidence of endometrial cancer in the United States. N Engl J Med 294:1259, 1976.
2. Lyon JL, Gardner JW: The rising frequency of hysterectomy: Its effect on uterine cancer rates. Am J Epidemiol 105:439, 1977.
3. Szekely DR, Weiss NS, Schweid AI: The incidence of endometrial carcinoma in King County, Washington: A standardized histologic review. J Natl Cancer Inst 60:985, 1978.
4. Gordon J, Reagan JW, Finkel WD, et al: Estrogen and endometrial carcinoma: An independent pathology review supporting original risk estimate. N Engl J Med 297:570, 1977.
5. Jick H, Walker AM, Rothman KJ: The epidemic of endometrial cancer: A commentary. Am J Public Health 70:264, 1980.
6. Doll R, Kinlen LJ, Skegg DCG: Incidence of endometrial carcinoma. Lancet 1:1071, 1976.
7. Austin DF, Roe KM: The decreasing incidence of endometrial cancer: Public health implications. Am J Public Health 72:65, 1982.
8. Waterhouse J, Muir C, Correa P, et al (eds): Cancer incidence in five continents, Vol. III. Lyon, IARC Scientific Publications No. 15, 1976.
9. Doll R, Muir CS, Waterhouse J, (eds): Cancer incidence in five continents, Vol. II. Geneva, UICC, 1970.
10. Ryser HJP: Chemical carcinogenesis. N Engl J Med 285:721, 1971.
11. Diddle AW: Granulosa and theca cell ovarian tumors: Prognosis. Cancer 5:215, 1952.
12. Larson JA: Estrogens and endometrial cancer. Obstet Gynecol 3:551, 1954.
13. Salerno LJ: Feminizing mesenchymomas of the ovary—An analysis of 28 granulosa-theca cell tumors and their relationship to coexistant carcinoma. Am J Obstet Gynecol 84:731, 1962.
14. Siiteri PK, MacDonald PC: The role of extra-glandular estrogen in human endocrinology. Handbook of Physiology 2:615, 1973.
15. Dockerty MB, Lovelady SB, Foust GT, Jr: Carcinoma of the corpus uteri in young women. Am J Obstet Gynecol 61:966, 1951.
16. Chamlian DL, Taylor HB: Endometrial hyperplasia in young women. Obstet Gynecol 36:659, 1970.
17. Stein IF: The Stein-Leventhal syndrome—a curable form of sterility. N Engl J Med 259:420, 1958.
18. Leventhal ML: The Stein-Leventhal syndrome. Am J Obstet Gynecol 76:825, 1958.
19. MacDonald PC, Siiteri PK: The relationship between the extraglandular production of estrone and the occurrence of endometrial neoplasia. Gynecol Oncol 2:259, 1974.
20. Judd HL, Davidson BJ, Frumar AM, et al: Serum androgens and estrogens in postmenopausal women with and without endometrial cancer. Am J Obstet Gynecol 136:859, 1980.
21. Damon A: Host factors in cancer of the breast and uterine cervix and corpus. J Nat Cancer Inst 24:483, 1960.
22. Wynder EL, Escher GC, Mantel N: An epidemiological investigation of cancer of the endometrium. Cancer 19:489, 1966.
23. Elwood JM, Cole P, Rothman KJ, et al: Endometrial cancer: Fertility and other factors. J Natl Cancer Inst 59:1055, 1977.
24. Weiss NS, Farewell VT, Szekely DR, et al: Oestrogens and endometrial cancer: Effect of other risk factors on the association. Maturitas 2:185, 1980.
25. LaVecchia C, Franceschi S, Gallus G, et al: Oestrogens and obesity as risk factors for endometrial cancer in Italy. Int J Epidemiol 11:120, 1982.
26. Spengler RF, Clarke EA, Woolever CA, et al: Exogenous estrogens and endometrial can-

cer: A case-control study and assessment of potential biases. Am J Epidemiol 114:497, 1981.

27. Stavraky KM, Collins JA, Donner A, et al: A comparison of estrogen use by women with endometrial cancer, gynecologic disorders, and other illnesses. Am J Obstet Gynecol 141:547, 1981.

28. Hausknecht RU, Gusberg SB: Estrogen metabolism in patients at high risk for endometrial carcinoma. II. The role of androstenedione as an estrogen precursor in postmenopausal women with endometrial carcinoma. Am J Obstet Gynecol 116:981, 1973.

29. Schindler AE, Agathe E, Friedrich E: Conversion of androstenedione to estrone by human fat tissue. J Clin Endocrinol Metab 35:627, 1972.

30. Forney JP, Milewich L, Chen GT, et al: Aromatization of androstenedione to estrone by human adipose tissue in vitro. Correlation with adipose tissue mass, age, and endometrial neoplasia. J Clin Endocrinol Metab 53:192, 1981.

31. Lucas WE: Causal relationships between endocrine-metabolic variables in patients with endometrial carcinoma. Obstet Gynecol Surv 29:507, 1974.

32. Logan WPD: Marriage and childbearing in relation to cancer of the breast and uterus. Lancet 2:1199, 1953.

33. Peterson EP: Endometrial carcinoma in young women: A clinical profile. Obstet Gynecol 31:702, 1968.

34. Gusberg SB: Precursors of corpus carcinoma estrogens and adenomatous hyperplasia. Am J Obstet Gynecol 54:905, 1947.

35. Kistner RW: Endometrial alterations associated with estrogen and estrogen-progestin combinations. In Norris HJ, Hertig AT, Abell MR (eds): The Uterus. Baltimore, The Williams and Wilkins Co., 1973.

36. Gusberg SB, Hall RE: Precursors of corpus cancer. III. The appearance of cancer of the endometrium in estrogenically conditioned patients. Obstet Gynecol 17:397, 1961.

37. Gusberg SB, Kaplan AL: Precursors of corpus cancer. IV. Adenomatous hyperplasia as stage 0 of carcinoma of the endometrium. Am J Obstet Gynecol 87:662, 1963.

38. Antunes CMF, Stolley PD, Rosenshein NB, et al: Endometrial cancer and estrogen use: Report of a large case-control study. N Engl J Med 300:9, 1979.

39. Gray LA, Christopherson WM, Hoover RN: Estrogens and endometrial carcinoma. Obstet Gynecol 49:385, 1977.

40. Hoogerland DL, Buchler DA, Crowley JJ, Carr WF: Estrogen use—Risk of endometrial carcinoma. Gynecol Oncol 6:451, 1978.

41. Hulka BS, Fowler WC, Kaufman DG, et al.: Estrogen and endometrial cancer: Cases and two control groups from North Carolina. Am J Obstet Gynecol 137:91, 1980.

42. Jelovsek FR, Hammond CB, Woodard BH, et al: Risk of exogenous estrogen therapy and endometrial cancer. Am J Obstet Gynecol 137:85, 1980.

43. Jick H, Watkins RN, Hunter JR, et al: Replacement estrogens and endometrial cancer. N Engl J Med 300:218, 1979.

44. McDonald TW, Annegers JF, O'Fallon WM, et al: Exogenous estrogen and endometrial carcinoma: Case-control and incidence study. Am J Obstet Gynecol 127:572, 1977.

45. Mack TM, Pick MC, Henderson BE, et al: Estrogens and endometrial cancer in a retirement community. N Engl J Med 294:1262, 1976.

46. Salmi T: Endometrial carcinoma risk factors, with special reference to the use of oestrogens. Acta Endocrinol 233:37, 1980.

47. Shapiro S, Kaufman DW, Slone D, et al: Recent and past use of conjugated estrogens in relation to adenocarcinoma of the endometrium. N Engl J Med 303:485, 1980.

48. Smith DC, Prentice R, Thompson DJ, et al: Association of exogenous estrogen and endometrial carcinoma. N Engl J Med 293:1164, 1975.

49. Weiss NS, Szekely DR, English DR, et al: Endometrial cancer in relation to patterns of menopausal estrogen use. JAMA 242:261, 1979.
50. Ziel HK, Finkle WD: Increased risk of endometrial carcinoma among users of conjugated estrogens. N Engl J Med 293:1167, 1975.
51. Ziel HK, Finkle WD: Association of estrone with the development of endometrial carcinoma. Am J Obstet Gynecol 124:735, 1976.
52. Schiff I, Sela HK, Cramer D, et al: Endometrial hyperplasia in women on cyclic or continuous estrogen regimens. Fertil Steril 37:79, 1982.
53. Cutler BS, Forbes AP, Ingersoll FM, et al: Endometrial carcinoma after stilbestrol therapy in gonadal dysgenesis. N Engl J Med 287:628, 1972.
54. Hoover R, Fraumeni JF, Everson R, et al: Cancer of the uterine corpus after hormonal treatment for breast cancer. Lancet 1:885, 1976.
55. Kelsey JL, LiVolsi VA, Holford TR, et al: A case-control study of cancer of the endometrium. Am J Epidemiol 116:333, 1982.
56. Robboy SJ, Bradley R: Changing trends and prognostic features in endometrial cancer associated with exogenous estrogen therapy. Obstet Gynecol 54:269, 1979.
57. Elwood JM, Boyes DA: Clinical and pathological features and survival of endometrial cancer patients in relation to prior use of estrogens. Gynecol Oncol 10:173, 1980.
58. Collins J, Allen LH, Donner A, et al: Oestrogen use and survival in endometrial cancer. Lancet 2:961, 1980.
59. Chu J, Schweid AI, Weiss NS: Survival among women with endometrial cancer: A comparison of estrogen users and nonusers. Am J Obstet Gynecol 143:569, 1982.
60. Weiss NS: Noncontraceptive estrogens and abnormalities of endometrial proliferation. Ann Intern Med 88:410, 1978.
61. Whitehead MI: The effects of oestrogens and progestogens on the postmenopausal endometrium. Maturitas 1:87, 1978.
62. Paterson MEL, Wade-Evans T, Sturdee DW, et al: Endometrial disease after treatment with oestrogens and progestogens in the climacteric. Br Med J 1:822, 1980.
63. Gambrell RD, Massey FM, Castaneda TA, et al: Reduced incidence of endometrial cancer among postmenopausal women treated with progestogens. J Am Geriatr Soc 27:389, 1979.
64. Hammond CB, Jelovsek FR, Lee K, et al: Effects of long-term estrogen replacement therapy. II. Neoplasia. Am J Obstet Gynecol 133:537, 1979.
65. Benjamin I, Block RE: Endometrial response to estrogen and progesterone therapy in patients with gonadal dysgenesis. Obstet Gynecol 50:136, 1977.
66. Weiss NS, Sayvetz TA: Incidence of endometrial cancer in relation to the use of oral contraceptives. N Engl J Med 302:551, 1980.
67. Kaufman DW, Shapiro S, Slone D, et al: Decreased risk of endometrial cancer among oral contraceptive users. N Engl J Med 303:1045, 1980.
68. Kay CR: The happiness pill? J R Coll Gen Pract 30:8, 1980.
69. Hulka BS, Chambless LE, Kaufman DG, et al: Protection against endometrial carcinoma by combination-product oral contraceptives. JAMA 247:475, 1982.
70. Silverberg SG, Makowski EL, Roche WD: Endometrial carcinoma in women under 40 years of age. Cancer 39:592, 1977.
71. Studd JWW, Thom MH, Paterson MEL, et al: The prevention and treatment of endometrial pathology in postmenopausal women receiving exogenous estrogens. In Pasetto N, Paoletti R, Ambrus JL (eds): The Menopause and Postmenopause. Lancaster, MTP Press, 1980.
72. Whitehead MI, King RJB, McQueen J, et al: Endometrial histology and biochemistry in climacteric women during oestrogen and oestrogen/progestogen therapy. J R Soc Med 72:322, 1979.

73. Whitehead MI, Townsend PT, Pryse-Davies J, et al: Effects of estrogens and progestins on the biochemistry and morphology of the postmenopausal endometrium. N Eng J Med 305:1599, 1981.

74. Kessler II: Cancer mortality among diabetics. J Nat Cancer Inst 44:673, 1970.

75. Ragozzino M, Melson LJ, Chu C-P, et al: Subsequent cancer risk in the incidence cohort of Rochester, Minnesota, residents with diabetes mellitus. J Chronic Dis 35:13, 1982.

76. Corscaden JA, Fertig JW, Gusberg SB: Carcinoma subsequent to the radiotherapeutic menopause. Am J Obstet Gynecol 51:1, 1946.

77. Stander RW: Irradiation castration: A follow-up study of results in benign pelvic disease. Obstet Gynecol 10:223, 1957.

78. Hunter RM, Ludwick NV, Motley JF, et al. The use of radium in the treatment of benign lesions of the uterus: A critical twenty-year survey. Am J Obstet Gynecol 67:121, 1954.

79. Doll R, Smith PG: The long-term effects of X irradiation in patients treated for metropathia haemorrhagica. Br J Radiol 41:362, 1968.

80. Daniell HW: Osteoporosis of the slender smoker: Vertebral compression fractures and loss of metacarpal cortex in relation to postmenopausal cigarette smoking and lack of obesity. Arch Intern Med 136:298, 1968.

81. Jick H, Porter J, Morrison AS: Relation between smoking and age of natural menopause. Lancet 1:1354, 1977.

82. Bailey A, Robinson D, Vessey M: Smoking and age of natural menopause. Lancet 2:722, 1977.

83. McNamara PM, Hjortland MC, Gordon T, et al: Natural history of menopause: The Framington Study. J Cont Ed Ob Gyn 20:27, 1978.

84. Lindquist O, Bengtsson C: The effect of smoking on menopausal age. Maturitas 1:171, 1979.

85. Kaufman DW, Slone D, Rosenberg L, et al: Cigarette smoking and age at natural menopause. Am J Public Health 70:420, 1980.

11 | Approaches to the Evaluation and Management of Endometrial Carcinoma

James Tate Thigpen

Cancer of the uterine corpus has now become the most common invasive malignancy of the female pelvis in the United States. Over 38,000 women will develop this disease each year.[1] The overall incidence, furthermore, has continued to increase. These facts, combined with the relatively high probability of cure (66 percent)[2] if the process is diagnosed early and managed properly, necessitate a thorough understanding on the part of the physician of the proper approach to these patients. The ensuing discussion will present relevant facts about the disease process and will then assimilate these facts into a rational approach to the patient. Because endometrial carcinomas represent an overwhelming majority of cancers of the uterine corpus, considerations will be confined to this group of neoplasms. Finally, the primary purpose of discussion will not be to provide detailed pathophysiology but rather a rational framework for patient management.

THE DISEASE PROCESS

Clinical Characteristics

Endometrial carcinoma is a disease which affects primarily menopausal and postmenopausal women with a median patient age of 61.[3] Only 25 percent of cases are diagnosed prior to the menopause, and less than 5 percent are diagnosed prior to age 40.[4,5] A number of personal risk factors have been noted: obesity,[6] nulliparity,[7] late menopause,[3] diabetes,[8] hypertension,[3] immunodeficiency, and exogenous estrogens.[9] A more detailed consideration of these associated factors can be found in the preceding chapter. The precise mechanisms which underlie these observed associations are largely unknown.

The cardinal presenting manifestation of endometrial carcinoma is dysfunctional uterine bleeding. Certainly not all cases of dysfunctional bleeding result from endometrial carcinoma, but nearly 20 percent of abnormal bleeding in the postmenopausal woman will result from malignancy with a majority of these malignancies being endometrial carcinoma.[10] Over 90 percent of endometrial carcinomas, furthermore, will present with dysfunctional bleeding.[10] Purulent discharge and pain, the latter usually a late manifestation, may also be presenting complaints.

In summary, the profile of a typical patient with endometrial carcinoma is that of an obese, diabetic, hypertensive, menopausal or postmenopausal woman who presents with dysfunctional uterine bleeding (Table 11-1). Any such patient with dysfunctional uterine bleeding, particularly if she demonstrates any of those factors associated with endometrial carcinoma, deserves thorough evaluation for possible malignancy.

Pathology

Evaluation of a patient with symptoms suggestive of endometrial carcinoma requires that tissue be obtained from the uterine cavity. If endometrial carcinoma is present, the most likely histologic finding is that of adenocarcinoma. Approximately

Table 11-1. Clinical Characteristics of the Patient
with Endometrial Carcinoma

Median Age
61 years
Associated Factors
Obesity
Nulliparity
Late menopause
Diabetes
Hypertension
Immunodeficiency
Exogenous estrogens
Presenting Manifestations
Dysfunctional uterine bleeding
Purulent vaginal discharge
Pain

Table 11-2. Frequency of Five Histologic Types
of Endometrial Carcinoma

Histology	Frequency
Adenocarcinoma	70%
Adenoacanthoma	10%
Adenosquamous carcinoma	20%
Clear cell carcinoma	<1%
Squamous cell carcinoma	<1%

70 percent of patients will have pure adenocarcinoma. The majority of the remaining 30 percent will show adenocarcinoma mixed with either areas of squamous metaplasia (adenoacanthoma) or elements of squamous carcinoma (adenosquamous carcinoma).[11–13] Rarely, clear cell carcinoma or pure squamous carcinoma is demonstrated (Table 11-2). Whether the histologic type makes any difference in terms of prognosis or response to therapy is not clear. Although adenosquamous carcinoma has been thought to carry a poorer prognosis than adenocarcinoma, there is little evidence to support this if data are corrected for stage and grade.[12] Adenoacanthomas, however, may well have a slightly better outlook.[12] Clear cell carcinoma, although rare, appears to bode a poor prognosis,[14–18] while pure squamous carcinoma is too rare to permit comment.[19] The major prognostic differences among these five types appear to relate mostly to the frequency with which the lesions are poorly differentiated or more advanced in stage.

Of greater significance than the histologic type is the degree of histologic differentiation or grade of the endometrial carcinoma (Table 11-3). Grade is usually described in three groups: well-differentiated (grade 1), moderately differentiated (grade 2), and poorly differentiated (grade 3). Grade one tumors are most common (45 percent of all cases), whereas grade two (35 percent) and grade three (20 percent) neoplasms occur less frequently.[20] The overall impact of grade or survival is well documented in a review of 15 series involving 3,990 patients with better differentiated neoplasms showing better survival (Table 11-3).[21] This difference persists if extent of disease is held constant by considering only clinical stage I cases (Table 11-4).

In summary, sampling of the endometrium is essential to establish a histologic diagnosis of endometrial carcinoma and the degree of differentiation or grade. Whereas the histologic type of endometrial carcinoma appears to make little or no difference, grade is an independent prognostic variable and hence an important factor in decisions regarding patient management.

Table 11-3. Histologic Grade: Overall Frequency and
Impact on Survival of Endometrial
Carcinomas

Grade	Frequency[20] (n = 12840)	5-Year Survival[21] (n = 3990)
1	45%	81%
2	35%	74%
3	20%	50%

Table 11-4. Histologic Grade: Impact on Survival of Clinical Stage I Endometrial Carcinoma

	5-Year Survival		
Grade	Stage I[23]	Stage IA[22]	Stage IB[22]
1	93%	93%	90%
2	87%	86%	76%
3	70%	68%	63%

Patterns of Spread

Carcinoma of the uterine corpus arises from the glandular component of the endometrial mucosa and may be preceded by endometrial hyperplasia which demonstrates dysplastic changes (adenomatous hyperplasia). Initial growth usually produces an exophytic, friable mass within the uterine cavity and results in spontaneous bleeding as the initial manifestation of the disease. Both vertical and horizontal extension of the neoplasm ensues with consequent invasion of the myometrium and involvement of the uterine cervix. Spread beyond the uterus can take place by any of three routes: lymphatic metastases to parametrial, pelvic, inguinal, and para-aortic lymph nodes; hematogenous dissemination most commonly to lungs and less frequently to liver or bone; and peritoneal implantation from either transtubal spread or vertical penetration of the entire thickness of the uterine wall.

These patterns of spread and the impact of the extent to which clinical evidence of such spread is present are reflected in the current clinical staging system developed by the International Federation of Gynecology and Obstetrics (FIGO) (Table 11-5).[24] This system reflects patient survival reasonably well (Table 11-6), but the value of the system in reaching management decisions is limited by the fact that 75 percent of all cases are clinical stage I.[25] An accurate and detailed evaluation of extent of dis-

Table 11-5. FIGO Clinical Staging System for Endometrial Carcinoma

Stage	Description
Stage 0	Carcinoma in situ. Histological findings suspicious of malignancy
Stage I	Carcinoma is confined to corpus including isthmus
IA	Length of uterine cavity ≤8 cm
IB	Length of uterine cavity >8 cm
Stage I should be subgrouped by grade.	
G1	Highly differentiated adenomatous carcinoma
G2	Differentiated adenomatous carcinomas with partly solid areas
G3	Predominantly solid or entirely undifferentiated carcinoma
Stage II	Carcinoma has involved corpus and cervix but has not extended outside uterus
Stage III	Carcinoma has extended outside uterus but not outside true pelvis
Stage IV	Carcinoma has extended outside true pelvis or has involved bladder or rectal mucosa. Bullous edema does not make a case stage IV
IVA	Spread to adjacent organs
IVB	Spread to distant organs

Table 11-6. Clinical Stage (FIGO): Frequency of
Each Stage and Impact on 5-year
Survival (17,021 patients)

Stage	Frequency	5-Year Survival
I	75%	76%
II	13%	50%
III	9%	30%
IV	3%	9%
Total	100%	66%

ease to a greater degree than that reflected by the clinical stage may well be critical to proper management of these clinical stage I patients. Observations relevant to determining the degree of detail required in evaluating clinical stage I disease will be presented later (see Prognostic Factors).

Patterns of Recurrence

Recurrence after initial treatment with surgery and/or radiotherapy is most commonly extrapelvic in such locations as lungs, liver, bone, and the abdominal cavity. Other areas in which recurrent disease is not uncommonly seen include lymph nodes (inguinal, para-aortic, and supraclavicular), vaginal vault, parametrium, and pelvic wall. Of these failures, 70 percent are diagnosed within the first 2 years after treatment.[26] Patients who recur later than 5 years after initial diagnosis tend to be those who presented with more favorable disease initially, e.g., stage I grade 1 adenocarcinoma.

DIAGNOSIS

Any patient who presents with dysfunctional uterine bleeding, particularly those in the peri-menopausal and postmenopausal age groups, should be evaluated carefully for evidence of endometrial carcinoma. An absolute requirement of such an evaluation is a microscopic examination of samples of endometrial tissue. The simplest approach is the Papanicolaou smear, but the diagnostic accuracy of this technique is only 40 percent,[27] significantly less than the accuracy in cervix carcinoma. Aspiration curettage in the outpatient setting by a variety of techniques yields a higher rate of accuracy (up to 70 percent),[28] but a negative result obviously does not rule out malignancy. For a more accurate and complete evaluation, dilatation and fractional curettage will be required and will permit assessment for endocervical involvement.

Additional techniques advocated in the diagnostic evaluation include hysteroscopy and hysterography. Hysteroscopy[29] offers the advantage of a more complete curettage of the endometrial lining and is useful primarily in the patient with persistent, unexplained dysfunctional bleeding after a negative fractional curettage. Hysterography,[30] on the other hand, should be viewed as a technique which can provide information about volume, location, and configuration of an intracavitary tumor as well as clues to the degree of myometrial penetration. The technique is not, however, a substitute for endometrial tissue sampling and the establishment of a definite histologic diagnosis.

In summary, the establishment of a diagnosis of endometrial carcinoma requires endometrial tissue sampling which may necessitate a fractional currettage. There is no substitute for a definite histologic diagnosis.

PRETREATMENT EVALUATION

Once a diagnosis of endometrial carcinoma has been established, accurate and detailed knowledge of the histology and extent of disease is an absolute necessity to appropriate patient management. The planning of such an evaluation should take into account major prognostic factors to be identified and appropriate techniques to assess these factors.

Prognostic Factors

Previous discussion has already identified histologic grade and extent of disease as two major prognostic variables. Because of the previously noted frequency of clinical stage I disease, a more detailed assessment of important clinical and pathologic features is needed to identify high-risk and low-risk patient subsets.

Clinical Factors. Two clinical factors appear to provide clues as to probable disease outcome (Table 11-7).

Age. Age of the patient at the time of diagnosis correlates with expected five year survival with patients younger than 70 years having a much better survival rate (84 percent versus 61 percent):[31] Closer analysis reveals this to be a difference related to stage, grade, and depth of myometrial penetration rather than age per se. Younger patients tended to have less advanced, better differentiated disease than older patients. These observations have subsequently been confirmed by two other series.[32–33]

Size of the uterine cavity. Size of the uterine cavity as determined by sounding the depth of the cavity has also been reported to predict survival. Patients with cavities less than or equal to 8 centimeters in depth have slightly better 5-year survival rates than those patients with larger uterine cavities in some series,[34–39] but other

Table 11-7. Impact of Patient Age and Depth of Uterine Cavity on Survival in Clinical Stage I Endometrial Carcinoma

Prognostic Factor	5-Year Survival
Age[31]	
<70 years (n = 512)	84%
≥70 years (n = 106)	61%
Depth of uterine cavity[34–39]	
≤8 cm (n = 722)	76%
>8 cm (n = 447)	66%

series[33,40] show no difference. One potential source of error is the presence of benign abnormalities which might distort and hence enlarge the uterine cavity.

In summary, the two clinical factors of age and depth of uterine cavity do offer clues as to prognosis but appear to be less important than specific pathologic factors as predictors of outcome.

Pathologic Factors. The medical literature is replete with retrospective studies and small prospective studies which assess the relative prognostic significance of a variety of pathologic features of endometrial carcinoma.[12,14-19,22-23,41-64] A number of features are identified as having prognostic significance: histologic grade, depth of myometrial penetration, involvement of the uterine cervix, vascular space invasion, and evidence of extrauterine extension to other pelvic organs, lymph nodes, peritoneal cavity, or distant sites. Accurate assessment of the relative importance of these factors is difficult, if not impossible, because of the relatively small numbers of patients in certain subgroups and the lack of uniformity of surgical technique and pathologic evaluation of tissue. Because of the potential importance of identifying subgroups of patients within clinical stage I at high risk for recurrence, prospective studies in clinical stage I cases on a small and subsequently a much larger scale were untaken by the Gynecologic Oncology Group (GOG).[65-68] Results of these prospective studies will be emphasized in the ensuing definition of significant prognostic factors. Five-year survival data are not yet available for the GOG patients, so results will be expressed as frequency of recurrence and death after a minimum of three years of follow-up.

The patient population in the initial GOG prospective study includes only clinical stage I cases of endometrial carcinoma. The distribution of histologic types and FIGO substage are shown in Table 11-8.[67] This distribution is typical of that reported in the literature and presented earlier. The relatively small number of adenoacanthomas and adenosquamous carcinomas renders statements regarding prognostic impact impossible.

Histologic grade. Histologic grade has already been presented as a major prognostic factor. This observation is supported by the results of the initial prospective study of the GOG. The frequency with which each grade is seen among clinical stage I cases parallels that reported in the literature,[67] as do the relative frequencies of recurrence and death by grade (Table 11-9).[68]

Depth of myometrial invasion. Depth of myometrial invasion is cited in vir-

Table 11-8. Composite of Study Population of GOG Prospective Trial of Clinical Stage I Endometrial Carcinomas with Regard to Histologic Type and FIGO Substages

Factor	Patients	Percent
Histologic type		
Adenocarcinoma	184	83%
Adenoacanthoma	15	7%
Adenosquamous carcinoma	23	10%
FIGO Stage		
IA	130	59%
IB	92	41%

tually all series in the literature as a major prognostic factor. As can be seen in Table 11-10, deep myometrial penetration (outer ⅓) was seen relatively uncommonly among clinical stage I patients in the initial prospective study.[67] The presence of deep invasion predicted for a high recurrence and death rate and thus confirms observations in numerous retrospective series.[68]

Table 11-9. Histologic Grade: GOG Prospective Study of Frequency and Impact on Recurrence and Death in Clinical Stage I Endometrial Carcinoma (n = 222)[67,68]

Grade	Frequency[67]	Recurrence Rate[68]	Death Rate[68]
Grade 1	42%	4%	5%
Grade 2	40%	15%	13%
Grade 3	18%	42%	29%

Table 11-10. Depth of Myometrial Penetration: GOG Study of Frequency and Impact on Recurrence and Death Rate in Clinical Stage I Endometrial Carcinoma (n = 222)[67,68]

Depth of Myometrial Invasion	Frequency	Recurrence Rate	Death Rate
Endometrium only	41%	8%	5%
Superficial muscle (inner ⅓)	36%	13%	11%
Intermediate muscle (middle ⅓)	8%	12%	12%
Deep muscle (outer ⅓)	15%	46%	36%

Table 11-11. Lymph Node Involvement: GOG Prospective Study of Frequency and Impact on Recurrence and Death Rate in Clinical Stage I Endometrial Carcinoma (n = 222)[67,68]

Nodes	Frequency	Recurrence Rate	Death Rate
Pelvic nodes			
Involved	10.4%	57%	52%
Not involved	89.6%	11%	5%
Para-aortic nodes			
Involved	7.6%	59%	53%
Not involved	92.4%	11%	8%

Table 11-12. Peritoneal Cytology: GOG Prospective Study of Frequency of Positivity and Impact on Recurrence and Death Rates in Clinical Stage I Endometrial Carcinoma (n = 171)[67,68]

Cytologic Findings	Frequency[67]	Recurrence Rate[68]	Death Rate[68]
Positive	15%	38%	50%
Negative	85%	10%	7%

Lymph node involvement.   Lymph node involvement has been reported in a surprising percentage of patients with clinical stage I disease.[50,53,69] Pelvic lymph nodes were found, in these retrospective series, to be involved in 9 to 12 percent of patients. The prospective GOG trial confirms these observations and notes a 7.6 percent incidence of para-aortic node involvement (Table 11-11).[67] A notably higher frequency of recurrence and death was seen in those patients with evidence of lymph node involvement.[68] The status of the pelvic nodes is an excellent indicator of para-aortic node involvement.[67] In those patients with negative pelvic nodes, only one percent had positive para-aortic nodes, whereas positive pelvic nodes were associated with positive para-aortic nodes in at least 50 percent of cases.

Positive peritoneal cytology.   Positive peritoneal cytology was evaluated in the GOG study and appeared to correlate with a high risk for recurrence and death (Table 11-12).[67,68] This finding also confirms previous data.[70]

Adnexal spread.   Adnexal spread was found in 7.2 percent of patients in the GOG study and likewise correlated with subsequent recurrence and death (Table 11-13).[67,68] Spread to other extra-uterine structures within the pelvis was less frequently observed (tubes 5 percent, ovaries 4.5 percent, pelvic wall 1 percent) but did predict for recurrence and death.[67]

Vascular invasion.   Vascular invasion in association with the primary tumor has been reported to influence the rate of recurrence and subsequent death. In one series of patients with clinical stage I endometrial carcinoma,[41] patients with evidence of vascular invasion had a death rate of 27 percent versus only 9 percent in those with no such finding. This observation is not uniformly reported, however, and agreement among pathologists as to what constitutes vascular invasion is difficult to achieve. In the GOG study, the number of cases with vascular invasion varied from 16 to 25 with the observer with radical differences among the lists of which patients had vascular invasion. The significance of the finding is therefore not clear at present.

Cervix involvement and gross extrauterine spread.   The significance of cervix involvement and gross extrauterine spread are apparent from the earlier discussion of

Table 11-13. Adnexal Spread: GOG Prospective Study of Frequency and Impact on Recurrence and Death Rate in Clinical Stage I Endometrial Carcinoma (n = 222)[67,68]

Adnexae	Frequency[67]	Recurrence Rate[68]	Death Rate[68]
Involved	7.2%	38%	50%
Not involved	92.8%	14%	10%

Table 11-14. Cervix Involvement: Prognostic Significance of the Nature of the Involvement[61,62]

Type of Involvement	3-Year Survival
Endocervical glands only	74%
Stromal invasion	47%

the FIGO staging system and its relation to survival (Table 11-6). In regard to cervix involvement, such involvement limited to the endocervical glands does not appear to worsen prognosis as compared to clinical stage I disease, whereas stromal invasion of the cervix significantly affects outcome (Table 11-14).[61,62]

Based on all of these considerations, a summary of major pathologic prognostic variables would include: histologic grade, depth of myometrial invasion, pelvic and para-aortic lymph node status, peritoneal cytology, cervix involvement, and additional evidence of extra-uterine spread (Table 11-15). A major consideration for the clinician is whether each of these parameters represents an independent prognostic variable and hence a parameter which must be evaluated in each patient. From a review of older literature[21,41–64,69] and the results of the initial and current GOG prospective studies on surgical-pathologic variables in endometrial carcinoma,[65–68,71] the interrelationship of the variables is apparent. Within clinical stage I cases, the correlation among depth of myometrial invasion, grade, and lymph node status (Table 11-16) allows the delineation of a group at high risk for lymph node involvement (those with deep myometrial invasion, those with intermediate invasion and grade two or three neoplasms, those with superficial invasion and grade three neoplasms) based on characteristics of the primary neoplasm.[67] Furthermore, as noted earlier, para-aortic node involvement almost never occurs in the absence of pelvic node involvement in this trial.[67] The impact of cervix involvement on lymph node involve-

Table 11-15. Pathologic Variables of Major Prognostic Significance in Patients with Endometrial Carcinoma

Histologic grade
Depth of myometrial invasion
Pelvic and para-aortic lymph node status
Peritoneal cytology
Cervix status
Extrauterine spread

Table 11-16. Correlation Among Grade, Depth of Myometrial Invasion, and Lymph Node Involvement in GOG Prospective Study of Clinical Stage I Endometrial Carcinoma (n = 222)[67]

Depth	Grade	Cases	Pelvic Nodes	Para-aortic Nodes
Endometrium	1	58	2%	2%
	2	27	4%	0%
	3	7	0%	0%
Superficial	1	27	0%	0%
	2	40	3%	0%
	3	13	23%	38%
Intermediate	1	4	0%	0%
	2	8	25%	12%
	3	5	20%	0%
Deep	1	4	25%	0%
	2	13	46%	38%
	3	16	44%	31%

ment is evident from a review of the literature (10.6 percent positive pelvic nodes in stage I versus 36.5 percent positive pelvic nodes in stage II),[21] and similarly grade and depth of invasion are closely interrelated with deep invasion uncommon in grade 1 neoplasms (12 percent) but quite common in grade 3 neoplasms (46 percent).[21]

Thus, certain variables have been delineated as significant predictors of outcome in patients with endometrial carcinoma. The most important of these variables are pathologic features and include: histologic grade, depth of myometrial invasion, stromal invasion of the cervix, pelvic and para-aortic lymph node status, peritoneal cytology, and other evidence of extra-uterine spread.

Patient Evaluation

The pretreatment evaluation of the patient should attempt to define the status of the major prognostic variables for that particular patient. This will include a determination of not only the clinical stage of the patient but also certain additional pathologic features of disease. This entire body of information will be essential to treatment planning.

Certain studies should be obtained in every patient with endometrial carcinoma. A thorough history and physical examination is essential to determine not only clues to possible extension of the carcinoma but, more importantly, the presence of other disease processes such as diabetes and hypertension which might adversely affect treatment tolerance and outcome. Along these same lines, a complete blood count, measurement of renal and liver function by blood tests (blood urea nitrogen, creatinine, SGOT, alkaline phosphatase, and bilirubin), and a blood glucose should be obtained. A chest x-ray should routinely be obtained both to look for metastases and to search for potential cardiopulmonary problems. Finally, a thorough sampling of endometrial tissue by fractional curettage should be carried out to establish the diagnosis, assess grade and cervix status, and acquire tissue for estrogen and progesterone receptor assays. The value of receptor assays is not as yet firmly established, but the assays do appear to be clinically useful[3] and may be unavailable later if all tumor tissue is removed by curettage. A more detailed consideration of these assays will be presented later.

Additional studies may be of value in specific circumstances. In those patients with high risk factors present on general evaluation such as high grade neoplasm, cervix involvement, or evidence of extrauterine extension, attempts to define further the extent of disease clinically should be undertaken. If a locally advanced lesion is present, intravenous pyelogram and cystoscopy plus barium enema may help to define local extent and should be done. Hysterography and hysteroscopy are recommended by some[72–74] to assess the size of the primary tumor and extent of involvement of the uterus, but these techniques carry a theoretical risk of producing transtubal spread and are not of unequivocal value.[10] Evaluation for possible distant spread, in addition to a chest x-ray to assess the most common site of distant dissemination, the lungs, should include radionuclide scans of liver and bone. Assessment for possible pelvic and intra-abdominal dissemination and/or spread to lymph nodes can be accomplished with sonography or computerized tomography of the abdomen and pelvis.[75,76] The relative merits of these two procedures are not currently known, but both

Table 11-17. Pretreatment Evaluation of Patients with Endometrial Carcinoma

Test	Applicability
History	G
Physical examination	G
Pelvic examination	G
Measurement of depth of uterine cavity	G
Complete blood count	G
Blood glucose	G
Renal function tests (BUN, creatinine)	G
Liver function tests (SGOT, alkaline phosphatase, bilirubin)	G
Endometrial tissue sampling	G
Dilatation and fractional curettage	G
Hormone receptor assay	G
Hysteroscopy	S
Cystoscopy	S
Chest x-ray	G
Intravenous pyelogram	S
Barium enema	S
Liver scan	S
Bone scan	S
Hysterography	S
Lymphangiogram	S
Abdominal sonography	S
Computerized tomography of abdomen	S

G = Generally applicable to all patients
S = Specific applicability to certain patients
   as explained in text

have the disadvantage of requiring gross nodal enlargement to two or three centimeters in order to demonstrate lymph node abnormalities. Some investigators[75] still employ lymphangiography with or without sonography or computerized tomography to evaluate nodal status.

In conclusion, Table 11-17 lists useful diagnostic studies and indicates whether each study is generally applicable to all patients or useful only in specific circumstances. Completion of such an evaluation allows the establishment of the clinical stage (Table 11-5) of the patient. This will allow an initial therapeutic plan to be set. More precise data regarding extent of disease and prognostic variables will be forthcoming after initial surgical therapy and will follow a more precise estimate of risk for recurrence. These data may necessitate further therapeutic planning as will be discussed.

MANAGEMENT OF EARLY DISEASE

Patients with FIGO stages I and II endometrial carcinoma are generally considered to have relatively early disease with a reasonable probability of cure. The vast majority of cases of endometrial carcinoma (78 percent) will present as early disease with most of these (75 percent) having clinical stage I disease. Proper treatment planning necessitates that groups at low and high risk for recurrence be distinguished on the basis of major prognostic variables and that therapeutic options for the groups be carefully assessed.

Identification of Risk Groups

The prospective studies of the GOG[65–68] have provided not only confirmation of pathologic variables of major prognostic importance (Table 11-15) but also a data base amenable to precise analysis as to efficacy of the ways in which the variables interrelate. For the individual patient, placement into a prognostic group requires information from the staging evaluation (Table 11-17) plus findings at laparotomy which is usually a part of the initial approach to treatment. This laparotomy should include a total hysterectomy and bilateral salpingo-oophorectomy, a sampling of peritoneal fluid for cytology, and an evaluation of pelvic lymph nodes. Whether para-aortic node sampling should be undertaken is debatable, but the relative infrequency of involvement of these nodes in the absence of positive pelvic nodes would suggest that such a procedure is necessary only if pelvic nodes are positive for tumor.

Patients to be considered at high risk for recurrence are those with less well-differentiated neoplasms, deeper myometrial invasion, stromal invasion of the cervix, positive pelvic and/or para-aortic nodes, positive peritoneal cytology, or other evidence of extrauterine spread. Other factors which may have a bearing on patient risk are age at diagnosis and the presence of other diseases such as diabetes and hypertension. In fact, these other aspects may limit the amount of information that can be obtained at laparotomy by increasing surgical risk. In such cases, the correlations observed between grade, depth of myometrial invasion, and cervix status on the one hand and the status of pelvic and para-aortic nodes on the other may guide designation of risk (Table 11-16). Any grade three lesion, a grade two lesion with intermediate to deep myometrial invasion, and a grade one lesion with deep myometrial invasion as well as any lesion associated with stromal invasion in the cervix are at high risk for lymph node involvement and should be considered at high risk for recurrence.

The division of patients with early disease into high risk and low risk groups (Table 11-18) permits an approach to patient management which reduces patient exposure to unnecessary and potentially harmful therapy in the case of the low risk group and provides for the possibility of additional therapy in the high risk group, therapy which may enhance chances for cure.

Therapeutic Options

Treatment which has been employed in the management of early endometrial carcinoma includes surgery alone[21,22,26,45,46,52,57,59,60,77], pre-operative radiotherapy followed by surgery[13,21–23,26,43,45,51,55–60,63,64,68,78–92], surgery followed by post-operative radiotherapy[21,22,26,41,43,46,47,56–60,63,68,91–93], and radiotherapy alone[21,94–97]. Whereas clinical stage I cases have been managed with all 4 approaches, clinical stage II cases have virtually all received some form of radiotherapy, usually in combination

Table 11-18. Determination of Risk for Recurrence Based on Pathologic Variables of Prognostic Significance in Patients with Early Endometrial Carcinoma (Clinical Stages I and II)[68]

Risk	Pathologic Features
High[a]	Grade 3 lesion
	Grade 2 lesion with intermediate or deep myometrial invasion
	Grade 1 lesion with deep myometrial invasion
	Positive pelvic and/or para-aortic lymph nodes
	Positive peritoneal cytology
	Stromal invasion of the cervix
	Extrauterine spread
Low[b]	Grade 1 lesion without deep myometrial invasion
	Grade 2 lesion without intermediate or deep myometrial invasion
	Negative peritoneal cytology
	No stromal invasion of the cervix
	No extrauterine spread

[a] One or more factors present
[b] All factors must be present

with surgery[48,61,62,98–103] At the risk of understatement, it can be concluded fairly that the optimal approach is not known. Consideration of the advantages and disadvantages of each option would therefore be a reasonable starting point for the evolution of therapeutic recommendations.

Surgery Alone. Surgery is regarded by most investigators as the primary treatment for early endometrial carcinoma. The standard surgical procedure has been and remains a total abdominal hysterectomy and bilateral salpingo-oophorectomy. Because of recent observations about important prognostic variables,[67,68] to this procedure must be added sampling of pelvic lymph nodes, peritoneal fluid, and, in selected cases, para-aortic lymph nodes. Controversy centers on whether this procedure alone is adequate treatment for most or all patients with early endometrial carcinoma or should be more radical or accompanied by radiation therapy.

Patients who met the criteria for the low-risk group (Table 11-18) appear to have an excellent 5-year disease-free survival when treated with standard surgery alone.[52] Greater than 90 percent of such patients remain disease-free beyond 5 years.[68] No good evidence exists to show that more radical surgery[77] or adjunctive radiation therapy[68] will improve on these results.

Patients who are in the high-risk group (Table 11-18) do not fare as well with surgery alone. In those cases where there is evidence of extrauterine spread (positive nodes or cytology or other evidence of such spread), 5-year disease-free survival is less than 60 percent[68] whether adjunctive radiotherapy is added to surgery or not. For those patients, surgery alone does not appear adequate therapy. The critical question is whether additional therapy with other modalities will alter this outlook. This question is the subject of a current GOG study of adjunctive chemotherapy in patients with high-risk early endometrial carcinoma.[104]

Radiotherapy Alone. Radiotherapy as the only treatment for early endometrial carcinoma is generally reserved for those patients who are deemed inoperable because of a high operative risk. The reason for this relates to the observation of poorer survival rates in operable patients so treated as compared to patients managed with some form of surgery (Table 11-19).[2,31,95,96] These observations cannot be refuted on the basis that only high-risk patients received radiotherapy alone since institutions using radiotherapy alone for all patients reported only a 46 percent 5-year survival rate in clinical stage I patients.[2]

Combined Therapy. A myriad of approaches to the use of combinations of surgery and radiotherapy have been reported. These include: surgery preceded by radium and/or external beam, surgery followed by radium and/or external beam, and surgery both preceded and followed by radiation therapy. Dosages of radiation have also varied widely, as have the intervals between surgery and radiotherapy. Despite the large number of reported studies and the readily apparent enthusiasm of a majority of investigators for combined therapy[10,21,25,105–107], no concurrently controlled studies and no good uncontrolled data are available to support the value of adjunctive radiotherapy in any of these patients. The rationale cited for the use of such therapy includes theoretical considerations and a proven ability for radiation to cure some patients with endometrial carcinoma.[25] Patients chosen to receive adjunctive radiotherapy vary from all stage I and II patients to those who meet the criteria for the high risk group (Table 11-18).

It should be remembered, on the other hand, that patients who receive radiotherapy in combination with surgery may experience a variety of adverse effects which may be seen in as many as 24 percent of the patients.[87] Complications include local inflammation and tissue necrosis, thrombophlebitis, and pulmonary embolus. These risks must be weighed carefully against expected benefit.

There does seem to be one well-established beneficial effect of adjunctive radiotherapy, a reduction of the frequency of vaginal recurrence with preoperative radiation (from 12 percent to 2 percent).[108] Whether this will translate to an enhanced cure rate or whether such an effect is a sufficient justification for the use of preoperative radiotherapy is debatable.

Recommendations

The optimal approach to patients with early endometrial carcinoma is not known. The best that can be achieved from a review of available data is the evolution of an arbitrary approach which seems rational in light of our present knowledge (Table 11-20). Great emphasis will be placed on the precise definition of major prognostic variables in each patient.

For patients with low-risk disease (Table 11-18), surgery alone in the form of a total abdominal hysterectomy and bilateral salpingo-oophorectomy should be curative in over 90 percent of cases. The use of adjunctive therapy subjects the patient to the risk of adverse effects with little or no expected benefit and cannot be condoned.

For patients with high-risk disease, optimal treatment is in all probability not yet

Table 11-19. Survival Rates in Patients with Operable Early Endometrial Carcinoma
Managed with Radiotherapy Alone

Series	Overall	5-Year Survival Radiation Alone	Surgery
Kottmeir[2]	70%	46%	
Nilsen and Koller[31]		68%	98%
Candiana et al[95]		50%	85%
Hernandez[96]		55%	70%

Table 11-20. Therapeutic Recommendations for Patients
with Early Endometrial Carcinoma

Risk Group	Recommendations
Low	Total abdominal hysterectomy Bilateral salpingo-oophorectomy
High	Total abdominal hysterectomy Bilateral salpingo-oophorectomy ? adjunctive radiotherapy

available. Surgery in the form of a total abdominal hysterectomy and bilateral salpingo-oophorectomy should certainly be performed. The rationale for the use of radiotherapy, particularly to prevent vaginal recurrence, seems compelling in these patients at high risk for recurrence. It must be remembered, however, that no proof of
efficacy other than possibly the prevention of vaginal recurrence exists and that adverse effects may be reasonably frequent. No firm recommendation can thus be made
regarding the use of adjunctive radiotherapy, much less the form that the radiotherapy
should take. Adjunctive systemic therapy has no proven role to play at present in
these patients and should be reserved for clinical trials. Close to half of these high-
risk patients can be expected to recur.

MANAGEMENT OF ADVANCED OR RECURRENT
DISEASE

Patients who demonstrate clinical stage III or IV disease at presentation or who
develop recurrence after initial management of early disease with surgery and/or radiotherapy have a significantly greater chance of dying of their disease process than
those patients with early disease. For these patients, endometrial carcinoma is any-
thing but the ''benign cancer'' that many have regarded it to be. The approach to
these patients, however, may differ according to the specific site or sites of involvement.

Prognostic Groups

Those patients with primary clinical stage III or IV disease will comprise approximately 15 percent of the entire primary patient population with endometrial carcinoma.[25] An additional 20 to 25 percent of the initial patient population can be ex-

Table 11-21. Advanced or Recurrent Endometrial Carcinoma:
Composition of Patient Population

Patient Characteristics	Frequency	Five-Year Survival
Localized disease only	40%	25–30%
Localized and distant disease	30%	<15%
Distant disease only	30%	<15%

pected to relapse, most within 2 years of diagnosis, after treatment with surgery and/or radiotherapy.[109] Within this overall group of patients, it is important to recognize two distinct groups: those with locoregional disease only (disease confined to pelvis) and those with distant spread with or without locoregional disease (Table 11-21).

Patients with locoregional disease only will account for approximately 40 percent of the overall patients with late disease.[109] Within this group of patients are 2 distinct clinical subgroups: those patients with disease confined to the ovaries and/or fallopian tubes and those patients with involvement of other pelvic structures. The former subgroup demonstrates a significantly higher 5-year survival than the latter (in one study, 80 percent versus 15 percent).[110] Patients who are surgically stage III but clinically stage I or II are generally not included in the advanced disease group, but the increased application of surgical staging to this disease has raised serious questions as to whether they should be included. It would appear that the expected 5 year survival of such patients is superior to that for clinical stage III patients (44 percent versus 12 percent in one trial).[111] Overall, patients with locoregionally advanced or recurrent disease will demonstrate a 25 to 30 percent five year survival.[112,113]

Patients with evidence of distant spread with or without locoregional disease will comprise approximately 60 percent of patients with late disease.[109] The most common site of distant spread is the lungs (40 percent of those patients with such spread).[109] Other not uncommon sites include liver, bone, lymph nodes, and peritoneal cavity. A small subgroup of the latter, those patients with clinical stage I or II disease but microscopic contamination of the peritoneal cavity, deserves special mention. The impact of such a finding on survival is not clearly known, but these patients appear to have a high risk of relapse which exceeds 50 percent.[114] Overall, patients with distant spread have a 5-year survival of less than 15 percent.[106]

Management of Locoregional Disease

The proper pretreatment evaluation of patients who present with recurrent or advanced disease limited to the pelvis is not completely settled.[106] Operative evaluation in addition to the usual clinical evaluation (Table 11-17) has been suggested and, if done, should include evaluation of pelvic and para-aortic nodes, peritoneal cytology, and the peritoneal surface with biopsy of any suspicious areas.[106] Careful assessment of those areas to which distant spread is likely to occur is also essential to proper treatment planning. Such an assessment should include, as a minimum, a chest x-ray, radionuclide scans of liver and bone, and probably a non-invasive study of the peritoneal cavity and retroperitoneal areas with computerized tomography or sonography. Additionally, tissue samples should be sent for assays of estrogen and proges-

Table 11-22. Treatment of Patients with Locoregionally Advanced or Recurrent
Endometrial Carcinoma

Patient Description	Therapeutic Recommendation
Adnexal involvement only evidence of extrauterine spread	Radical hysterectomy plus bilateral pelvic lymphadenopathy plus postoperative radiotherapy
Evidence of pelvic disease outside uterus and adnexae	Radiotherapy (external beam and/or local radiation)[a]

[a]Those patients with complete regression with radiation and those with vaginal
metastases without other extrauterine spread should be considered for post-radiation
hysterectomy.

terone receptors since these values may prove valuable in deciding on appropriate
systemic therapy at some future juncture. In short, the pretreatment evaluation as outlined in Table 11-17 is applicable to these patients and should be augmented with
operative evaluation where feasible and appropriate.

The mainstay of the treatment of patients with locoregional disease only is radiotherapy with or without surgery. Those patients who have extension confined clinically to ovaries and/or fallopian tubes only should be approached surgically with
postoperative whole-pelvis radiation to follow surgery. The surgical procedure most
commonly employed is a radical hysterectomy and bilateral pelvic lymphadenectomy.[25,106] Five-year survival in such cases is generally reported as 50 percent.[10]

For those patients who have clinical evidence of parametrial extension, vaginal
metastases, or more extensive pelvic disease, radiotherapy represents the modality of
choice for initial management. Various combinations of external beam and local radiotherapy have been employed.[25,106,111–113] In those cases which demonstrate complete regression of bulk disease and those which have vaginal metastases as the only
evidence of extrauterine disease, some authorities advocate hysterectomy in combination with radiotherapy.[10] Expected 5-year survival rates range from 25 to 50 percent in this group of patients. Those who have only vaginal metastases as extrauterine
disease fare better than the rest of the group with overall survival of 50 percent at 5
years.[113]

In summary (Table 11-22), radiotherapy is the treatment of choice for most patients with advanced or recurrent endometrial carcinoma limited to the pelvis. In those
selected patients with extrauterine disease confined to ovaries and/or fallopian tubes,
radical hysterectomy and bilateral pelvic lymphadenectomy should probably precede
radiotherapy. In those cases with clinically complete regression of disease on radiotherapy or with vaginal metastases only, hysterectomy should be considered after radiotherapy.

Management of Disseminated Disease

Evaluation.   Patients with evidence of distant spread should be carefully evaluated to establish extent of disease at the onset of treatment. Precise information will
permit an accurate assessment of response to therapy later in the course of patient
management. The evaluation should again include most of those items listed in Table

11-17 with an emphasis on sites of potential distant spread: lungs, liver, bone, nodes, and peritoneal cavity. In general, operative evaluation of these patients is neither necessary nor appropriate, but tissue sampling for estrogen and progesterone receptor assays and documentation of recurrence is appropriate and helpful. Pretreatment assessment of renal and hepatic function and of specific systems which might be adversely affected by certain systemic agents, e.g., adriamycin and cardiotoxicity, should also be included.

Information obtained from this evaluation will permit an intelligent choice of therapy. Although surgery and radiotherapy may on occasion play a role in palliating specific localized problems, the primary choices for therapy center on systemic therapy with either hormonal agents or chemotherapy.

Hormonal Therapy.   Endometrial carcinoma has long been recognized as a hormonally sensitive neoplasm.[115] Progestational agents have been the most commonly used form of hormonal therapy in patients with endometrial carcinoma.[116] The relative lack of toxicity of these agents has made them a favored approach to systemic treatment of disseminated disease almost to the exclusion of any other form of systemic therapy.

Contrary to popular misconception, however, objective studies document that progestins, while useful, are effective in only one third of the patients so treated (Table 11-23).[116] More recent studies suggest even lower frequencies of objective response (Table 11-24).[117,118] The frequency with which response is seen appears to correlate well with histologic grade and with length of time from initial diagnosis to start of progestin therapy (Table 11-25).[116,117] Other factors examined with no apparent relationship to response rate include age, site of disease, and prior or concomitant radiotherapy.[116] Median survival of patients treated with progestins ranges from 9 months[118] to 20 months[119], the latter a selected group of patients with a disease course of greater than 3 years at the time of initiation of hormonal therapy.

Table 11-23. Composite Data on Three Progestational Agents in the Treatment of Endometrial Carcinoma[116]

Progestational Agent	Patients	Responses	Frequency
Medroxyprogesterone	151	52	34%
Megestrol acetate	125	40	33%
Medrogestrone	56	17	30%

Table 11-24. Recent Studies of Progestational Agents in Treatment of Endometrial Carcinoma

Progestational Agent	Patients	Responses	Frequency
Delalutin[117]	114	18	16%
Depo-provera C. T. Provera[118]	109	13	12%

Table 11-25. Correlation of Tumor Responses to Progestins with Grade and Length of Disease Course

Parameter	Response
Histologic grade	
Well differentiated	52%
Poorly differentiated	16%
Length of disease	
More than three years	33%
Less than three years	8%

Table 11-26. Correlation Between Histologic Grade and Receptor Status in Endometrial Carcinoma

Tumor Characteristic	ER + PR +	
	Ehrlich [122]	Creasman [121]
Grade 1	84%	83%
Grade 2	55%	58%
Grade 3	22%	31%
Recurrent	23%	36%
Irradiated	21%	—

Table 11-27. Correlation Between Receptor Status and Response to Progestins in Endometrial Carcinoma

Study	ER + PR + Response	ER − PR − Response
Creasman [121]	3/5 (60%)	1/8 (12%)
Ehrlich [122]	7/8 (88%)	1/16 (7%)
Benraad [125]	5/6 (83%)	0/5 (0%)
Martin [126]	13/13 (100%)	1/7 (14%)
McCarty [127]	4/5 (80%)	0/8 (0%)
Total	32/37 (86%)	3/44 (7%)

Table 11-28. Results of Treatment of Disseminated Endometrial Carcinoma with Tamoxifen

Regimen	Patients	Response
Tamoxifen 60 mg/m^2/day [134]	17	9 (53%)
Tamoxifen 20 mg/day [135]	10	3 (30%)
Tamoxifen 20 mg/day [136]	25	0 (0%)
Total	52	12 (24%)

Recent studies have suggested a possible predictive value for estrogen and progesterone receptor assays in endometrial carcinoma.[120–124] A distinct correlation between histologic grade and the frequency of receptor positivity was observed (Table 11-26).[121,122] Since grade appears to relate to frequency of response, such a correlation between receptor status and response would be predicted. Similarly, this correlation would be predicted from data supporting a relationship between receptor status and response in breast carcinoma. The few studies of receptor status and hormonal response in endometrial carcinoma do indeed point to a strong predictive value of receptor assays (Table 11-27)[121,122,125–127] and support the use of such assays to determine which patients should be treated with progestins for disseminated disease.

A variety of different progestational agents has been used in the management of endometrial carcinoma.[116,128–131] A relevant question to consider is whether one agent has any advantages over others. There is no definitive evidence of the superiority of one agent over others. A possible distinguishing characteristic, however, might relate to ease of administration. Oral preparations would appear to offer an advantage in this regard over agents that require parenteral administration. Adequate absorption from the gastrointestinal tract would have to be ensured, however, in comparison with drug availability of parenteral preparations. Studies of medroxyprogesterone plasma levels resulting from oral and intramuscular administration reveal no significant difference.[132,133] Oral agents would therefore appear to be progestins of choice in the hormonal treatment of disseminated endometrial carcinoma. Usual daily doses are C.T. Provera (Upjohn) 150 mg or Palace (Bristol) 160 mg.

An alternative hormonal agent which has been evaluated in endometrial carcinoma is the anti-estrogen, tamoxifen.[134–137] Although the number of cases so treated is small, there is reasonable evidence of drug efficacy (Table 11-28). Doses ranged from 20 mg daily[135,136] to 60 mg/m² daily.[134] In at least one study, all responders were noted to have previously responded to oral progestins.[134] A single case known to be receptor positive (ER + PR +) did display a complete response of pulmonary metastases with tamoxifen.[137] Tamoxifen thus appears to be a reasonable second-line hormonal manipulation in patients who are known to be receptor positive or who have previously responded to progestins.

Chemotherapy.   The widely held views that endometrial carcinoma is a "benign malignancy" not requiring aggressive management and that progestins are the treatment of choice for patients with advanced or recurrent disease have hampered the development of effective chemotherapy for patients who encounter disseminated disease.[138,139] In a 1976 review of chemotherapy in gynecologic cancer,[140] only three drugs could be cited as having been studied in a sufficient number of cases to suggest the possibility of activity (Table 11-29). These data are collected from multiple studies with varying response definitions and hence are of questionable validity.

More recent studies of *single agents* have clarified the activity of certain agents. Among these, the most definite evidence of activity is found with adriamycin (Table 11-30).[141,142] In the GOG trial in particular,[142] adriamycin was noted to induce responses in disease confined to previously irradiated pelvic areas as well as extrapelvic sites and to result in 25 percent clinically complete responses with a median survival of 14 months as compared to 7 months for all other patients.

A second drug with some evidence of activity is hexamethylmelamine (Table

Table 11-29. Single Agents with Probable Activity in
Endometrial Carcinoma as of 1976[140]

Drug	Patients	Response
Adriamycin	18	7 (38%)
Cyclophosphamide	33	7 (21%)
5-Fluorouracil	43	10 (23%)

Table 11-30. Active Single Agents in the Treatment of Endometrial Carcinoma

Regimen	Patients	Response
Adriamycin 50 mg/m^2/3 weeks[141]	21	4 (19%)
Adriamycin 60 mg/m^2/3 weeks[142]	43	16 (37%)
Hexamethylmelamine 8 mg/kg/day[143]	20	6 (30%)

Table 11-31. Cis-platinum as a Single Agent in the Treatment of Endometrial Carcinoma

Regimen	Prior Chemotherapy	Patients	Response
3 mg/kg/3 weeks[144]	Yes	13	4 (31%)
50–100 mg/m^2/3 weeks[145]	No	26	11 (42%)
50 mg/m^2/3 weeks[146,147]	Yes	25	1 (4%)
50 mg/m^2/3 weeks[148]	No	11	4 (36%)

Table 11-32. Additional Single Agents Tested in Treatment of Endometrial
Carcinoma

Regimen	Patients	Response
Piperazinedione 9 mg/m^2/3 weeks[149]	20	1 (5%)
VP-16 100 mg/m^2 days 1,3,5/4 weeks[150]	29	1 (3%)

11-30).[143] Only a single trial has been conducted to date, and independent confirmation of activity would be desirable. The drug nevertheless appears to possess reasonable activity in the treatment of endometrial carcinoma. All responses were partial responses with a median duration of response of 3.5 months (range 1 to 7 months).

Most confusing is evidence related to the level of efficacy of cis-platinum (Table 11-31).[144–148] Of the four triaals reported, three suggest significant activity.[144,145,148] Only one of these three studies, however, contains sufficient patients to allow a reasonable conclusion to be drawn.[145] The fourth trial suggests little or no activity in a reasonable number of patients. The major differences between the two larger trials relate to prior chemotherapy and dose levels. In the positive study,[145] all but 5 patients had received no prior chemotherapy. Furthermore, 20 of the 26 patients received larger drug doses (70–100 mg/m^2). An attempt to clarify this situation is now in progress by the GOG and employs cis-platinum 50 mg/m^2/3 weeks in patients with no prior chemotherapy.

Other drugs that have been tested in a concerted fashion as single agents in endometrial carcinoma have shown no evidence of activity (Table 11-32).[149,150] These include piperazinedione[149] and VP-16.[150] The GOG is continuing a series of studies of single agents in endometrial carcinoma in the hope that other active drugs will be forthcoming.

Despite the lack of a plethora of active drugs, studies of combination chemotherapy have been conducted (Table 11-33).[151–160] These trials have generally involved relatively small numbers of patients and, lacking concurrent controls, have provided little evidence of results superior to the use of single-agent adriamycin. Two attempts at controlled studies involving large numbers of patients have been undertaken by the GOG.

The first of these larger trials[161] was based on promising results with two combinations (Table 11-34) consisting of cyclophosphamide plus adriamycin plus 5-fluorouracil plus medroxyprogesterone acetate (CAF-M)[155] versus melphalan plus 5-fluorouracil plus medroxyprogesterone acetate (MF-M).[159] Not only did the trial fail to show a difference between the two combinations, but also the individual response rates of the two regimens were drastically lower than those reported in the smaller trials and no better than that seen in the GOG study of adriamycin alone.[142]

Table 11-33. Uncontrolled Trials of Combination Chemotherapy in Endometrial Carcinoma

Regimen	Patients	Response
Adriamycin plus cyclophosphamide	8[151]	5 (62%)
	26[152]	8 (31%)
	29[153]	10 (34%)
Adriamycin plus cyclophosphamide plus medroxyprogesterone	55[154]	15 (27%)
Adriamycin plus cyclophosphamide plus BCG	27[153]	10 (37%)
Adriamycin plus cyclophosphamide plus 5-fluorouracil plus medroxyprogresterone	56[154]	9 (16%)
	20[155]	15 (75%)
	29[156]	13 (45%)
Adriamycin plus cyclophosphamide plus 5-fluorouracil plus vincristine	20[157]	10 (50%)
Adriamycin plus cyclophosphamide plus cis-platinum	20[158]	9 (45%)
Melphalan plus 5-fluorouracil plus medroxyprogesterone	15[159]	14 (93%)
	11[160]	6 (55%)
Chlorambucil plus 5-fluorouracil plus medroxyprogesterone	12[154]	2 (17%)

Table 11-34. GOG Comparative Trial of Two Promising Combinations in Treatment of Endometrial Carcinoma[161]

Regimen	Patients	Response
Cyclophosphamide 400 mg/m²/3 weeks Adriamycin 40 mg/m²/3 weeks 5-fluorouracil 400 mg/m²/3 weeks Medroxyprogesterone acetate 160 mg/day	77	29 (38%)
Melphalan 7 mg/m² days 1–4/4 weeks 5-fluorouracil 525 mg/m² days 1–4/4 weeks Medroxyprogesterone acetate 160 mgs/day	78	28 (36%)

Table 11-35. GOG Comparative Trial of Adriamycin With or Without Cyclophosphamide in Endometrial Carcinoma—Preliminary Results[162]

Regimen	Patients	Response
Adriamycin 60 mg/m²/3 weeks	62	20 (32%)
Adriamycin 60 mg/m²/3 weeks plus Cyclophosphamide 500 mg/M²/3 weeks	60	17 (28%)

Table 11-36. Therapeutic Agents Tested to Date in Disseminated Endometrial Carcinoma

Agent	Status
Hormonal agents	
Progestins	Active
Tamoxoifen	Probably active
Chemotherapy	
Adriamycin	Active
Hexamethylmelamine	Probably active
Cis-platinum	Probably active
5-fluorouracil	Possibly active
Cyclophosphamide	Possibly active
Piperazinedione	Inactive
VP-16	Inactive

The second large GOG trial is still underway.[162] This study compares directly adriamycin alone to adriamycin plus cyclophosphamide (Table 11-35). No differences between the two regimens have appeared as yet.

Conclusions. Great strides have not as yet been realized in the management of·patients with disseminated disease (Table 11-36). The hormonal agents, progestins and tamoxifen, appear to have reasonable activity in patients who are receptor positive (ER + PR +) or, if receptor status is unknown, who have better differentiated neoplasms or longer duration of disease. Responses are neither as frequent nor as well-maintained as has been commonly accepted to be the case.

Only adriamycin among the various cytotoxic agents has unequivocal activity in endometrial carcinoma. There is reason to believe that both hexamethylmelamine and cis-platinum will prove to be useful agents. Whether cyclophosphamide and 5-fluorouracil are truly active remains doubtful. No combination of these agents, with or without progestins, has been shown to offer any advantage over adriamycin as a single agent in disseminated endometrial carcinoma.

FUTURE DIRECTIONS

The prognosis for the majority of patients with endometrial carcinoma who present with low-risk stage I disease is excellent with five-year survival rates that exceed 90 percent. It is unlikely that the near future will see the improvement of treatment results in these patients. For the remaining one-third of patients with endometrial carcinoma, significant advances in treatment are urgently needed to prevent the majority of these unfortunate women from dying as a result of their disease.

High-Risk Early Disease

The capability to identify patients with early endometrial carcinoma who are at great risk to recur has improved markedly as a result of prospective studies[67,68,71] of this group of patients and will continue to improve with additional information from the largest of these trials.[71] The major problem now concerns the identification of therapeutic options that can improve the outlook for this group at high risk for recurrence. No solid evidence exists at present that radiotherapy offers such improvement. Reasonable studies of radiotherapy as a surgical adjuvant in such patients are desperately needed but are unlikely to evolve because of preconceptions about not only the need for but also the optimal approach to the use of radiation therapy in these patients.

Alternatives or additions to the use of adjuvant radiotherapy also need to be evaluated. While progestins have been unsuccessfully used as adjuvant therapy in early endometrial carcinoma,[163–166] none of these studies have been carried out in only receptor positive (ER + PR +) patients who can reasonably be expected to respond to hormonal manipulation. Such a trial is needed before adjuvant hormonal therapy can be judged of no value.

A second systemic option for high-risk patients is the use of chemotherapy in combination with surgery and/or radiotherapy. One such trial is in progress (Fig. 11-1)[104] and seeks to determine the value of adriamycin as an adjuvant to surgery followed by radiotherapy. Such trials, to have meaning, will have to be concurrently controlled and will require large numbers of patients with relatively uncommon disease characteristics. A cooperative group setting will virtually be required to complete the study. Such a study is also limited at present by the lack of effective combination chemotherapy. The identification of additional active drugs and subsequent combinations with enhanced efficacy thus is a priority even in the management of early endometrial carcinoma.

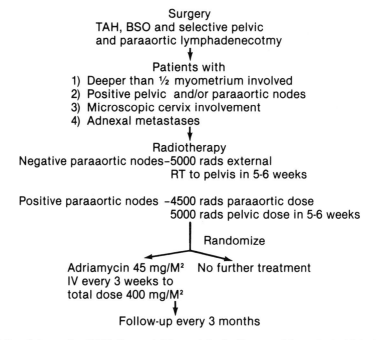

Fig. 11-1. Schema for GOG Protocol 34, a trial of adjuvant adriamycin in high-risk early endometrial carcinoma.

Advanced or Recurrent Disease

Further improvement in current abilities to deal with late endometrial carcinoma depends almost entirely on the development of more effective systemic therapy. Interest has increased considerably in the last 7 years in this line of clinical research so that progress can be reasonably expected. Among specific objectives are included new drug development, identification of active drug combinations, and the development of new methods of delivery of systemic therapy such as intracavitary infusions[167] and vehicles to enhance agent delivery to target cells.[168] Totally different approaches to the treatment of disseminated disease such as hyperthermia and various biologic response modifiers are also under evaluation. Whether these novel options will actually prove of value is highly speculative, but the development of effective combination chemotherapy and more effective application of hormonal therapy through use of receptor assays are both objectives almost certain to be realized in the near future.

REFERENCES

1. Cancer statistics—1980. Ca-Cancer Journal for Clinicians 30:23, 1980.
2. Kottmeier HR (ed): Annual Report on the Results of Treatment in Carcinoma of the Uterus, Vagina, and Ovary. Radiumhemment, Stockholm, vol. 15, 1974.
3. Creasman W, Weed J: Cancer of the endometrium. Current Problems in Cancer 5, No. 2, 1980.

4. Mattingly RF: Malignant tumors of the uterus. In Telinde (ed): Operative Gynecology. ed 5. Philadelphia, JB Lippincott, 1977.

5. Crissman J, Azoury R, Barnes A, et al: Endometrial carcinoma in women 40 years of age or younger. Obstet Gynecol 57:699, 1981.

6. Wynder EL, Escher GC, Mantel W: An epidemiological investigation of cancer of the endometrium. Cancer 19:489, 1966.

7. MacMahon B: Risk factors for endometrial cancer. Gynecol Oncol 2:122, 1974.

8. Friek HC, Munnell EW, Richart RM, et al: Carcinoma of endometrium. Amer J Obstetr Gynecol 115:663, 1973.

9. Gusberg SB: The changing nature of endometrial cancer. N Engl J Med 302:729, 1980.

10. Morrow CP, Townsend DE (eds): Synopsis of Gynecologic Oncology. ed 2. New York, John Wiley and Sons, 1981.

11. Landgren R, Fletcher G, Gallagher S, et al: Treatment failure sites according to irradiation technique and histology in patients with endometrial cancer. Cancer 40:131, 1977.

12. Salazar O, DePapp E, Bonfiglio T, et al: Adenosquamous carcinoma of the endometrium. Cancer 40:119, 1977.

13. Underwood P, Lutz M, Kreutner A, et al: Carcinoma of the endometrium: Radiation followed immediately by operation. Amer J Obstet Gynecol 128:86, 1977.

14. Crum C, Fechner R: Clear cell adenocarcinoma of the endometrium. Am J Diag Gyne Obst 3:261, 1979.

15. Giri S, Schneider V, Belgrad R: Clear cell carcinoma of the endometrium: an uncommon entity with a favorable prognosis. Int J Radiat Oncol Biol Phys 7:1383, 1981.

16. Kurman R, Scully R: Clear cell carcinoma of the endometrium. An analysis of 21 cases. Cancer 37:872, 1976.

17. Photopoulos G, Carney C, Edelmend A, et al: Clear cell carcinoma of the endometrium. Cancer 43:1448, 1979.

18. Silverberg S, DiGiorgi L: Clear cell carcinoma of the endometrium. Clinical, pathologic and ultrastructural finds. Cancer 31:1127, 1973.

19. Melin JR, Wanner L, Schula D, et al: Primary squamous cell carcinoma of the endometrium. Obstetr Gynecol 53:115, 1979.

20. Walton L: Diagnosis and management of early carcinoma of the endometrium. J Nat Med Assoc 70:309, 1978.

21. Jones HW III: Treatment of adenocarcinoma of the endometrium. Obstetr Gynecol Survey 30:147, 1975.

22. Malkasian G, Annegers J, Fountain K: Carcinoma of the endometrium: Stage I. Amer J Obstet Gynecol 136:872, 1980.

23. Salazar O, Feldstein M, DePapp E, et al: The management of clinical stage I endometrial carcinoma. Cancer 41:1016, 1978.

24. Classification and staging of malignant tumors in the female pelvis. ACOG Technical Bulletin No. 47, June, 1977.

25. Berman M, Balloon S, Lagasse L, et al: Prognosis and treatment of endometrial cancer. Amer J Obstet Gynecol 136:679, 1980.

26. Salazar O, Feldstein M, DePapp E, et al: Endometrial carcinoma: Analysis of failures with special emphasis on the use of initial preoperative external pelvic radiation. Int J Radiat Oncol Biol Phys 2:1101, 1977.

27. Naib AM: Exfoliative Cytology. Boston, Little Brown and Co, 1970.

28. Glassburn JR: Carcinoma of the endometrium. Cancer 48:575, 1981.

29. Stock RJ, Kambour A: Prehysterectomy curettage. Obstetr Gynecol 45:537, 1975.

30. Edinger D, Watring W, Anderson B: Hysterography as a diagnostic technique in endometrial carcinoma. Clin Obstet Gynecol 22:729, 1979.

31. Nilsen PA, Koller O: Carcinoma of the endometrium in Norway 1957–1960 with special reference to treatment results. Amer J Obstetr Gynecol 105:1099, 1969.
32. Ng A, Reagan J: Incidence and prognosis of endometrial carcinoma by histologic grade and extent. Obstetr Gynecol 35:437, 1970.
33. Wade ME, Kohorn EI, Morris JM: Adenocarcinoma of the endometrium; evaluation of preoperative irradiation and factors influencing prognosis. Amer J Obstetr Gynecol 99:869, 1967.
34. Anderson JE, Mettzar HD, Scarbrough JE, et al: Adenocarcinoma of the endometrium. Cancer 18:955, 1965.
35. Austin JH, MacMahon B: Indicators of prognosis in carcinomas of the corpus uteri. Surg Gynecol Obstetr 128:1247, 1969.
36. Cheon HK: Prognosis of endometrial carcinoma. Obstetr Gynecol 34:680, 1969.
37. DeMuelenaere GFGO: Prognostic factors in endometrial carcinoma. S Afr Med J 49:1695, 1975.
38. Graham JB: The value of preoperative or postoperative treatment by radium for carcinoma of the uterine body. Surg Gynecol Obstetr 132:855, 1971.
39. Gusberg SB, Yannopoulos D: Therapeutic decisions in corpus cancer. Amer J Obstetr Gynecol 83:157, 1964.
40. Shah CA, Green TJ: Evaluation of current management of endometrial carcinoma. Obstetr Gynecol 39:500, 1972.
41. Aalders J, Abeler V, Kolstad P, et al: Postoperative external irradiation and prognostic parameters in stage I endometrial carcinoma. Obstet Gynecol 56:419, 1980.
42. Beck R: Experience in treating two hundred and eighty-eight patients with endometrial carcinoma from 1968 to 1972. Amer J Obstet Gynecol 133:260, 1979.
43. Chung C, Stryker J, Nahhas W, et al: The role of adjunctive radiotherapy for stage I endometrial carcinoma: preoperative vs. postoperative irradiation. Int J Radiat Oncol Biol Phys 7:1429, 1981.
44. Connelly P, Alberhasky R, Christopherson W: Carcinoma of the endometrium III. Analysis of 865 cases of adenocarcinoma and adenoacanthoma. Obstet Gynecol 59:569, 1982.
45. Homesley H, Boronow R, Lewis J Jr: Treatment of adenocarcinoma of the endometrium at Memorial-James Ewing Hospitals, 1949–1965. Obstet Gynecol 47:100, 1976.
46. Iversen T, Holter J: Radical surgery in stage I carcinoma of the corpus uteri. Brit J Obstet Gynecol 88:1135, 1981.
47. Joslin C, Vaishampayan G, Mallik A: The treatment of early cancer of the corpus uteri. Brit J Radiol 50:38, 1977.
48. Kinsella T, Bloomer W, Lavin P, et al: Stage II endometrial carcinoma: 10-year follow-up of combined radiation and surgical treatment. Gynecol Oncol 10:290, 1980.
49. Mainsaet M, Brigati D, Boyce J, et al: The significance residual disease after radiotherapy in endometrial carcinoma: clinicopathologic correlation. Amer J Obstet Gynecol 138:557, 1980.
50. Masubuchi S, Fujimoto I, Masubuchi K: Lymph node metastasis and prognosis of endometrial carcinoma. Gynecol Oncol 7:36, 1979.
51. McCabe J, Sagerman R: Treatment of endometrial cancer in a regional radiation therapy center. Cancer 43:1052, 1979.
52. Morrow P: Endometrial carcinoma stages I and II: Is surgery adequate? Int J Radiat Oncol Biol Phys 6:365, 1980.
53. Morrow CP, Disaia P, Townsend D: Current management of endometrial carcinoma. Obstet Gynecol 42:399, 1973.
54. Musumeri R, DePalo G, Conti U, et al: Are retroperitoneal lymph node metastases a major problem in endometrial adenocarcinoma? Cancer 46:1887, 1980.

55. Nussbaum H, Kagan A, Chan P, et al: Stage I grade III endometrial carcinoma: Evaluation of treatment and recommendation for management. Gynecol Oncol 11:50, 1981.
56. Ohlsen J, Johnson G, Stewart R, et al: Combined therapy for endometrial carcinoma: Preoperative intracavitary irradiation followed promptly by hysterectomy. Cancer 39:659, 1977.
57. Paterson E, Spratt D, Tomkiewisz Z, et al: Management of Stage I carcinoma of the uterus. Obstet Gynecol 59:755, 1982.
58. Piver S: Stage I endometrial carcinoma: the role of adjunctive radiation therapy. Int J Radiat Oncol Biol Phys 6:367, 1980.
59. Piver S, Yazizi R, Blumenson L, et al: A prospective trail comparing hysterectomy, hysterectomy plus vaginal radium, and uterine radium plus hysterectomy in Stage I endometrial carcinoma. Obstet Gynecol 54:85, 1979.
60. Prem K, Adcock L, Okagaki T, et al: The evolution of a treatment program for adenocarcinoma of the endometrium. Amer J Obstet Gynecol 133:803, 1979.
61. Surwit E, Fowler W, Rogoff E: Stage II carcinoma of the endometrium. Obstet Gynecol 52:97, 1978.
62. Surwit E, Fowler W, Rogoff E, et al: Stage II carcinoma of the endometrium. Int J Radiat Oncol Biol Phys 5:323, 1979.
63. Wharam M, Phillips T: The role of radiation therapy in clinical stage I carcinoma of the endometrium. Int J Radiat Oncol Biol Phys I:1081, 1976.
64. Wilson F, Cox J, Chahbazian C, et al: Time dose relationships in endometrial adenocarcinoma: Importance of the interval from external pelvic irradiation to surgery. Int J Radiat Oncol Biol Phys 6:597, 1980.
65. Lewis G, Mortel R, Slack N: Endometrial cancer. Cancer 39:959, 1977.
66. Creasman W, Boronow R, Morrow P, et al: Adenocarcinoma of the endometrium: Its metastatic lymph node potential. A preliminary report. Gynecol Oncol 4:239, 1976.
67. Boronow R, Morrow P, Creasman W, et al: Surgical staging in endometrial cancer: Clinical-pathologic findings of a prospective study. Obstet Gynecol (in press).
68. DiSaia P, Creasman W, Boronow R, et al: Risk factors and recurrence patterns in stage I endometrial cancer. Submitted to Amer J. Obstet Gynecol.
69. Lewis DV, Stallworthy JA, Cowdell R: Adenocarcinoma of the body of the uterus. J Obstetr Gynaecol Br Commonw 77:343, 1970.
70. Creasman WT, Rutledge FN: The prognostic value of peritoneal cytology in gynecologic malignant disease. Amer J Obstetr Gynecol 110:773, 1971.
71. Lewis G: Personal communication regarding GOG, protocol 33.
72. Anderson B: Diagnosis and staging of endometrial carcinoma. Clin Obstet Gynecol 25:75, 1982.
73. Anderson B, Marchant D, Munzenrider J, et al: Routine noninvasive hysterography in the evaluation and treatment of endometrial carcinoma. Gynecol Oncol 4:354, 1976.
74. Johnson J, Norman O: Relation between prognosis in early carcinoma of the uterine body and hysterographically assessed localization and size of tumor. Gynecol Oncol 7:71, 1979.
75. Bernardino M, Dodd G: Imaging of the pelvic contents in the female oncologic patient. Cancer 48:504, 1981.
76. Chen S, Kumari S, Lee L: Contribution of abdominal computed tomography (CT) in the management of gynecologic cancer: Correlated study of CT image and gross surgical pathology. Gynecol Oncol 10:162, 1980.
77. Patricio M, Tavares M, Vilhena M, et al: Radiosurgical treatment of endometrial carcinoma: the value of simple surgery versus extended surgery. Int J Radiat Oncol Biol Phys 5:355, 1979.
78. Baker H, Makk L, Morrissey R, et al: Stage I adenocarcinoma of the endometrium. Obstet Gynecol 54:146, 1979.

79. Cheung A: Prognostic significance of negative hysterectomy specimen following intra-cavitary irradiation in stage I endometrial carcinoma. Brit J Obstet Gynecol 88:548, 1981.

80. Chung C, Stryker J, Nakkas W, et al: Analysis of residual disease following preoperative radiotherapy versus initial surgery in endometrial carcinoma. Int J Radiat Oncol Biol Phys 8:213, 1982.

81. Draca P, Tesic M, Valeek M, et al: On the value of preoperative intracavital irradiation in carcinoma of the uterus. Gynecol Oncol 9:1, 1980.

82. Fayos J: Pre-operative external radiation therapy. Int J Radiat Oncol Biol Phys 6:369, 1980.

83. Fayos J, Maroles P: Carcinoma of the endometrium. Results of treatment. Int J Radiat Oncol Biol Phys 6:571, 1980.

84. Gagnon J, Moss W, Gabourel L, et al: External irradiation in the management of stage II endometrial carcinoma. Cancer 44:1247, 1979.

85. Gusberg S, Yannopoulos D: Therapeutic decisions in corpus cancer. Amer J Obstet Gynecol 88:157, 1964.

86. Nolan J, Huen A: Prognosis in endometrial cancer. Gynecol Oncol 4:384, 1976.

87. Park R, Patow W, Petty W, et al: Treatment of adenocarcinoma of the endometrium. Gynecol Oncol 2:60, 1974.

88. Ritcher N, Lucas W, Yon J, et al: Preoperative whole pelvic external irradiation in stage I endometrial cancer. Cancer 48:58, 1981.

89. Tak W, Marchant D, Munzenrider J, et al: Preoperative irradiation for carcinoma of the endometrium: Indications and results. Gynecol Oncol 5:18, 1977.

90. Underwood P, Fenn J, Wallace K, et al: Adenocarcinoma of the Endometrium: Role of preoperative radiation in stage I disease. Amer J Obstetr Gynecol 128:86, 1977.

91. Surwit E, Joelsson I, Einhorn N: Adjunctive radiation therapy in the management of stage I cancer of the endometrium. Obstet Gynecol 58:590, 1981.

92. Tak W: Carcinoma of the endometrium with cervical involvement (stage II). Cancer 43:2504, 1979.

93. Onsurd M, Aalders J, Abeler V, et al: Endometrial carcinoma with cervical involvement (stage II): prognostic factors and value of combined radiological-surgical treatment. Gynecol Onxol 13:76, 1982.

94. Abayomi O, Enami B, Anderson B: Treatment of endometrial carcinoma with radiation therapy alone. Cancer 49:2466, 1982.

95. Candiani G, Mangioni C, Marzi M: Surgery in endometrial cancer: Age, route, and operability rate in 854 stage I and II fresh consecutive cases: 1955–1976. Gynecol Oncol 6:363, 1978.

96. Hernandez W, Nolan J, Morrow P, et al: Stage II endometrial carcinoma: two modalities of treatment. Amer J Obstet Gynecol 13:171, 1978.

97. Kjellgren O, Sigurd J: Efficacy of primary radiation in carcinoma of the endometrium. Acta Obstet Gynecol Scand (Suppl) 66:69, 1977.

98. Boronow R: Carcinoma of the corpus: Treatment at M. D. Anderson Hospital. In Cancer of the Uterus and Ovary. Year Book Medical Publishers, Chicago, 1969.

99. Bruckman J, Goodman R, Murthy A, et al: Combined irradiation and surgery in the treatment of stage II carcinoma of the endometrium. Cancer 42:1146, 1978.

100. Greenberg S, Glassbrun J, Antoniades J, et al: Management of carcinoma of the uterus stage II. Cancer Clin Trials 4:183, 1981.

101. Homesley H, Boronow R, Lewis J: Stage II endometrial adenocarcinoma. Memorial Hospital for Cancer, 1949–1965. Obstet Gynecol 49:604, 1977.

102. Madoc-Jones H: Adenocarcinoma of the endometrium, stage II problems in definition and management. Int J Radiat Oncol biol Phys 6:887, 1980.

103. Nakkas W, Whitney C, Stryker J, et al: Stage II endometrial carcinoma. Gynecol Oncol 10:303, 1980.
104. Lewis G: Personal communication of GOG preliminary data.
105. Berman M: The treatment of stage I carcinoma of the endometrium. In Ballon S (ed): Controversies in Gynecologic Oncology. GK Hull, Boston, 1981.
106. Berman M, Ballon S: Treatment of endometrial cancer. Cancer Treatment Reviews 6:165, 1979.
107. Johnson G: The treatment of stage I carcinoma of the endometrium. In Ballon S (ed): Controversies in Gynecologic Oncology. GK Hull, Boston, 1981.
108. Brady L, Lewis G, Antoniades J, et al: Evolution of radiotherapeutic techniques. Gynecol Oncol 2:314, 1974.
109. Yoonessi M, Anderson D, Morley G: Endometrial carcinoma. Cancer 43:1944, 1979.
110. Bruckman J, Bloomer W, Marck A, et al: Stage III adenocarcinoma of the endometrium: Two prognostic groups. Gynecol Oncol 9:12, 1980.
111. Danoff B, McDay J, Louka M, et al: Stage III endometrial carcinoma: Analysis of patterns of failure and therapeutic implications. Int J Radiat Oncol Biol Phys 6:1491, 1980.
112. Antoniades J, Brady L, Lewis G: The management of stage III carcinoma of the endometrium. Cancer 38:1838, 1976.
113. Purtoli Ľ, Ciatto S, Cionini L, et al: Salvage with radiotherapy of postsurgical relapses of endometrial cancer. Tumori 66:475, 1980.
114. Fountain K, Malkasian G: Radioactive colloidal cold in the treatment of endometrial cancer. Cancer 47:2430, 1981.
115. Kistner RW: Histologic effect of progestins on hyperplasia and carcinoma in situ of the endometrium. Cancer 12:1106, 1959.
116. Kohorn E: Gestagens and endometrial carcinoma. Gynecol Oncol 4:398, 1976.
117. Piver S, Barlow J, Lurain J, et al: Medroxyprogesterone acetate (Depo-Provera) vs. hydroxyprogesterone caproate (Delalutin) in women with metastatic endometrial adenocarcinoma. Cancer 45:268, 1980.
118. Thigpen T: Personal communication of preliminary Gynecologic Oncology Group data.
119. Reifenstein EC: Hydroxyprogesterone caproate therapy in advanced endometrial cancer. Cancer 27:485, 1971.
120. Billiet G, DeHertogh R, Bonte J, et al: Estrogen receptors in human uterine adenocarcinoma: Correlation with tissue differentiation, vaginal karyopyenotic index, and effect of progestogen on anti-estrogen treatment. Gynecol Oncol 14:33, 1982.
121. Creasman W, McCarty K, Barton T: Clinical correlates of estrogen- and progesterone-binding proteins in human endometrial adenocarcinoma. Obstet Gynecol 55:363, 1980.
122. Ehrlich C, Young P, Cleary R: Cytoplasmic progesterone and estradiol receptors in normal, hyperplastic and carcinomatous endometria: Therapeutic implications. Amer J Obstet Gynecol 141:539, 1981.
123. Freedman M, Hoffman P, Jones W: The clinical value of hormone receptor assays in malignant disease. Cancer Treatment Reviews 5:185, 1978.
124. Janne O, Kauppila A, Kontula K, et al: Female sex steroid receptors in normal hyperplastic, and carcinomatous endometrium. The relationship to serum steroid hormones and gonadotropins and changes during medroxyprogesterone acetate administration. Int J Cancer 24:545, 1979.
125. Benraad T, Finberg L, Koenders A, et al: Do estrogen and progesterone receptors in metastasizing endometrial cancers predict the response to gestagen therapy? Acta Obstet Gynecol Scand 59:155, 1980.
126. Martin P, Rolland P, Ganxamerre M, et al: Estradiol and progesterone receptors in nor-

mal and neoplastic endometrium correlation between receptors, histopathologic examination and clinical responses under progestin therapy. Int J Cancer 23:321, 1979.

127. McCarty K JR, Barton T, Fetter B, et al: Correlation of estrogen and progesterone receptors with histologic differentiation in endometrial adenocarcinoma. Amer J Pathol 96:171, 1979.

128. Bonte J, Decoster J, Ide P, et al: Hormonoprophylaxis and hormonotherapy in the treatment of endometrial adenocarcinoma by means of medroxyprogesterone acetate. Gynecol Oncol 6:60, 1978.

129. Kelly R, Baker W: The role of progesterone in human endometrial cancer. Cancer Res 25:1190, 1965.

130. Kennedy B: Progestagens in the treatment of carcinoma of the endometrium. Surg Gynecol Obstet 103:114, 1968.

131. Rozier J, Underwood P: Use of progestational agents in endometrial adenocarcinoma. Obstet Gynecol 44:60, 1974.

132. Laatikainen T, Nieminen U, Adlercreutz H: Plasma medroxyprogesterone acetate levels following intramuscular or oral administration in patients with endometrial adenocarcinoma. Acta Obstet Gynecol Scand 58:95, 1979.

133. Sall S, DiSaia P, Morrow P, et al: A comparison of medroxyprogesterone serum concentrations by the oral or intramuscular route in patients with persistent or recurrent endometrial carcinoma. Amer J Obstet Gynecol 135:647, 1979.

134. Bonte J, Ide P, Billiet G, et al: Tamoxifen as a possible chemotherapeutic agent in endometrial adenocarcinoma. Gynecol Oncol 11:140, 1981.

135. Swenerton K: Treatment of advanced endometrial adenocarcinoma with tamoxifen. Cancer Treatment Rep 64:805, 1980.

136. Slavik M: Personal communication of Gynecologic Oncology Group data.

137. Kauppila A, Vikko R: Endometrial carcinoma insensitive to progestin and cytotoxic chemotherapy may respond to tamoxifen. Acta Obstet Gynecol Scand 60:589, 1981.

138. Deppe G: Chemotherapeutic treatment of endometrial carcinoma. Clin Obstet Gynecol 25:93, 1982.

139. Thigpen T, Vance R, Balducci L, et al: Chemotherapy in the management of advanced or recurrent cervical and endometrial carcinoma. Cancer 48:658, 1981.

140. DeVita VT, Wasserman TH, Young RC, et al: Perspectives on research in gynecologic oncology. Cancer 38:509, 1976.

141. Horton J, Begg C, Arseneau J, et al: Comparison of adriamycin with cyclophosphamide in patients with advanced endometrial cancer. Cancer Treatment Rep 62:159, 1978.

142. Thigpen T, Buchsbaum H, Mangan C, et al: Phase II trial of adriamycin in the treatment of advanced or recurrent endometrial carcinoma: A gynecologic oncology group study. Cancer Treatment Rep 63:21, 1979.

143. Seski J, Edwards C, Copeland L, et al: Hexamethylmelamine chemotherapy for disseminated endometrial cancer. Obstet Gynecol 58:361, 1981.

144. Deppe G, Cohen C, Bruckner H: Treatment of advanced endometrial adenocarcinoma with cis-dichlorodiammineplatinum (II) after intensive prior therapy. Gynecol Oncol 10:51, 1980.

145. Seski J, Edwards C, Herson J, et al: Cisplatin chemotherapy for disseminated endometrial cancer. Obstet Gynecol 59:225, 1982.

146. Thigpen T, Shingleton H, Homesley H, et al: Cisplatin in the treatment of advanced or recurrent cervix and uterine cancer. In Prestayko A, Crooke S, Carter S (eds): Cisplatin: Current Status and New Development. New York, Academic Press, 1980.

147. Thigpen T, Blessing J, DiSaia P, et al: Phase II trial of cisplatin in the management of advanced or recurrent endometrial carcinoma. Proc ASCO 22:469, 1981.

148. Trope, C, Grundsell H, Johnson J, et al: A phase II study of cisplatinum for recurrent corpus cancer. Eur J Cancer 16:1025, 1980.

149. LaGasse L, Thigpen T, Morrison F: Phase II trial of Piperazinedione in treatment of advanced endometrial carcinoma, uterine sarcoma, and vulvar carcinoma. Proc ASCO 20:388, 1979.

150. Slayton R, Blessing J, Delago G: Phase II trial of etoposide in the management of advanced or recurrent endometrial carcinoma. Cancer Treat Rep 66:1669, 1982.

151. Muggia F, Chia G, Reed J, et al: Doxorubicin cyclophosphamide: Effective chemotherapy for advanced endometrial adenocarcinoma. Amer J Obstet Gynecol 128:314, 1977.

152. Seski J, Edwards C, Gershenson D, et al: Doxorubicin and cyclophosphamide chemotherapy for disseminated endometrial cancer. Obstet Gynecol 58:88, 1981.

153. Alberts D: Personal communication of Southwest Oncology Group, preliminary data.

154. Horton J, Elson P, Gordon P, et al: Combination chemotherapy for advanced endometrial cancer. Cancer 49:2441, 1982.

155. Bruckner HW, Deppe G: Combination chemotherapy of advanced endometrial adenocarcinoma with adriamycin, cyclophosphamide, 5-fluorouracil, and medroxyprogesterone acetate. Obstetr Gynecol 50:105, 1977.

156. Deppe G, Jacobs A, Bruckner H, et al: Chemotherapy of advanced and recurrent endometrial carcinoma with cyclophosphamide, doxorubicin, 5-fluorouracil, and megesterol acetate. Amer J Obstet Gynecol 140:313, 1981.

157. Kauppila A, Jamne O, Kujamsure E, et al: Treatment of advanced endometrial adenocarcinoma with a combined cytotoxic therapy. Cancer 46:2162, 1980.

158. Turbow M, Thornton J, Ballon S, et al: Chemotherapy of advanced endometrial carcinoma with platinum, adriamycin, and cyclophosphamide (PAC). Proc ASCO 1:108, 1982.

159. Cohen CJ, Deppe G, Bruckner HW: Treatment of advanced adenocarcinoma of the endometrium with melphalan, 5-fluorouracil, and medroxyprogesterone acetate. Obstetr Gynecol 50:415, 1977.

160. Piver S, Lele S, Barlow J: Melphalan, 5-fluorouracil, and medroxyprogesterone acetate in metastatic or recurrent endometrial carcinoma. Obstet Gynecol 56:370, 1980.

161. Cohen C, Bruckner H, Deppe G, et al: A randomized study comparing multi-drug chemotherapeutic regimens in the treatment of advanced or recurrent endometrial carcinoma. Amer J Obstet Gynecol (in press).

162. Thigpen T: Personal communication of preliminary GOG data.

163. Bokhman J, Chepick O, Volkova A, et al: Adjuvant hormone therapy of primary endometrial carcinoma with oxyprogesterone caproate. Gynecol Oncol 11:371, 1981.

164. Bonte J: Radium therapy and medroxyprogesterone treatment in the management of primary and recurrent or metastatic uterine adenocarcinoma. In Brush W et al (ed): Endometrial Cancer. London, William Heinemann Medical Books, 1973.

165. Decoster J, Bonte J, Marcq A: Medroxyprogesterone acetate release from silastic devices as replacement for local irradiation by redium tubes in preoperative intrauterine packing for endometrial adenocarcinoma. Gynecol Oncol 5:189, 1977.

166. Lewis G, Clack N, Mortel R, et al: Adjuvant progestagen therapy in the primary definitive treatment of endometrial cancer. Gynecol Oncol 2:362, 1974.

167. Roloz J, Jacobs A, Holland J, et al: Intraperitoneal infusion of doxorubicin in the treatment of gynecologic carcinomas. Med Ped Oncol 9:245, 1981.

168. Gal D, Ohaski M, MacDonald P, et al: Low density liproprotein as a potential vehicle for chemotherapeutic agents and radionecleotides in the management of gynecologic neoplasms. Amer J Obstet Gynecol 139:877, 1981.

12 | Gestational Trophoblastic Disease: Prognostic Factors and Management

Walter Burnett Jones

Hydatidiform mole, chorioadenoma destruens (invasive mole), and choriocarcinoma are neoplasms that originate in the fetal chorion. Hertz developed the concept of "gestational trophoblastic disease" to emphasize the interrelationship among these abnormalities.[1] In his view, the morphologic characterization of hydatidiform mole, invasive mole, and choriocarcinoma delineates successive phases in the evolution of a disease continuum. The benign hydatidiform mole represents the beginning, while the highly malignant choriocarcinoma represents the end of the spectrum.

Prior to 1956, patients who developed metastatic gestational trophoblastic disease faced an almost uniformly fatal outcome. Li, Hertz, and Spencer's report in 1956 of three patients with metastases who achieved complete sustained remission after therapy with methotrexate was therefore a landmark in the development of successful chemotherapy in this disease.[2] Hertz, Lewis, and Lipsett in 1961 reported 47 percent complete and sustained remissions in 63 consecutive patients with metastatic disease using methotrexate and vincaleukoblastine sulfate.[3] Following this achievement, Ross and co-workers in Dr. Hertz's group in 1966 reported a complete and sustained remission rate of 74 percent in 50 consecutive patients with metastatic disease who were treated with sequential methotexate and actinomycin D.[4] The continued improvement in prognosis for these patients is reflected in reports from major treatment centers where sustained remissions are currently being achieved in approximately 90 percent of patients with metastatic disease, and virtually 100 percent of patients with localized disease.[5-10]

Because most patients who develop malignant gestational trophoblastic disease do so as a sequel of a hydatidiform mole, the diagnosis and management of this condition will be discussed first. Following this, an outline of current therapy as related to a therapeutic classification based on an individual patient's risk of developing a drug-resistant tumor is presented. Patients are separated into four categories which take into account the initial hCG level, duration of disease, sites of metastases if present, and whether or not previous unsuccessful chemotherapy has been given. Hammond and associates utilized similar criteria to divide their patients with metastases into "good" and "poor" prognostic groups.[11] A more comprehensive scoring system has been devised by Bagshawe in which twelve factors affecting prognosis are assigned numerical values. The totals are then used to divide patients into low-, medium-, and high-risk categories.[12]

Finally, a brief review of the chemistry and techniques for measurement of hCG are presented. This hormone functions as a specific tumor marker in cases of gestational trophoblastic disease and is relied upon to monitor response to therapy. Advances in hCG assay methodology have made it possible to detect minimal amounts of viable tumor in patients who otherwise would be considered free of disease. The recognition of the need for additional therapy in such patients has been a significant factor in the overall improvement in prognosis for patients with gestational trophoblastic disease.

HYDATIDIFORM MOLE

Diagnosis

The early stages of hydatidiform mole may be very similar to those of a normal pregnancy. Because of this, a high degree of suspicion is required to arrive at the correct diagnosis. An abnormal gestation is suggested clinically by vaginal bleeding, uterine growth more rapid than gestational age, hyperemesis, toxemia before the 24th week of pregnancy, and theca lutein cysts of the ovaries. In a review of 347 cases of hydatidiform mole reported by Curry et al.[13] symptoms of abnormal bleeding were present in 89 percent of patients, nausea and vomiting in 14 percent, and preeclampsia in 12 percent. Significantly, 46 percent of their patients had uterine size increased over that expected for the duration of pregnancy and approximately 15 percent of patients had enlarged ovaries.

Markedly elevated levels of hCG frequently accompany an in situ hydatidiform mole and may suggest this diagnosis. However, in view of the very high levels of hCG seen in some cases of normal gestation, it is important to stress that the height of the hCG titer should not be considered diagnostic evidence of a molar pregnancy. Although rarely a mole can occur in the presence of a fetus,[14] as shown in Figure 12-1, the usual absence of a fetus as evidenced by a lack of fetal electrocardiogram tracing and the absence of fetal heart tones when expected are helpful signs in establishing the diagnosis.

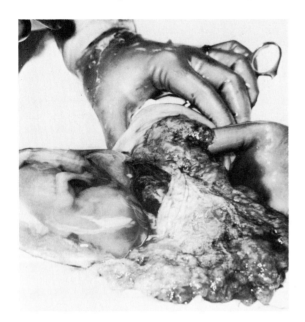

Fig. 12-1. Mole and coexistent fetus treated by hysterotomy showing marked hydatidiform degeneration of the placenta.

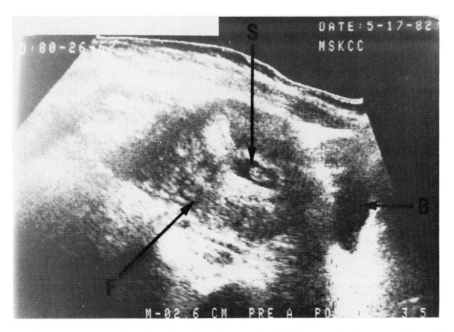

Fig. 12-2. Sonogram of patient thought to have a hydatidiform mole because of large-for-dates uterus, but found to have a normal intrauterine pregnancy and fibroids.

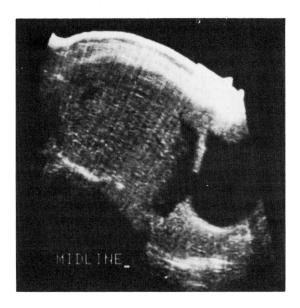

Fig. 12-3. Sonogram of large-for-dates uterus showing characteristic echoes of hydatidiform mole.

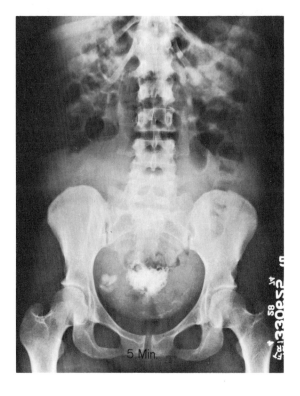

Fig. 12-4. Amniogram showing honeycombed, moth-eaten pattern of hydatidiform mole.

The initial diagnostic procedure when a patient is suspected of having an in situ molar pregnancy should be pelvic ultrasound. The observation by Donald that ultrasonography is not associated with any known hazards becomes important whenever the differential diagnosis includes a normal pregnancy.[15] In a patient with a large for dates uterus, the correct diagnosis may be an intrauterine pregnancy associated with uterine myomata (Fig. 12-2). The sonogram can establish this diagnosis and also provide an early diagnosis of hydatidiform mole when the expected fetal sac is absent and characteristic echoes of molar tissue are observed (Fig. 12-3). In cases where the sonogram shows no evidence of fetal parts but is inconclusive for molar pregnancy, an intra-amniotic injection of contrast medium can be diagnostic.[16] The characteristic image of molar vesicles surrounded by opaque contrast medium is commonly described as honeycombed or moth-eaten (Fig. 12-4). It should be noted, however, that some authors find the radiation exposure of an amniogram unacceptable when the differential diagnosis includes a normal intrauterine gestation.[17] Recent experience with the hysteroscope, an endoscopic instrument primarily used to study abnormalities related to uterine bleeding in non-pregnant women, has been recommended for differential diagnosis of hydatidiform mole. According to Baggish and Barbot,[18] in molar disease, direct observation of the gestation with a 6mm contact hysteroscope can be performed safely and represents a direct atraumatic technique for making a positive diagnosis. While this method of diagnosis may prove to be of value in the future, at present its use in this condition is still experimental.

Treatment of Hydatidiform Mole

Once the diagnosis is made, evacuation of the mole should be carried out promptly. First, the patient should be medically stabilized with strict attention given to fluid management. Correction of anemia, actual or dilutional should be carefully monitored because transfusion of large quantities of whole blood can result in vascular overload and acute pulmonary edema. Approximately 10 percent of patients with molar pregnancy reported by Twiggs et al.[19] experienced severe acute respiratory embarassment during hospitalization. In their study the majority of patients were thought to have developed trophoblastic embolization, but thyrotoxicosis and iatrogenic fluid overload were also significant etiologic factors. This complication appears to occur primarily in patients with a uterus large for dates and more than 16 weeks gestational size. For this reason central venous pressure monitoring or the use of the Swan-Ganz catheter to measure pulmonary wedge pressure is advisable in such patients.

Dilatation and curettage is recommended when the uterus is 12 weeks gestational size or smaller, while suction curettage is the method of choice when the uterus is larger. The procedure should be carried out during an infusion of an oxytocic agent so as to enhance contractility of the uterus and to decrease inadvertent perforations. Tow documented the safety of vaginal evacuation in more than 300 patients who had the procedure without a single instance of uterine perforation, regardless of uterine size.[20] Once the mole is evacuated by suction curettage, most authorities recommend a gentle curettage of the uterine wall with a blunt curette so as to reduce the amount of retained tissue. It should be noted that oxytocin infusion is not recommended as a primary means of evacuating a hydatidiform mole because of the risk of massive deportation of trophoblastic tissue to the lungs. For similar reasons it is ill-advised to evacuate an in situ mole by means of intrauterine injection of hypertonic saline solution. Frost reported the death of a patient following this treatment.[21] At autopsy, aggregates of trophoblastic cells were found in multiple arterioles of the lungs. The role of vaginal prostaglandins in emptying the uterus is uncertain. This is because of the increased blood loss that sometimes follows the procedure and the observation that many patients will ultimately require a curettage after delivery of the mole. Since there is no extra-amniotic space in molar pregnancies attempts at "extra-amniotic" injection of prostaglandins are clearly contraindicated. Such a procedure may result in the solution entering the maternal circulation producing severe systemic reactions and cardiovascular collapse.[22]

Hysterotomy and hysterectomy are also effective methods of evacuating an in situ hydatidiform mole. Indeed, either may be the procedure of choice in situations where profuse hemorrhage is encountered. In current clinical practice, however, hysterotomy is rarely indicated because of the safety of suction curettage when the uterus is enlarged. Hysterectomy on the other hand may be recommended as primary therapy in women over 40 years of age and those of high parity. Analyses of malignancy rates in relation to age and parity have shown a two- to three-fold increase in frequency of proliferative sequelae in such patients. Hysterectomy appears to decrease this risk in these patients. For similar reasons hysterectomy is also considered appropriate therapy in patients who have completed their desired child bearing regardless of age or parity. It should be noted, however, that removal of the uterus does not decrease the requirement for close post operative follow-up. Curry et al.[13] reported that their patients with moles encountered a 20 percent chance of malignant sequelae despite removal of the uterus.

The temporal combination of chemotherapy and surgery was advocated by Lewis et al.[23] in 1965 to treat any cells left behind in the uterus or pushed into the circulation by the surgical procedure. Goldstein documented the effectiveness of this approach when actinomycin D was given at the time of curettage.[24] Although metastatic disease was eliminated and local proliferative sequelae diminished by this technique, most authors do not recommend its use as routine practice. Objections center around the following observations: (1) most patients are cured by evacuation alone; (2) essentially all patients who develop malignant sequelae in the immediate post-evacuation period can be cured by present modalities; (3) minimal drug toxicity is experienced by most patients, but severe reactions or even death may occur in an unusually sensitive patient; (4) cytotoxic agents are teratogens, and therefore recessive mutagenic changes may occur; (5) responsiveness to subsequent therapy is decreased in patients who develop persistent disease after adjunctive chemotherapy. Authorities agree that this treatment should be limited to use by experienced clinicians who have access to laboratory facilities for the appropriate monitor of drug toxicity. When adjunctive chemotherapy is used, it should be given on an individualized basis and limited perhaps to patients such as those with a history of prior molar pregnancy, older and high parity patients or to those whose follow-up is uncertain.

Follow-up

Post-molar follow-up practices have changed very little since Delph's careful study of the decline of hCG after molar evacuation. While incomplete involution of the uterus and vaginal bleeding may be signs of persistent trophoblastic disease, she documented that measurement of subsequent hCG levels is the most reliable method of identifying patients who require additional therapy.[25] For this reason weekly gonadotropin determinations are recommended until normal values are obtained. Delph further observed that approximately 1 in 4 patients had a positive hCG assay at 8 weeks and of this group approximately 50 percent developed a clinically or histologically malignant condition. Similarly, Curry et al.[13] recently reported that 40 percent of their patients with elevated titers after 60 days required chemotherapy. On the other hand Pastorfide et al.[26] utilizing a sensitive beta subunit assay for hCG have shown that the hormone may be detected in the serum of successfully treated patients for periods extending to 15 weeks depending on the method of evacuation. In some centers chemotherapy is withheld for even longer periods of time so long as hCG levels are declining. Most authorities, however, institute chemotherapy in all patients who have detectable serum hCG levels 12 weeks after evacuation of the mole. Current recommendations for chemotherapy therefore include:

1. Persistence of serum hCG 12 weeks after evacuation of the mole;
2. Plateau of hCG levels for 2 consecutive weeks; and
3. hCG level rises during the follow-up period.

While the incidence of malignant sequelae following a molar pregnancy averages approximately 10 percent in collected series, the risk for an individual patient is quite variable.[27] As indicated previously age and parity are significant risk factors. Additional risk factors include the presence of ovarian enlargement and large for dates uteri (50 percent),[13,28] excessive bleeding after evacuation, acute pulmonary symptoms,[19,29–31] and the use of oral contraceptives before negative hCG titers are attained[32] and the history of a prior mole.[33]

Vassilakos and Kajii and Szulman and Surti have classified hydatidiform moles into two distinct entities: "partial" and "complete" moles and have indicated that certain morphologic and cytogenetic features of moles may also be predictive of subsequent trophoblastic neoplasia.[34,35] In their studies, complete moles were characterized by the absence of normal villi, the lack of an embryo, cord or amniotic membranes, the presence of marked trophoblastic hyperplasia and anaplasia and the exclusive occurence of the female karyotype, 46xx. Partial moles were associated with a fetus, cord and/or amniotic membrane, the absence of trophoblastic cell anaplasia and marked hyperplasia, and karyotypes which included trisomies, triploidy, and tetraploidy. According to their findings, only complete moles constitute the potential for proliferative sequelae. Although the view that complete moles carry a higher risk of malignancy than partial moles is supported by the findings of several authors, these authorities emphasize the need to also closely monitor patients with partial moles because the actual risk in these cases is yet to be defined.[14,36,37]

Of interest are the recent reports establishing the origin of the female karyotype in complete moles. Kajii and Ohama, Wake et al. and Jacobs et al. from analyses using polymorphic chromosome markers have determined that complete moles receive only paternal chromosomes and are thus androgenetically derived.[38-40] The mechanism of androgenesis, according to Yamashita et al.[41] who studied histocompatibility specificities (HLA) of complete moles and parents and Lawler et al.[42] who employed biochemical markers, involves fertilization by a haploid sperm followed by duplication of its chromosomes after meiotic devision.

Recent studies have shown that the slope of the hCG regression after the evacuation may provide yet another method of identifying patients who are likely to develop malignant sequelae. Schlaerth et al.[43] observed that the regression of hCG levels followed a log-normal distribution in patients with truly benign disease. In contrast, the majority of patients with malignancy manifested an abnormal hCG regression curve that could be identified in many patients by 3 weeks and in 87 percent of patients by 6 weeks after evacuation.

TREATMENT OF GESTATIONAL TROPHOBLASTIC DISEASE

Group I Non-Metastatic

1. Tumor confined to the uterus
2. Titer and duration of disease less important
3. All histopathologic diagnoses

Patients in this category are found to have their disease confined to the uterus after complete history, physical examination, and chest x-ray. Pre-treatment evaluation includes the following laboratory studies: hemoglobin, hematocrit, white blood cell count, differential count, serum glutamic oxaloacetic transaminase, bilirubin, alkaline phosphatase, and plasma fibrinogen. Routine urinalysis and quantitative test for hCG are also performed.

The more commonly encountered clinical situations include: (1) Rising serum concentrations of hCG, plateau of hCG levels or persistence of hCG in the serum following evacuation of a mole (2) choriocarcinoma following abortion or full-term delivery.

Specific and sensitive assays are required to monitor hCG regression after evacuation of a hydatidiform mole in order to facilitate the early identification of patients who require additional therapy. Techniques to accomplish this are discussed in detail elsewhere in this presentation. Because approximately half of all choriocarcinoma and invasive moles occur following a molar pregnancy, early diagnosis is possible in most of these cases. The benefit to the patient can be seen in the results from the Southeastern Regional Center for Trophoblastic Disease where 69 patients treated for persistent disease all achieved complete and sustained remission.[13] The adverse effect of late diagnosis is apparent from the report by Bagshawe et al.[44] who observed an increasing mortality as the interval between evacuation of the mole and start of chem-

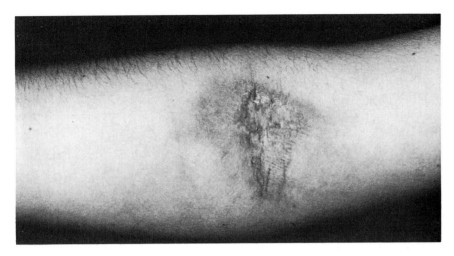

Fig. 12-5. Slough and necrosis of skin following extravascular infiltration of actinomycin D.

otherapy increased. In patients treated within 6 months, the mortality was 5 percent whereas a mortality rate of 60 percent occurred when treatment was started after 12 months.

Early diagnosis of choriocarcinoma following a term pregnancy, abortion, or ectopic pregnancy is more difficult because the symptom-free interval may not suggest a temporal relationship to the antecedent pregnancy. The correct diagnosis can be arrived at early, however, if the gynecologic history reveals a previous ectopic pregnancy, recent term pregnancy, or irregular vaginal bleeding and the patient has a positive test for hCG.

The dose and schedule of chemotherapeutic agents for patients with non-metastatic disease is Methotrexate (10–30 mg IM daily x5) or Actinomycin-D (8–13 micrograms/kg body weight IV daily x5).

Both drugs appear to be equally effective in the treatment of non-metastatic dis-

Table 12-1. The Methotrexate/Citrovorum Protocol

Day	Time	Therapy
1	8 a.m.	CBC, Platelet count, SGOT
	4 p.m.	Mtx, 1.0–1.5 mg/kg, IM
2	4 p.m.	CF, 0.1–0.15 mg/kg, IM
3	8 a.m.	CBC, platelet count, SGOT
	4 p.m.	Mtx, 1.0–1.5 mg/kg, IM
4	4 p.m.	CF, 0.1–0.15 mg/kg, IM
5	8 a.m.	CBC, platelet count, SGOT
	4 p.m.	Mtx, 1.0–1.5 mg/kg, IM
6	4 p.m.	CF, 0.1–0.15 mg/kg, IM
7	8 a.m.	CBC, platelet count, SGOT
	4 p.m.	Mtx, 1.0–1.5 mg/kg, IM
8	4 p.m.	CF, 0.1–0.15 mg/kg, IM
11, 15, 18, 21		CBC, platelet count, SGOT

ease and there does not appear to be significant cross resistance between these agents. Actinomycin-D is the obvious drug of choice if hepatic impairment is present. It should be noted that actinomycin-D should be given through the tubing of a previously started intravenous infusion because extravascular infiltration causes necrosis and slough (Fig. 12-5). Therapy is given at intervals of approximately 2 weeks until hCG is undetectable.

The use of methotrexate with citrovorum factor (CF) rescue as primary therapy for non-metastatic disease was reported by Goldstein et al.[45] in 1976. The main advantage of this regimen is its applicability for ambulatory treatment based on the lack of significant toxicity despite the use of a much higher dose of methotrexate than the dose employed when methotrexate is used alone. The methotrexate/citrovorum protocol is given in Table 12-1.

According to Goldstein et al.[45] the initial course of methotrexate (Mtx) in non-metastatic disease should be 1.0 mg/kg, CF always being one tenth of Mtx dose. With response use the same dose. Without response-increase Mtx by 0.5 mg/kg and CF by 0.05 mg/kg. If there is no response for 2 consecutive courses, change the drug. This regimen according to these authors has provided complete and sustained remission rates of more than 90 percent in patients with non-metastatic disease. Smith et al.[46] on the other hand compared methotrexate alone with a similar methotrexate/citrovorum rescue regimen in non-metastatic disease patients and found that methotrexate-resistant disease developed in 7.7 percent of the first group and in 27.5 percent in the latter group. They concluded that methotrexate with folinic acid while less toxic than methotrexate alone is less effective than methotrexate alone in the induction of remission of non-metastatic gestational trophoblastic disease.

Group II Metastatic (Low Risk)

1. Apparent metastases in sites other than liver or brain
2. Titer less than 100,000 IU/24 hr (20,000 ng/ml) duration of disease greater than 4 months
3. All histopathologic diagnoses

Workers at the National Cancer Institute (NCI) first reported that in patients with metastatic disease who had an initial hCG titer of less than 100,000 IU/24 hours and who were treated within 4 months of apparent onset of their disease the remission rate with single-agent chemotherapy was 94 percent.[4] Certain patients could therefore be identified who by virtue of the location of metastases (lungs or vagina), duration of their disease, and initial hCG titer shared a favorable prognosis despite the presence of metastases. Such patients are at low risk of developing resistance to sequential single-agent chemotherapy consisting of methotrexate and actinomycin-D.

The dose and schedule of these agents is Methotrexate (10–30 mg IM daily x5) or Actinomycin-D (8–13 micrograms/kg body weight IV daily x5).

The drugs are administered sequentially, that is when resistance to the first drug occurs the second drug is then begun. Criteria for changing to the second drug are:

CHEMOTHERAPY OF MGTD (LOW RISK) PATIENTS

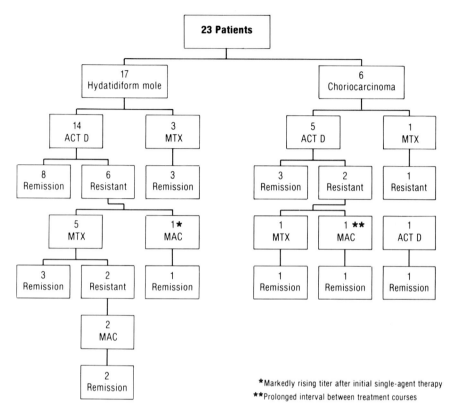

Fig. 12-6. Treatment and outcome in patients with low-risk metastatic (Gr II) gestational trophoblastic disease.

1. Plateau of gonadotropin above normal after two or more courses of the agent
2. Rising gonadotropin titer during treatment
3. Unusually severe or prolonged toxicity preventing repetition of therapy

In a report of 23 low risk metastatic disease patients from Memorial Hospital all of the patients achieved complete and sustained remission.[47] Sixty-one percent of the patients were successfully treated with one drug. Sequential treatment with the second agent was required in 21.5 percent of the patients before full remission was achieved. The remaining patients required combination chemotherapy (methotrexate, actinomycin D, and chlorambucil) prior to entering complete remission. The outline of chemotherapy and results of treatment in these patients is shown in Figure 12-6. In view of the finding in this study that approximately half of the patients developed resistance to the first agent, it becomes important to carefully monitor these patients for signs of drug resistance so as to begin the second agent at the earliest possible time. Evidence of a plateau or rising hCG titer or the development of new metastases is a clear indication of treatment failure and should result in prompt institution of a new agent. Following this approach to therapy, complete remission can be expected in 80 to 90 percent of patients treated with sequential methotrexate and actinomycin-D and virtually 100 percent of patients when combination chemotherapy is added.

Group III Metastatic (Moderate Risk)

1. Apparent metastases in sites other than liver and brain
2. Titer greater than 100,000 IU/24 hr (20,000 ng/ml) duration of disease greater than 4 months
3. All histopathologic diagnoses

Ross et al.[4] at the NCI also demonstrated the adverse effect on prognosis of an initially high hCG titer and long duration of disease in patients with metastases when treatment consisted of single-agent chemotherapy. Whereas 94 percent of their patients achieved remission when treated early, as previously indicated the comparable rate was 36 percent when treatment was delayed and titers were high. Clearly, such patients are at high risk of not responding to sequential single-agent chemotherapy. Hammond et al.[11] documented, on the other hand, that a high cure rate could be achieved in this group of patients when combination chemotherapy was given as initial treatment. In 1974, a remission rate of 100 percent in a small group of patients with an initially high hCG titer and/or long duration of disease was reported from Memorial Hospital when combination chemotherapy was utilized as initial treatment.[10] Over the past 15 years complete and sustained remission in more than 90 percent of patients meeting these criteria has been achieved at this institution. Based on this experience we pointed out the importance of separating out patients with regard to hCG level and/or duration of disease from those at ''high risk'' on the basis of the site of metastases. While these patients are at high risk of failing single-agent chemotherapy their risk of failing initial combination therapy is considered to be moderate, and we have classified them accordingly. In a recent review from the John I. Brewer Trophoblastic Disease Center, Lurain et al.[48] also found that time and hCG titer alone or in combination did not have a statistically significant effect on outcome in their patients with metastatic choriocarcinoma.

Recommended initial therapy in this group of patients consist of the following drugs given simultaneously for 5 days: Methotrexate (15 mg IM), Actinomycin D (0.5 mg IV), Chlorambucil (10 mg P.O.). When hepatic impairment is present use Actinomycin D (0.5 mg IV) and 6-Mercaptopurine (100 mg P.O.). When resistant cases are encountered, patients proceed to multi-agent regimens which are discussed with respect to therapy for patients in group IV.

Group IV Metastatic (High Risk)

1. Apparent metastases to brain or liver
2. Titer and duration of disease less important
3. All histopathologic diagnoses
4. Previous unsuccessful chemotherapy elsewhere

Patients in this group are found to have metastases to the brain or liver or have received prior unsuccessful treatment.

It is worth noting here that an initial response to conventional single-agent chemotherapy is a common clinical finding in almost all patients with metastases including those categorized as group III or IV. Physicians should be made aware, however, that such responses are unlikely to be sustained, and the use of combination chemotherapy after the development of resistance is unlikely to be successful.

Brain and liver metastases present special problems. Although they are rare sites of first metastases, symptoms of tumor in these locations may be the first sign of trophoblastic disease. Significantly, patients who present with primary hepatic or cerebral manifestation of their disease enjoy a more favorable prognosis than patients who develop these complications after resistance has occurred in other systemic locations. The initial symptoms of metastatic tumor in the brain may occur in the absence of gynecologic complaints or abnormal pelvic findings. When the tumor causes intracerebral hemorrhage an acute syndrome may occur, which is characterized by sudden headache, vomiting, and loss of consciousness. A radionuclide or CAT scan of the brain may initially be negative, but evidence of a space-occupying intracranial lesion as shown in Figure 12-7 in the presence of a positive test for hCG supports the diagnosis of metastatic choriocarcinoma. Bagshawe has provided evidence to show that a serum/CSF ratio of hCG of more than 1 in 60 is strongly suggestive of brain

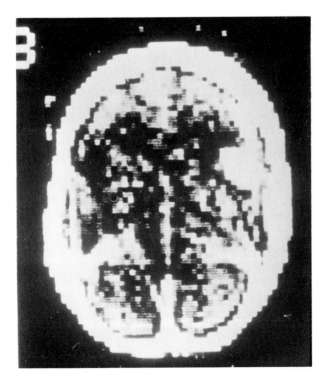

Fig. 12-7.   CT scan showing space occupying lesion (Gr IV) of metastatic choriocarcinoma.

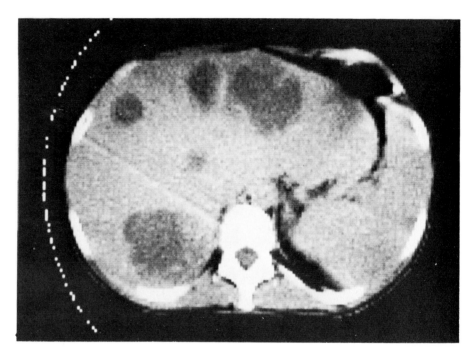

Fig. 12-8. CT scan of liver showing multiple areas of metastatic choriocarcinoma.

metastases.[49] This ratio should be measured in all patients when there is doubt since it may be diagnostic at a time when computerized tomography and radionuclide scans are negative.

Occult metastases in the liver rarely cause symptoms until extensive involvement of the parenchyma has occurred. Tumor in this site may then cause pain by the stretching of Glisson's capsule or intraabdominal hemorrhage if rupture of the capsule occurs. Transient increases in hepatic enzymes frequently follow drug therapy and are therefore not relied upon for early diagnosis of liver metastases. Persistently abnormal liver function tests however may be the first sign of abundant metastases in this site. Fortunately, tumor in the liver can often be adequately defined by ultrasound, isotope scanning or computerized tomography (Fig. 12-8). The management of patients in group IV is outlined below.

Brain Metastases.   Combination chemotherapy is the same as that for Group III. Additional therapy includes (for acutely decompensated patients) Mannitol (1.5–2.0 grams IV over 30 to 60 minutes) and Dexamethasone (10 mg IV, then 4 mg q 6 hrs. 4 mg P.O. q 6 hrs when patient is stable).

Radiation therapy begins after 72 hours of steroid treatment at 300 rads × 10 over 10 days to 2 week period. Taper steroids as tolerated after radiation therapy is completed.

Liver Metastases.   Combination chemotherapy is the same as that for Group III.

Radiation therapy begins immediately at 300 rads × 10 over 10 days to 2 week period.

Chemotherapy of Resistant Disease. Despite the success resulting from the use of combination chemotherapy as initial treatment of patients in Group III and IV, the relative lack of success in altering the outcome of patients who become resistant to initial therapy continues to be a major challenge to the therapist. This may also include some patients who are begun on single-agent therapy by virtue of their lower risk status (Gr II). In an effort to improve the prognosis in these situations, protocols have been planned that incorporate multiple agents with differing spectrums of toxicity and differing mechanisms of action with the intent of diminishing drug resistance and at the same time lessening toxic morbidity. Bagshawe introduced the CHAMOCA regimen in the mid 1970's and documented its effectiveness in patients who had developed drug resistance after single-agent or simple combination therapy.[50] He further observed that the use of this regimen as initial therapy in patients at "high risk" (Group IV, "poor prognosis") was more successful in preventing drug resistance than initial combination chemotherapy although often at the expense of increased toxicity. The dosages and schedule of drugs utilized in this regimen are shown in Table 12-2.

In patients with cerebral metastases on presentation Begent and Bagshawe[51] reported complete and sustained remission in 7 of 12 patients when the CHAMOCA regimen was employed as initial chemotherapy. It should be noted that in these patients the dosage of intravenous methotrexate was increased to 1 gram/m2 on day 2 of the regimen with folinic acid dosage increased to 30 mg every 12 hours for 3 days, starting 32 hours after the beginning of the infusion. Intrathecal methotrexate, 12.5 mg, was also given on day 2 of the regimen. The authors also stressed the importance of maintaining the urinary output above 2.5 liters per day.

Surwit et al.[52] modified the CHAMOCA protocol essentially by the incorporation of additional actinomycin D, and with its use they were able to obtain complete remission in five of six patients who had developed resistance to triple therapy (methotrexate, actinomycin D, and chlorambucil). The modified Bagshawe protocol is given in Table 12-3.[52] In a subsequent report by Weed et al.[53] a remission rate of 56 percent was achieved with this protocol.

Table 12-2. CHAMOCA—Bagshawe

Day 1		Hydroxyurea 1 g q.d.s. for 24 hr
Day 2	10:00 a.m.	Vincristine 1.0 mg/sq m Stat i.v.
	3:00 p.m.	Methotrexate 100 mg/sq m Stat i.v.
		Methotrexate 200 mg/sq m 12-hr infusion i.v.
Day 3	3:00 p.m.	Folinic acid 15 mg i.m. or p.o.
Day 4	8:00 a.m.	Folinic acid 15 mg i.m. or p.o.
	10:00 a.m.	Cyclophosphamide 600 mg/sq m i.v.
		Actinomycin-D 0.5 mg i.v.
	8:00 p.m.	Folinic acid 15 mg i.m. or p.o.
Day 5	8:00 a.m.	Folinic acid 15 mg i.m. or p.o.
	10:00 a.m.	Actinomycin-D 0.5 mg i.v.
Day 6	10:00 a.m.	Actinomycin-D 0.5 mg i.v.
Day 7		No treatment
Day 8		No treatment
Day 9[a]		Adriamycin 30 mg/sq m i.v.
		Cyclophosphamide 400 mg/sq i.v.

[a]Check WBC and platelets before giving.

Table 12-3. Bagshawe 8-Day Multiagent Chemotherapy-Surwit & Hammond

Day	Time	Agents
1		500 mg hydroxyurea PO q.i.d.
	1900 hrs	Actinomycin D 0.2 mg IV
2	0700 hrs	Vincristine 1 mg/M^2 IV
		Methotrexate 100 mg/M^2 IV push
	1900 hrs	Methotrexate 200 mg/M^2 IV over 12 hrs
		Actinomycin D 0.2 mg IV
		Actinomycin D 0.2 mg IV
3	1900 hrs	Cyclophosphamide 500 mg/M^2 IV
		Folinic acid 14 mg IM
4	0100 hrs	Folinic acid 14 mg IM
	0700 hrs	Folinic acid 14 mg IM
	1300 hrs	Folinic acid 14 mg IM
	1900 hrs	Folinic acid 14 mg IM
		Actinomycin D 0.5 mg IV
5	0100 hrs	Folinic acid 14 mg IM
	1900 hrs	Actinomycin D 0.5 mg IV
6		No treatment
7		No treatment
8	1900 hrs	Adriamycin 30 mg/M^2
		Cyclophosphamide 300 mg/M^2

A modification of Bagshawe's CHAMOMA protocol[5] in which the same drugs are used in a different sequence with additional vincristine (ITMA) has been used at our institution in the treatment of eight patients who were resistant to triple therapy (Table 12-4). All of the patients experienced an initial response, but only two patients achieved complete remission. In a smaller group of resistant patients, all with brain or liver metastases, high-dose methotrexate with CF rescue has been utilized at our institution. A starting dose of 100 mg/kg given by intravenous infusion over a 24-hour period followed by CF was given initially. After approximately 1 week, the patients were recycled on high-dose methotrexate during which time the dosage of methotrexate was escalated up to 300 mg/kg when no response to lesser dosages was observed. Four patients received 16 courses of this therapy and while initial responses were observed, none were sustained.

Recently, VP16, a semisynthetic derivative of podophyllotoxin, has been shown to have considerable activity in patients with drug-resistant choriocarcinoma. When administered as a single agent, Newlands et al.[54] achieved a combined response and improvement rate of 57 percent in 37 evaluable patients. These authors defined response as greater than a log fall in serum hCG concentration following a single course of therapy. An improvement was defined as a greater than 50 percent fall in the hCG concentration following a single course of therapy. The drug was given in a dosage of 100 mg/M^2 IV for five consecutive days as a short infusion in 200 ml of saline over 30 minutes. Because this drug is clinically well-tolerated and based on its proven activity in drug-resistant patients, these authors have recommended it for use in patients classified according to Bagshawe's scoring system as "medium risk." These patients are then cycled to a sequence of agents as shown in Table 12-5. Of 38 patients treated, all showed some reduction in hCG concentration with 13 responses and

Table 12-4. Gestational Trophoblastic Disease Intensive Treatment Multiple Agent (ITMA)

Day	Time	Therapy
1	6 p.m.	Hydroxyurea 500 mg b.i.d. for 24 hours
2	10 a.m.	Vincristine 1 mg/M^2 IV
	5 p.m.	Mtx 100 mg/M^2 stat IV
		200 mg/M^2 IV over 12 hours
3	5 p.m.	Folinic Acid 24 mg IV stat
4	8 a.m.	Folinic Acid 12 mg PO
	10 a.m.	Cyclophosphamide 25 mg/kg IV
	8 p.m.	Folinic Acid 12 mg PO
5	8 a.m.	Folinic Acid 12 mg PO
	8 p.m.	Folinic Acid 12 mg PO
6		Rest
7	10 a.m.	Vincristine 1 mg/M^2 IV
	5 p.m.	Actinomycin D 0.5 mg IV
8	10 a.m.	Actinomycin D 0.5 mg IV
9		Rest
10	10 a.m.	Adriamycin 10 mg/M^2 IV
		Melphalan 6 mg/M^2 IV

Table 12-5. Sequential Chemotherapy for Medium Risk Patients—Newlands and Bagshawe[a]

a. VP16 (Etoposide)	100 mg/M^2 in 200 ml of saline i.v.
	for 5 consecutive days
b. MTX/FA (Hydroxyurea and 6-MP)	
Day 1	Hydroxyurea (HU) 500 mg p.o. 12 hourly for two doses
Day 2	MTX 50 mg i.m. at noon
Day 3	FA 6 mg i.m. at 6:00 p.m.; 6-MP 75 mg p.o.
Day 4	MTX 50 mg i.m. at noon
Day 5	FA 6 mg at 6:00 p.m.; 6-MP 75 mg p.o.
Day 6	MTX 50 mg i.m. at noon
Day 7	FA 6 mg i.m. at 6:00 p.m.; 6-MP 75 mg p.o.
Day 8	MTX 50 mg i.m. at noon
Day 9	FA 6 mg i.m. at 6:00 p.m.; 6-MP 75 mg p.o.

c. Actinomycin D—This is given on days 1–5 in a dose of 0.5 mg (total dose) i.v. for 5 consecutive days.

[a]The courses of therapy are alternated according to the following sequence: a b c b a b c. If resistance occurs, then the ineffective regimen is replaced by Vincristine and Cyclophosphamide.

17 improvements observed. At the time of their report, 30 (79 percent) of the patients were in complete remission.

Recent attention has been directed toward the evaluation of cis-platinum in drug-resistant patients. Newlands reported the Charing Cross Hospital experience in the treatment of 24 drug-resistant patients utilizing cis-platinum with vincristine and methotrexate.[55] The combined response and improvement rate was 62 percent. Cis-platinum has been utilized at Memorial Hospital in the treatment of four heavily pre-treated patients. One patient with brain and liver metastases achieved complete remission when cis-platinum was given with VP16. Surwit and Hammond recently reported on two drug-resistant patients who achieved full remission after treatment with a new regimen consisting of vinblastine sulfate, bleomycin and cis-platinum (VBC).[52]

These responses suggest that cis-platinum was the active agent in the regimen in view of our experience with four patients treated with vinblastine, actinomycin D and bleomycin (VAB) who did not respond.

Finally, Vindesine (desacteyl vinblastine amide sulfate), a chemically-derived structural analog of the vinca alkaloid, vinblastine sulfate, when utilized as secondary therapy in three resistant patients at Memorial Hospital showed clear evidence of tumor activity as determined by hCG response. In one patient, the pretreatment hCG serum concentration of 110,000 ng/ml decreased to 6,000 ng/ml 8 days after the therapy. Unfortunately, the patient died within 2 weeks of her treatment of severe pulmonary insufficiency. While the hCG responses in the other patients were not as striking, these observations suggest that further studies are indicated to assess the value of this agent in patients with gestational trophoblastic disease.

In summary, studies at various treatment centers are directed toward the goal of matching treatment schedules and drugs to the individual patient's risk of developing a resistant tumor. The results of these efforts indicate that administering appropriate therapy to low and moderate risk patients can decrease the frequency with which these patients enter into the high risk, drug-resistant category. Future prospects for an improved prognosis in drug-resistant patients center around the search for new active chemotherapeutic agents.

Because of the central role played by hCG in the diagnosis and management of patients with gestational trophoblastic disease, some characteristics of the hormone and techniques for its measurement are considered next.

MEASUREMENT OF HCG

Gestational trophoblastic neoplasms are unique in that they consistently produce hCG when viable tumor is present. The value of hCG testing in early diagnosis has previously been discussed with respect to the follow-up of patients after a molar pregnancy. In this situation a plateau or rising hCG titer can signal the presence of proliferative sequelae weeks or months prior to clinical or roentgenographic evidence of disease. In the management of patients undergoing chemotherapy the response of the hCG titer is a direct measure of therapeutic effectiveness, thus permitting cytotoxic agents or schedules to be changed well in advance of the usual clinical signs of disease progression. Assay reports of minimal levels of hCG indicate minimal remaining viable tumor and the need for additional chemotherapy.[56] This is of importance to the clinician when recommending therapy to the asymptomatic patient without evidence of metastatic disease, who would prefer to avoid further treatment. Alternatively, the complete disappearance of hCG from the plasma and urine can provide a basis for withholding treatment and furnish a tentative diagnosis of remission. These are some of the reasons that hCG has been characterized as an ideal tumor marker.[57] Because of its function as a specific tumor marker in patients with GTD, special consideration must be given to the methods used to measure the hormone. First a brief review of some structural and functional relationships of hCG.

Human chorionic gonadotropin is a glycoprotein consisting of two dissimilar noncovalently linked polypeptide subunits with attached carbohydrate side chains.[58-60] The subunits designated alpha and beta are essentially without biologic activity as individual free subunits. The primary structure of alpha subunits of all human gly-coprotein hormones are nearly identical and consist of 89 to 92 amino acid residues in identical sequences. The beta subunits, on the other hand, have similar yet dis-tinctive amino acid contents and sequences and confer both immunologic and bio-logic specificities.[61,62] It is noteworthy that 80 percent of the first 115 amino terminal residues of the hCG beta subunit are identical to those of the human luteinizing hor-mone (hLH) beta subunit. This similarity in structure accounts for the well-known cross-reaction between hCG and hLH in all biologic and non-specific radioimmu-noassays. The beta subunit of hCG, however, also differs by containing an additional 30 aminoacid residue carboxy terminal sequence which is distinctive.[63–65]

It is useful to separate the development of methodologies for measuring hCG into basically three types: the biologic, immunologic, and radioimmunologic. The biologic assay utilized in all the early studies in the National Institute of Health (NIH) series was the Klinefelter mouse uterine weight assay.[66] This assay was based on kaolin acetone extracts of 24-hour urine specimens concentrated according to the technique of Albert and Berkson.[67] While this method measured total gonadotropins (hFSH, hLH) it also made it possible to detect elevated levels of hCG by virtue of the biologic cross-reactivity between hCG and LH. In the NIH series, a patient was considered to be in complete remission when three weekly urinary hCG titers were within the range that could be accounted for by pituitary LH. Lewis reported that when these criteria were met, 90 percent of such patients required no further therapy, whereas 8 percent experienced relapse within 2 months, 1 percent within the year and 1 percent after 1 year.[68]

Functionally, hCG has both biologic and immunologic activity and can therefore be measured also by immunologic techniques. Indeed, the intact molecule, free alpha and beta subunits, and natural fragments of hCG have all been reported to be im-munogenic and antigenic.[69] Wide et al.[70] reported on the immunological determina-tion of hLH in 1961. Advantage has now been taken of these properties to produce reagents and assays to rapidly detect and quantify hCG. In a recent symposium on early diagnosis of pregnancy, comparative data were presented on 8 slide tests and 9 tube tests currently available for measuring hCG.[71] Sensitivity levels of the various test ranged between 250 mIU/ml and greater than 3000 mIU/ml. Physicians should be made aware, therefore, that such tests cannot be relied upon to detect low levels of hCG. Since the amount of gonadotropin excreted in the urine of women with func-tioning gonads is usually less than 10 mIU/ml an assay may be reported as negative at a time when values are distinctly above normal pituitary levels of the cross-react-ing hLH. This becomes of great importance when one considers that approximately 30 percent of patients with malignant disease have a titer less than that detected by such tests.[6,13,72] When routine pregnacy tests become negative, the utilization of more sensitive assays becomes mandatory in the follow-up of patients with GTD.

Odell et al.[73] developed a radioimmunoassay for hLH which cross-reacted with hCG and was sensitive enough to measure gonadotropin to a level that could be ac-counted for by pituitary LH. This assay while not capable of differentiating hCG from LH significantly simplified the collection and processing of samples for assay. Of greater importance, however, was its reliability in measuring hCG throughout the full range of levels found in the serum of patients with GTD.

In 1972, Vaitukitis et al.[74] developed a radioimmunoassay specific for HCG and its beta subunit in serum and plasma which allowed clinicians to differentiate for the first time low levels of HCG from pituitary LH. Because this assay utilizes an anti-serum generated against hCG beta, it is commonly referred to as a "beta subunit assay." As Vaitukitis pointed out such a designation is misleading since it implies that only hCG beta is measured when in fact both hCG and hCG beta are detected in this assay.[75] Moreover, since the plasma half-life of hCG is approximately 100-times longer than that of hCG beta, hCG is the predominant molecular species measured. The value of this assay in the monitor of patients with GTD has been confirmed over the past decade by several investigators.[56,76,77]

The radioreceptorassay for hCG developed by Saxena et al.[78] in 1974, has provided a rapid and reliable test for measuring low levels of the hormone. This assay utilizes plasma membranes containing specific receptor for LH-hCG prepared from fresh bovine corpora lutea and requires only 15 minutes of incubation time. While this assay is sensitive, reliable, and capable of providing prompt results it does not overcome the one important limitation of the other biologic and non-specific RIA systems, namely, the inability to measure low concentrations of hCG specifically in the presence of hLH.[79]

Since the concentrations of hCG in urine and serum are approximately equivalent, i.e. the amount of hCG excreted by the kidney in a 24 hr urine specimen contains approximately as much hCG as 1000ml serum, Schreiber et al.[80] reasoned that assays of urine concentrates were potentially more effective than serum assays for detecting persistence of minute amounts of hormone-secreting trophoblastic tissue. Utilizing a new specific RIA for hCG in human urinary extracts previously described by Chen et al.[81] they reported on two patients with recurrent GTD who had no detectable levels of hCG in the serum as determined by the beta subunit assay but did have measurable tumor activity which could be detected in the new urinary RIA. The details of this assay as reported by Ayala and associates exploits ability to absorb hCG from a kaolin acetone urine concentrate to concanavalin A covalently linked to agarose. This procedure gives a final concentration benefit ratio of between 500 and 1000 depending on the amount of urine excreted per 24 hours.[82] This concentrate is assayed with the use of the standard beta subunit RIA or a newly developed RIA based on the 23-amino acid carboxy-terminal peptide chain of the beta subunit of hCG. Although this assay has great advantages in sensitivity, it has the added complication that the urine of normal subjects contains as much as 6 to 52 ng hCG/24 hour urine specimen. However, in the range between 50 and 500 ng/24 hour urine specimen, it is clearly possible to detect low levels of hCG excretion which indicate tumor activity which would not be measured in the beta-subunit assay with serum.

Recently, attention has been directed to the need for assays responsive to isolated subunits for use in diagnosing and monitoring therapeutic response of gestational trophoblastic neoplasms. Vaitukitis and Ebersole, for example, have shown that the presence of free alpha and free beta subunits in serum, urine or tumor extracts to be an expression of more severe malignancy in patients with GTD.[83] Dawood et al.[84] reported that alpha subunit levels increased while hCG and hCG beta decreased or became undetectable in patients with choriocarcinoma in whom cerebral metastases eventually developed. Quigley et al.[85] suggested that routine measurement of alpha subunit in patients successfully treated for GTD may help identify patients who require additional chemotherapy or more intensive follow-up.

Future prospects suggest that the improved assays for hCG will exploit the rapidly expanding monoclonal antibody technology. Monoclonal antibodies to hCG have been utilized by Stenman and co-workers to develop a rapid, and specific serum RIA but this assay lacks the sensitivity of previously available RIA's.[86] Ehrlich et al.[87], on the other hand, have reported an increased binding of hCG with the use of a monoclonal antibody specific for hCG beta and a monoclonal antibody that binds the alpha subunit. Their observation that mixtures of monoclonal antibodies increases the apparent affinity for hCG relative to that of the individual antibodies could potentially result in the development of assays of greater sensitivity and specificity than those currently available.

Finally, increased interest in possible new markers in patients with GTD has centered around the recently discovered placenta-specific tissue proteins. Pregnancy-specific B1-glycoprotein (SP1) has received the most attention because of the similarity between the regression profile of this protein and that of hCG. In addition evidence that SP1 can be detected in the blood of patients in remission as judged by the absence of demonstrable hCG for 3 months suggest that assays for this protein may identify patients with minimal remaining tumor.[88] While the study of these markers has provided new insights into the biosynthesis of glycoproteins by the trophoblast, they have not been employed in the routine management of GTD patients. This is because low levels of hCG in some patients have not been accompanied by detectable concentrations of SP1, and isolated peaks of SP1 detected in patients in remission have not been associated with later recurrence of disease.[89] Furthermore, Serale et al. report of measurable levels of SP1 in the blood of 13 percent of healthy volunteers and non-pregnant healthy women suggest that the presence of SP1 in the blood of some GTD patients may be a non-specific finding and not a sign of tumor activity.[90]

In summary, the beta subunit assay for hCG performed on serum or plasma has proven over the past decade to be a specific and sensitive monitor of tumor activity. When routine tests for hCG are negative, the utilization of such an assay becomes imperative to rule out the presence of viable trophoblastic tissue.

REFERENCES

1. Hertz R: Biological aspects of gestational neoplasms derived from trophoblasts. Ann NY Acad Med 172:279, 1971.
2. Li MC, Hertz R, Spencer DB: Effect of methotrexate therapy upon choriocarcinoma and chorioadenoma. Proc Soc Exp Biol Med 93:361, 1956.
3. Hertz R, Lewis JL, Jr, Lipsett MB: Five year's experience with the chemotherapy of metastatic choriocarcinoma and related trophoblastic tumors in women. Am J Obstet Gynecol 82:631, 1961.
4. Ross GT, Goldstein DP, Hertz R, et al: Sequential use of methotrexate and actinomycin D in the treatment of metastatic choriocarcinoma and related trophoblastic diseases in women. Am J Obstet Gynecol 93:223, 1965.
5. Bagshawe KD: Treatment of trophoblastic tumors. Recent Results in Cancer Res 62:192, 1977.
6. Brewer JI, Eckman TR, Dolkart RE, et al: Gestational trophoblastic disease: A Comparative study of the results of therapy in patients with invasive mole and with choriocarcinoma. Am J Obstet Gynecol 109:335, 1971.

7. Goldstein DP: The chemotherapy of gestational trophoblastic disease: Principles of clinical management. JAMA 220:209, 1972.
8. Hammond CB, Parker RT: Diagnosis and treatment of trophoblastic disease: A report from the Southeastern Regional Center. Obstet & Gynecol 35:132, 1970.
9. Brewer JI, Halpern B, Torok EE: Gestational trophoblastic disease: Selected clinical aspects and chorionic gonadotropin test methods. In Current Problems in Cancer, Vol 8. Chicago, Yearbook Medical Publishers, Inc., 1979.
10. Jones WB, Lewis JL Jr: Chemotherapy of gestational trophoblastic neoplasms. Am J Obstet Gynecol 120:14, 1974.
11. Hammond CB, Borchert LG, Tyrey L, et al: Treatment of metastatic trophoblastic disease: Good and poor prognosis. Am J Obstet Gynecol 115:451, 1973.
12. Bagshawe KD: Risk and prognostic factors in trophoblastic neoplasia. Cancer 38:1373, 1976.
13. Curry SL, Hammond CB, Tyrey L, et al: Hydatidiform mole: Diagnosis, management and long-term follow-up of 347 patients. Obstet Gynecol 45:1, 1975.
14. Jones WB, Lauersen NH: Hydatidiform mole with coexistent fetus. Am J Obstet Gynecol 122:267, 1975.
15. Donald I: Diagnostic uses of sonar in obstetrics and gynecology. In Greenhill JP (ed): Yearbook of Obstetrics and Gynecology 1967–1968. Chicago, Yearbook Medical Publishers Inc., 1968.
16. Torres AH and Pelegrina IA: Transabdominal intrauterine contrast medium injection: Cen and in the early diagnosis hydatidiform mole. Am J Obstet Gynecol 94:936–938, 1966.
17. Birnholz JC: Amniography in the early diagnosis of hydatidiform mole. J Rad 49:812, 1976.
18. Baggish MS and Barbot J: Contact hysteroscopy for easier diagnosis. Contemp Obstet Gynecol 16:3, 1980.
19. Twiggs LB, Morrow CP and Schlaerth JB: Acute pulmonary complications of molar pregnancy. Am J Obstet Gynecol 135:189–194, 1979.
20. Tow WSH: The influence of the primary treatment of hydatidiform mole on its subsequent course. J Obstet Gynaecol Br Cwlth 73:544–552, 1966.
21. Frost ACG: Death following intrauterine injection of hypertonic saline solution with hydatidiform mole. Am J Obstet Gynecol 101:342, 1968.
22. McNocole, Gray H: Adverse reaction to extra-amniotic prostaglandin E_2. Br J Obstet Gynaecol 84:229, 1977.
23. Lewis JL Jr, Gore H, Hertig AT, et al: Treatment of trophoblastic disease with rationale for the use of adjunctive chemotherapy at the time of indicated operation. Am J Obstet Gynecol 96:710, 1966.
24. Goldstein DP: Prevention of gestational trophoblastic disease by the use of actinomycin-D in molar pregnancies. Obstet Gynecol 43:475, 1974.
25. Delfs E: Quantitative chorionic gonadotropin: Prognostic value in hydatidiform mole and chorionepitheioma. Obstet Gynecol 9:1, 1957.
26. Pastorfide GB, Goldstein DP, Kosasa TS, et al: Serum chorionic gonadotropin activity after molar pregnancy, therapeutic abortion, term delivery. Am J Obstet Gynecol 118:293, 1974.
27. Jones WB: Treatment of chorionic tumors. Clin Obstet Gynecol 18:247, 1975.
28. Morrow CP, Kletzky OA, Disaia PS, et al: Clinical and laboratory correlates of molar pregnancy and trophoblastic disease. Am J Obstet Gynecol 128:424, 1977.
29. French W, Freund U, Carlson RN, et al: High output failure associated with pulmonary edema complicating hydatidiform mole. Arch Intern Med 137:376, 1977.
30. Kohorn EI, McGinn RC, Benard J, et al: Pulmonary embolyation of trophoblastic tissue in molar pregnancy. Obstet Gynecol 51:16, 1968.

31. Orr JW Jr, Austin JM, Hatch KD, et al: Acute pulmonary edema associated with molar pregnancies: A high-risk factor for development of persistent trophoblastic disease. Am J Obstet Gynecol 136:412, 1980.

32. Stone M, Dent J, Kardana A, et al: Relationship of oral contraception to development of trophoblastic tumor after evacuation of a hydatidiform mole. Br J Obstet Gynaecol 83:913, 1976.

33. Federschneider JM, Goldstein DP, Berkowitz RS, et al: Natural history of recurrent molar pregnancy. Obstet Gynecol 55:457, 1980.

34. Vassilakos P, Kajii T: Hydatidiform mole: Two entities. Lancet 1:259, 1976.

35. Szulman AE, Surti U: The syndrome of hydatidiform mole. I. Cytogenetic and morphologic correlations. Am J Obstet Gynecol 131:665, 1978.

36. Berkowitz RS, Goldstein DP, Marean AR, et al: Proliferative sequelae after evacuation of partial hydatidiform mole. Lancet 2:804, 1979.

37. Stone M, Bagshawe KD: An analysis of the influence of maternal age, gestational age, contraceptive method, and the mode of primary treatment of patients with hydatidiform moles on the incidence of subsequent chemotherapy. Br J Obstet Gynaecol 86:782, 1979.

38. Kajii R, Ohama K: Androgenetic original of hydatidiform mole. Nature 268:633, 1977.

39. Wake N, Takagi N, Sasaki M. Androgenesis as a cause of hydatidiform mole. J Natl Cancer Inst 60:51, 1978.

40. Jacobs, PA, Hassold TJ, Matsuyama AM, et al: Chromosomal constitution of gestational trophoblastic disease. Lancet 2:49, 1978.

41. Yamashita K, Wake N, Araki R, et al: Human lymphocytic antigen expression in hydatidiform mole: Androgenesis following fertilization by a haploid sperm. Am J Obstet Gynecol 135:597, 1979.

42. Lawler SD, Povey S, Evans MW, et al: Genetic studies of complete and partial hydatidiform moles. Lancet 2:580, 1979.

43. Schlaerth JB, Morrow CP, Kletzky OA, et al: Prognostic characteristics of serum human chorionic gonadotropin titer regression following molar pregnancy. Obstet Gynecol 58:478, 1981.

44. Bagshawe KD, Golding PR, Orr AH: Choriocarcinoma after hydatidiform mole: Studies related to effectiveness of follow-up practice after hydatidiform mole. Br Med J 2:733, 1969.

45. Goldstein DP, Goldstein PR, Bottomley P, et al: Methotrexate with citrovorum factor rescue for nonmetastatic gestational trophoblastic neoplasms. Obstet Gynecol 48:321, 1976.

46. Smith EB, Weed JC, Tyrey L, et al: Treatment of nonmetastatic gestational trophoblastic disease: Results of methotrexate alone versus methotrexate-folic acid. Am J Obstet Gynecol 144:88, 1982.

47. Jones WB: Management of low-risk metastatic gestational trophoblastic disease. J Reprod Med 26:213, 1981.

48. Lurain JR, Brewer JI, Torok EE, et al: Gestational trophoblastic disease: The effect of duration of disease and hCG titer on response to therapy. J Reprod Med 27:401, 1982.

49. Bagshawe KD, Harland S: Detection of intracranial tumours with special reference to immunodiagnosis. Proc R Soc Med 69:51, 1976.

50. Bagshawe KD: Treatment of trophoblastic tumours. Proc First Interntl Cong Asia Fed Obstet & Gynecol, Singapore, 1976, pp. 109–116.

51. Begent RHJ, Bagshawe KD: The management of high-risk choriocarcinoma. Sem in Oncol 9:198, 1982.

52. Surwit EA, Hammond CB: Treatment of metastatic trophoblastic disease with poor prognosis. Obstet Gynecol 55:565, 1980.

53. Weed JC, Barnard DR, Currie JL, et al: Chemotherapy with the modified Bagshawe protocol for poor prognosis metastatic trophoblastic disease. Obstet Gynecol 59:377, 1982.

54. Newlands ES, Bagshawe KD: The role of VP16-213 (Etoposide: NSC-141540) in gestational choriocarcinoma. Cancer Chemother Pharmacol 7:211, 1982.
55. Newlands ES: New chemotherapeutic agents in the management of gestational trophoblastic disease. Sem Oncol 9:239, 1982.
56. Jones WB, Lewis JL Jr, Lehr M: Monitor of chemotherapy in gestational trophoblastic neoplasm by radioimmunoassay of the beta-subunit of human chorionic gonadotropin. Am J Obstet Gynecol 121:669, 1975.
57. Jones WB: Human chorionic gonadotropin: The ideal tumor marker? In Ballon SC (ed): Controversies in Gynecologic Oncology. Boston, G.K. Hall, 1981, pp. 367–375.
58. Canfield RE, Agosto GM, Bell JJ: In Butt WR, Crooke AC, Ryle M (eds): Gonadotropins and Ovarian Development. Edinburgh, 1970, E&S Livingstone Ltd., p. 161.
59. Swaminathan N, Bahl OP: Dissociation and recombination of the subunits of human chorionic gonadotropin. Biochem Biophys Res Commun 40:422, 1970.
60. Morgan FJ, Canfield RE: Nature of the subunits of chorionic gonadotropin. Endocrinol 88:1045, 1971.
61. Pierce JG (Eli Lilly Lecture): The subunits of pituitary thyrotropin: Their relationship to other glycoprotein hormones. Endocrinol 89:1331, 1971.
62. Vaitukaitis JL: Glycoprotein hormones and their subunits: Immunological and biological characterization. In McKerns KW (ed): Structure and Function of the Gonadotropins. New York, Plenum Press, 1978, pp. 339–360.
63. Bahl OP, Carlsen RB, Bellisario R, et al: Human chorionic gonadotropins: Amino acid sequence of the alpha and beta subunits. Biochem Biophys Res Commun 48:416, 1972.
64. Ross GT: Clinical relevance of research on the structure of human chorionic gonadotropin. Am J Obstet Gynecol 129:795, 1977.
65. Morgan FJ, Birken S, Canfield RE: The amino acid sequence of human chorionic gonadotropin: The alpha subunit and the beta subunit. J Biol Chem 250:5247, 1975.
66. Klinefelter HF, Albright F, Griswold GC: Experience with quantitative test for normal or decreased amounts of follicle-stimulating hormone in urine in endocrinological diagnosis. J Clin Endocrin Metab 3:529, 1943.
67. Albert A, Berkson J: Clinical bioassay for chorionic gonadotropin. J Clin Endocrin Metab 11:805, 1951.
68. Lewis JL Jr: Chemotherapy of gestational choriocarcinoma. Cancer 30:1517, 1972.
69. Ross GT: Clinical relevance of research on the structure of human chorionic gonadotropin. Am J Obstet Gynecol 129:795, 1977.
70. Wide DL, Rios P, Gemzell C: Immunological determination of human pituitary hormone (LH). Acta Endocrinol 37:445, 1961.
71. Derman R: Early diagnosis of pregnancy: A symposium. J Reprod Med 26:149, 1981.
72. Ross GT, Hammond CB, Lipsett MB: Chemotherapy of metastatic and nonmetastatic gestational trophoblastic neoplasms. Tex Rep Biol Med 24:326, 1966.
73. Odell WD, Ross GT, Rayford PL: Radioimmunoassay for human luteinizing hormone. J Clin Invest 46:248, 1967.
74. Vaitukaitis JL, Braunstein GD, et al: A radioimmunoassay which specifically measures human chorionic gonadotropin in the presence of human luteinizing hormone. Am J Obstet Gynecol 113:751, 1972.
75. Vaitukaitis JL: Practical considerations of specific hCG assays for clinical use. Ligand Rev 3:45, 1981.
76. Goldstein DP, Kosasa TS, Skarim AT: The clinical application of a specific radioimmunoassay for human chorionic gonadotropin in trophoblastic and nontrophoblastic tumors. Surg Gynecol Obstet 138:1, 1974.
77. Pastorfide GB, Goldstein DP, Kosasa TS: The use of a radioimmunoassay specific for

human chorionic gonadotropin in patients with molar pregnancy and gestational tropho-blastic disease. Am J Obstet Gynecol 120:1025, 1974.

78. Saxena BB, Hasan SH, Haour F, et al: Radioreceptorassay of human chorionic gonado-tropin: Early detection of pregnancy. Science 184:793, 1974.

79. Landesman R, Saxena BB: Results of the first 1000 radioreceptorassays for the determi-nation of human chorionic gonadotropin: A new, rapid, reliable and sensitive pregnancy test. Fertil Steril 27:357, 1976.

80. Schreiber JR, Rebar RW, Chen HC, et al: Limitation of the specific serum radioimmu-noassay for human chorionic gonadotropin in the management of trophoblastic neoplasms. Am J Obstet Gynecol 125:705, 1976.

81. Chen HC, Ayala AR, Hodgen GD, et al: First specific assay for chorionic gonadotropin in human urinary extracts. Clin Res 24:375A, 1976.

82. Ayala AR, Nisula BC, Chen HC, et al: Highly sensitive radioimmunoassay for chorionic gonadotropin in human urine. J Clin Endocrinol Metab 47:767, 1978.

83. Vaitukaitus JL, Ebersole ER: Evidence for altered synthesis of human chorionic gonado-tropin in gestational trophoblastic tumors. J Clin Endocrinol Metab 42:1048, 1976.

84. Dawood MY, Saxena BB, Landesman R: Human chorionic gonadotropin and its subunits in hydatidiform mole and choriocarcinoma. Obstet Gynecol 50:172, 1977.

85. Quigley MM, Tyrey L, Hammond CB: Utility of assay of alpha subunit of human cho-rionic gonadotropin in management of gestational trophoblastic malignancies. Am J Obstet Gynecol 138:545, 1980.

86. Stenman UH, Tanner P, Ranta T, et al: Monoclonal antibodies to chorionic gonadotropin: Use in a rapid radioimmunoassay for gynecologic emergencies. Obstet Gynecol 59:375, 1982.

87. Ehrlich PH, Moyle WR, Moustafa ZA, et al: Mixing two monoclonal antibodies yields enhanced affinity for antigen. J Immunol 128:2709, 1982.

88. Rutanen E, Seppala M: Pregnancy-specific B1-glycoprotein in trophoblastic disease. J Clin Endocrinol Metab 50:57, 1980.

89. O'Brien TJ, Enguall E, Schlaerth JB, et al: Trophoblastic disease monitoring: Evaluation of pregnancy-specific B1-glycoprotein. Am J Obstet Gynecol 138:313, 1980.

90. Serale FB, Leake A, Bagshawe KD, et al: Serum SP1 pregnancy-specific B-glycoprotein in choriocarcinoma and other neoplastic disease. Lancet 1:579, 1978.

13 | Second Malignancies After Alkylating Agent Therapy or Radiation Therapy

Henry Gerad

Secondary cancer occurring as a delayed complication of primary antineoplastic therapy has been described after chemotherapy, irradiation, and the combination of chemotherapy and irradiation.[1-3] In order that iatrogenic neoplasms become apparent, the primary tumor must occur in a patient population which has either a high cure rate or a high percentage of long-term survivors. Advances in the diagnosis and treatment of gynecologic malignancies have prolonged survival such that there are increasing reports of both solid tumors and leukemia developing after treatment of the primary tumor. This chapter will provide an overview of the clinical characteristics and types of tumors that occur subsequent to therapy for gynecologic malignancy. An attempt will be made to integrate current knowledge about the carcinogenic potential of anticancer therapy and recommendations which have been made to prevent future iatrogenic cancer.

Irradiation has long been known to be oncogenic,[4] and is thought to induce malignant disease in a single cell or single small focus of cells.[5] Factors involved in radiation carcinogenesis have included dose rate, type of irradiation, radiation port, the specific organ irradiated, and age at exposure.[6,7] As detailed by Messerschmidt et al.,[7] at low levels of irradiation, little or no increase in tumor formation is seen which may be due to the fact that chromosomal DNA damage is not extensive and is repairable. As the dose is increased, chromosomal damage by irradiation increases, and tumor formation becomes more prevalent, often in a linear fashion. With further increase in dose, cell death occurs, eventually balancing the mutagenic effects. The curve for tumorigenicity will plateau at this level. Still higher doses produce more cell death than sublethal injury, and carcinogenic potential decreases. However, when two tissues of different radiation sensitivity are in a specified radiation port, the given dose may kill most of one tissue but be tumorigenic to the other tissue. This may in part explain the lack of excess leukemia compared to the increase in solid tumors after irradiation for cervical carcinoma. Further evidence supporting this observation will be presented later in the chapter.

Alkylating agents, the most commonly used chemotherapeutic agents in gynecologic cancer, have had their mutagenic effects demonstrated in a variety of experimental models.[8] The carcinogenic potential of alkylating agents as contrasted to the noncarcinogenicity of antimetabolites may relate to the fact that alkylators bind tightly to DNA.[3] These drugs then spontaneously, or after metabolic conversion, form highly reactive metabolites known as electrophilic reactants which damage cells by binding to macromolecules including DNA, RNA and proteins.[9] In patients with cancer, damage occurs in both neoplastic and normal cells. If nonlethal damage in normal cells can be fully repaired, they will return to normal. If cellular damage cannot be repaired, then malignant transformation may occur. A complete description of the mechanisms involved in chemical carcinogenesis can be found in previous reviews.[9–11]

Because secondary tumors can occur years after initial treatment, they must be differentiated from the random natural occurrence of malignancies in cured patients who have again become part of the population at risk.[12,13] The statistical term most often used in the literature to assess for an increased chance of a new malignancy is the relative risk. This term refers to the ratio of observed to expected (O/E) numbers of cases. In general, when this ratio is large, and the 95 percent confidence intervals around the estimate of relative risk do not include 1.0, then the estimate of relative risk is often statistically significant at the 5 percent level ($p < 0.05$). When confidence interval information has not been included in published studies, then the statistical significance of any increase in relative risk cannot be assumed.[7]

A problem with using the relative risk ratio to assess treatment risks is that this ratio assumes comparability between the observed and general populations. In such studies, patients with a specific primary malignancy should be compared to other such patients and not to the general population, of which only a very small portion has cancer.[12] Many studies have based their estimates of therapeutically induced neoplasms on inadequate or noncomparable populations as controls or estimates of expected values. This often makes conclusions of significance difficult to interpret.[7]

In gynecologic malignancies, a higher than expected incidence has been reported for a number of secondary tumors which could not be related to prior anti-cancer therapy. These included breast cancer,[13,14] thyroid cancer,[13,14] lung cancer,[15,16] bladder cancer,[16] and cancer of the oral cavity.[16] The possible reasons for the increase in these tumors have included smoking, hormonal imbalance and other factors.[13,14,16]

Several studies have not found an increase in the incidence of new tumors in patients treated with irradiation for gynecologic malignancies.[17–19] However, in the studies with longer follow-up or with larger numbers of patients, it was noted that subsequent tumors of the rectum, sigmoid colon, urinary bladder, endometrium, ovary, vagina, vulva, and overlying skin could occur in significant numbers.[18,19] An increase in the number of secondary tumors after radiation for gynecological cancer is further suggested by reports of a higher than expected incidence of cancer developing after irradiation for benign pelvic disease.[20,21] Buchler has reported that patients irradiated for cervical cancer are at greater risk for a second tumor than patients irradiated for other genital cancers.[22]

To follow will be a compilation of secondary solid tumors occurring after radiation therapy for gynecologic malignancies. The majority of this information is derived from reports of patients initially treated for cervical cancer. When possible, data considering expected incidence rates of second tumors will be presented. However, it must be remembered that conclusions drawn from this data may have come from less than optimal analysis.[12] Following the sections dealing with secondary solid tumors, the reported data for post-therapeutic acute leukemia will be presented.

CERVICAL CANCER AND SECONDARY TUMORS

Uterine Cancer

Ninety-seven cases of uterine cancer developing after irradiation of primary cervical cancer have been compiled from the literature.[20,23–43] The histologic diagnosis was mixed mesodermal tumor in 41 cases, adenocarcinoma in 46 cases, and unknown in 10 cases. Radiation therapy for the primary cervical cancer consisted of both internal radium implants and external irradiation in all but five cases in whom only radium implants were used. For all cases there was no estimation of absorbed uterine radiation dose. An average exposure would be impossible to calculate since these patients were treated over a 40-year time span, with differing radiation sources and therapeutic techniques. The dosage range for the internal radium implants was 1,000–9,000 mg. hr., with most patients receiving between 3,000–7,000 mg. hrs. The range for external radiation was 600–7,000 rads, with most patients receiving between 3,000–6,000 rads. For all cases, the mean latency time from initial irradiation until the development of uterine cancer was 11.9 years with a range of 1.5–29 years (Table 13-1). When subdivided by histologic diagnosis, the mean latency times were 12.2 years (range 3–29 years) and 11.2 years (range 1.5–29 years) until the occurrence of mixed mesodermal tumors and adenocarcinomas respectively.

Survival after the diagnosis of a secondary uterine cancer was available for 27 cases of mixed mesodermal tumor and for 17 cases of adenocarcinoma. Mean survival for mixed mesodermal tumors was 7.7 months (range 1–36 months) compared to a mean survival of 2.9 years (range 0.5–9+ years) for the adenocarcinomas. Therapy for both secondary tumors was similar and consisted of surgery and/or radiation. Radiation effects which obscure the diagnosis of cancer have been felt to be contributory to the short survival in secondary uterine tumors. Specifically, the lack of abnormal uterine bleeding secondary to postirradiation fibrosis and stenosis of the cervical canal has helped to create a low index of suspicion to investigate for a new cancer.[37,43] Consequently, the presentation of many of these patients was caused by abdominal distension which indicated already advanced intra-abdominal disease.[41,43]

Since prognosis of uterine cancer is influenced by the extent of tumor involvement at the time of diagnosis,[34] and since postirradiation tumors may have a greater propensity for rapid growth and intra-abdominal spread,[41] it is readily apparent how delay in diagnosis could contribute to poor survival. Although it is suggested that secondary mixed mesodermal tumors may have a poorer prognosis than secondary adenocarcinomas, the small number of patients available for review does not provide sufficient information to say this with any degree of certainty.

A large review of mixed mesodermal tumors has revealed an occurrence of approximately 10 percent in a postirradiation setting.[49] However, in other series of mixed mesodermal tumors, postirradiation occurrence has ranged from 4 to 38 percent.[50] Additional data suggesting that mixed mesodermal tumors were more likely to occur after radiation was presented by Varela-Duran et al.[41] In their series, the average age of patients developing mixed mesodermal tumors postirradiation was 7 years less than in patients with spontaneously occurring mixed mesodermal tumors. They theorized that there might have been a cause and effect relationship between pelvic irradiation and the earlier tumor development.[41]

Irradiation as an etiologic factor leading to the development of uterine malignancies remains a source of controversy in the literature.[20,29,44–48] Both affirmative and non-affirmative conclusions from these studies must be considered questionable due to the lack of proper control groups, the insufficient follow-up time after radiation and the small numbers of patients evaluated.[43] Bearing this in mind, the available statistical information can now be considered.

The relative risk reported for uterine cancer developing after irradiation for cervical cancer varies widely. Risk was found to be unchanged (O/E 3/3.2, relative risk 0.94) by Palmer and Spratt,[20] decreased (O/E 5.8/15.6, relative risk 0.37) by Czesnin and Wronkowski,[40] and increased (O/E 5/1.5, relative risk 3.33) by Morton and Villasanta.[35] By specific histologic diagnosis, Czesnin and Wronkowski[40] found a statistically significant increase in uterine sarcomas after previous cervical radiotherapy (O/E 4.3/0.8, relative risk 5.37). For adenocarcinomas, the incidence rate reported after cervical irradiation has ranged from 0.1 to 0.96 percent.[20,29,37,43] The 0.52 percent incidence reported by Fehr and Prem[37] was said to be twice the expected spontaneous incidence in their study population. The 0.1 percent incidence reported by Palmer and Spratt[20] may be misrepresentative since these data were obtained by questionnaire 12 or more years after treatment, and only 43 percent of the original patient population returned an adequate reply. Although the highest incidence of secondary uterine cancer was observed by Kwon et al.,[43] they could not explain its occurrence. Their report did not include the expected incidence (hence relative risk) of uterine cancer for their study population. Furthermore, they stated that comparisons of the widely differing reported incidence rates would not be meaningful because many variables, including the proportion of long-term survivors following radiation therapy for cervical carcinoma were not given in the original papers.

In summary, it is still inconclusive as to whether or not there is an increased risk for uterine cancer after cervical irradiation. However, it is uniformly agreed that careful clinical follow-up after cervical irradiation is mandatory because of the possibility that radiation effects may obscure the later diagnosis of uterine cancer which would worsen the prognosis of patients in whom this tumor does occur.

COLORECTAL CANCER

The development of colorectal cancer is a rare but well-recognized late complication of pelvic irradiation.[20,44,48,51] Three principle criteria have been suggested by Black and Akerman[52] to diagnose radiation-induced colorectal cancer. These are:

1. A minimum of 10 years between exposure to radiation and subsequent tumor development;
2. Severe irradiation-induced changes in the vicinity of the tumors; and
3. A relatively great exposure of the large bowel to irradiation.

Since the original report of two cases by Slaughter and Southwick,[53] at least 88 additional cases of colorectal cancer have been reported after cervical irradiation.[20,35–38,40,53–69]

The latency time from initial irradiation until the occurence of colorectal cancer was available for 65 of the 90 cases reviewed. Overall, there was a mean interval of 16.5 years with a range of 1 to 46 years (Table 13-1). When subdivided by location, mean latency time until appearance of anal squamous cell carcinoma was 10.0 years (range 7 to 12 years) in three of four cases. For 56 of 68 cases of rectosigmoid adenocarcinoma, mean latency time was 17.2 years (range 1 to 46 years), and in six of 18 cases of colon carcinoma, mean latency time was 10.5 years (range 2 to 29 years). In this larger series, 76 percent of the tumors developed in the rectosigmoid area. This finding supported the data of Castro et al.,[61] in which 73 percent of 26 tumors developed in the rectosigmoid area. The latency time was greater than ten years in 73 percent of all cases, which is also similar to the 69 percent figure reported by Castro et al.[61]

For nearly all cases where radiation dosage was reported, the dose range for in-

Table 13-1. Latency Times After Radiation Therapy For Cervical Cancer Until Occurrence of New Tumors[a]

Tumor	# Cases	Mean Latency (years)	Range (years)
All Sarcomas	38	13.3	3–27
Soft tissue sarcomas	15	12.1	4–26
Bone sarcomas	23	14.0	3–27
All Colorectal cancer	65	16.5	1–46
Anal squamous cell	3	10	7–12
Colon	6	10.5	2–29
Rectosigmoid	56	17.2	1–46
All Uterine Cancer	93	11.9	1.5–29
Mixed mesodermal tumors	41	12.2	3–29
Adenocarcinoma	43	11.2	1.5–29
Unknown histology	9	12.9	6–16
Bladder Cancer	19	13.3	0.5–31
Ovarian Cancer	8	13.8	7–31
Vaginal Cancer	21	14.1	6–26

[a]Latency times for cases of renal and vulvar cancer are included in the text.

ternal implantation was between 3,000 to 6,000 mg. hr., and for external irradiation was between 2,000 to 6,000 rads. Although these levels of irradiation are in the standard therapeutic range for cervical carcinoma, most patients in whom secondary colorectal cancer developed had clinical and/or pathological evidence of radiation-induced proctocolitis.[53–55,58,61,63–68] A 62 percent incidence of clinical and/or histological evidence of radiation-induced proctocolitis has previously been reported.[61] The high frequency of observed proctocolitis has supported the suggestion by MacMahon and Rowe that the occurrence of proctocolitis is a high risk factor for the later development of colon cancer.[58]

Overall, it is estimated that there is 5 to 10 percent incidence of radiation reactions in the bowel. Originally termed "factitial proctitis,"[70] these clinical and pathological radiation-induced changes have been previously reviewed.[71,72] Potentially increasing the risk for tumor development are the relatively fixed anatomic positions of the rectum and sigmoid colon which predispose these structures to continuous heavy irradiation. Additionally, post-operative pelvic adhesions or colonic malposition may also increase the local dosage of irradiation.[65]

The most common symptoms of irradiation-associated colonic cancer were found to be bleeding and abdominal pain.[61] Diarrhea was also said to occur in 50 percent of patients. The frequency of radiation associated colorectal cancers has been difficult to determine. This has been partially due to the previously limited survival of patients with pelvic cancer[52] and because irradiation damaged bowel is frequently removed before carcinoma can develop.[55,65]

The observed to expected risk of colorectal cancer developing after irradiation for cervical cancer has been reported with differing results. Risk was found to be decreased (O/E 5.8/21.7, relative risk 0.27) by Czesnin and Wronkowski,[40] unchanged (O/E 4/4.4, relative risk 0.91) by Morton et al.,[35] and slightly increased (O/E 2/1.4, relative risk 1.4) by Palmer and Spratt.[20] Dickson et al.[59] found increased risk independently for both colon (O/E 13/9.94, relative risk 1.3) and rectal carcinomas (O/E 12/4.35, relative risk 2.75).

Survival of patients developing irradiation-induced colorectal carcinomas has been reported to be poorer than in patients with spontaneously occurring tumors.[67] Data from Castro et al.[61] have tended to support this observation. In their series, there was a 20 percent five-year survival rate for patients who had surgery for irradiation associated colon cancer. Fifty-eight percent of the irradiation associated carcinomas in this series had the appearance of mucinous adenocarcinoma. The five-year survival rate was 44 percent for all patients with mucinous adenocarcinoma of the colon developing in the absence of prior irradiation. Thus it appeared that patients with irradiation associated colon adenocarcinoma had a poorer prognosis than other patients who spontaneously developed mucinous or non-mucinous adenocarcinomas.

Because of the potential risk of cancer for patients in whom irradiation-induced proctocolitis occurs, it is essential that they have close follow-up for life.[57,58,61,63,65] This may be made more difficult by intestinal stenosis which can prevent adequate proctoscopic or colonoscopic examination, and a carcinoma developing above a stricture may not be recognized. In all cases, any ulcerated or suspicious appearing lesions should be biopsied exclude the development of a carcinoma.

The need for aggressive diagnostic management is further suggested by two other factors. Irradiation-induced colon cancer may arise in flat non-polypoid mucosa, making it another condition besides ulcerative colitis in which large bowel cancer can arise outside of preformed polyps.[68] Secondly, there have been two cases in which two separate tumors occurred 3 and 5 years apart.[56,57] Thus, it appears that a continuing carcinogenic potential may exist for some patients. The precise type and timing of gastrointestinal evaluation for patients who develop radiation proctocolitis has yet to be determined. Such patients may need barium enemas at regular intervals.[65] Sequential determinations of the CEA level might also be beneficial.

BONE AND SOFT TISSUE SARCOMAS

The criteria defining the entity of postirradiation sarcoma in bone was first established by Cahan et al.[73] in 1948. These are:

1. The sarcomas should appear within the treated area;
2. Normal roentgen appearance of the bone region must be established prior to radiation treatment;
3. A relatively long latent period must exist between radiation therapy and the appearance of bone sarcoma (this period must exceed the so-called five-year cure period);
4. The existence of a malignant tumor must be histologically confirmed.

In 1971, Arlen et al.[74] modified the criteria to include malignant tumors devoid of osteoblastic activity such as Ewing's tumor and malignant lymphoma of bone. They also proposed that a latent period of 3 to 4 years was possible. While accepting that in many cases adequate radiologic examination prior to the development of a bone tumor was not available, they suggested a fifth criterion of pre-existing radiation osteitis. These modifications[74] along with Cahan's et al.[73] original criteria have become generally accepted for the diagnosis of postirradiation sarcoma of bone.[75] Excluding the criteria specific to bone, the remainder are also applicable to diagnose radiation induced soft tissue sarcomas.

Twenty-three bone and 17 soft tissue sarcomas have been reported after irradiation for cervical cancer.[39,40,59,76–90] The mean latency period for secondary bone sarcomas was 14.0 years (range 3 to 27 years) and for soft tissue sarcomas was 12.1 years (range 4 to 26 years) (Table 13-1). Histological diagnosis of the bone sarcomas included 11 osteogenic sarcomas, eight fibrosarcomas, and four chondrosarcomas. Histology of the soft tissue sarcomas included one each of malignant fibrous histiocytoma, rhabdomyosarcoma, leiomyosarcoma, reticulum cell sarcoma, malignant mesenchymoma, liposarcoma, neurofibroma, lymphangiosarcoma, mesothelioma, two spindle cell sarcomas, and six undefined sarcomas. Similar to the occurrence of sarcomas after radiation for other tumors, osteosarcoma and fibrosarcoma were the most common forms of radiation induced sarcoma, with chondrosarcoma and soft tissue sarcomas less frequently observed.[39]

Radiation dosage for the primary cervical cancer ranged between 2,000–7,000 rads delivered externally and 4,500–7,750 mg. hr. implanted internally. The dosage of radiation absorbed by bone was estimated for five cases, and ranged between 3,660–6,900 rads.[77,81,88] These dose ranges of radiation administered, or absorbed prior to the development of a secondary sarcoma are comparable to other series. Kim et al.[87] reported that none of their 47 radiation-related sarcomas occurred at administered doses less than 3,000 rads. Cahan et al.[73] listed bone exposures ranging from 1,510 to 25,000 R in their 11 postirradiation sarcomas. Mindell et al.[39] listed absorbed doses ranging from 1,500 to 8,100 rads in their 20 cases of postirradiation sarcoma.

The risk of postirradiation sarcoma is said to increase with higher initial doses of radiation.[39,75,88] The higher radiation dose is also thought to account for the long latency period that precedes tumor development. Postirradiation sarcoma is more likely to occur in bone because the dense mineral content of bone results in a greater proportion of the radiation energy being absorbed as compared with soft tissue. Hence, the bone dose is higher than in the surrounding soft tissue.[85,87,88]

The incidence of naturally occurring osteosarcoma in the pelvic girdle has been estimated to be one in four to five million population.[39,83] Phillips and Sheline[78] found an overall incidence of postirradiation sarcoma to be 0.03 percent. For patients who survived 5 or more years, the incidence rose to 0.1 percent. A similar incidence of 0.06 percent for survivors of 5 or more years was reported by Tountas et al.[88] In the series of Fehr and Prem,[83] for patients surviving 10 or more years, the incidence of postirradiation sarcoma was 0.64 percent, which was 650 times the expected natural occurrence of sarcoma. Increased risk was also noted by Czesnin et al.[40] In their series, the observed number of sarcomas per 100,000 population was 5.8 with only 0.4 cases expected. Relative risk was 14.5 which suggested a statistically significant risk of sarcoma after irradiation for cervical cancer.

The prior usage of orthovoltage equipment was felt to be contributory to the observed increase in risk for sarcoma. It was speculated that high energy megavoltage equipment would reduce this risk.[80] However, even with this change, a significant decrease in the number of postirradiation bone sarcomas has not been observed.[75]

Clinically, irradiation-induced sarcoma most commonly presents with pain, swelling, and radiographic changes.[39,75] In up to 50 percent of cases, the diagnosis of a bone tumor can be made more difficult by the occurrence of radiation osteitis in immediately adjacent bone.[91] Survival is usually short because radiation-induced sarcomas metastasize quickly and are relatively radioresistant.[39,75] Even with prompt radical surgical resection, the prognosis remains poor.[80] In this series, mean survival after diagnosis for eight bone sarcomas was 8½ months. This was similar to the 8-month mean survival reported by Mindell et al.[39] It is probable that the axial location of secondary pelvic sarcomas has contributed to their poor prognosis.[75] This is due to surgical inability to perform a complete resection. Only with extremity lesions has up to a 30 percent five-year survival been observed.[39,75]

Therefore, any patient surviving greater than 10 years and previously treated with radiation who is later suspected of having radiation osteitis should be considered at risk of developing osteogenic sarcoma.[85] Although many neoplasms may produce solitary osseous metastases after a relatively long and clinically quiescent period, such lesions occurring within the radiation field should not be merely assumed to be metastases. Biopsy is essential in these cases because the diagnosis of postirradiation sarcoma will have different therapeutic implications. Routine pelvic radiographs have also been recommended for patients surviving 10 or more years after primary irradiation in order to facilitate early diagnosis and possibly improve prognosis.[83]

UROLOGICAL CANCER

Twenty-six cases of bladder cancer, three cases of urethral cancer and one case each of ureteral and renal cancer have been reported after irradiation for cervical cancer.[20,35–38,40,58,59,92–94] The mean latency period until occurrence of secondary urological cancer was 13.3 years (range 0.5–31 years) (Table 13-1). The latency period until development of the single case of renal adenocarcinoma was 17 years.

In nearly all patients, radiation reactions which included cystitis and excessive fibrosis or papillomata at the base of the bladder occurred several years prior to the diagnosis of urological cancer.[59,93] Gross hematuria was the most common symptom which led to the diagnosis of bladder cancer. A change in ability to urinate was also present in some patients.[59,93,94] Interestingly, tumor location was not necessarily on the posterior bladder wall which is the most common site of bladder radiation reactions. The therapeutic approach for irradiation-induced bladder cancer has been the same as the therapeutic approach for spontaneously occurring bladder cancer, and has yielded similar results.[93]

After irradiation for cervical cancer, the risk of bladder cancer has been reported to be slightly decreased (0.29 E 3.5, relative risk 0.83) by Czesnin et al.[40] Increased risk (O/E 1.0/0.5, relative risk 2.0) was noted by Palmer and Spratt.[20] Dickson[59] reported a statistically significant increase in risk of death due to bladder cancer with p equal to 0.019 (O/E 5/1.49, relative risk 3.4). At the time of this report, five other patients with radiation reactions and papillomas were still being followed. For patients surviving 10 or more years, Kennedy et al.[94] reported a statistically significant increase in risk for bladder cancer (O/E 4/0.24, relative risk 16.6). Additionally, Duncan et al.[93] reported that 0.29 percent of their study population developed secondary bladder cancer. This figure was calculated to be 57 times the expected natural incidence in a comparable non-irradiated female population.

In long-term survivors who developed radiation reactions, careful follow-up is considered essential because of the risk of urological cancer.[93] Even though hematuria following radiation is usually due to vesical telangiectasia, this may be due to tumor and cystoscopy has been recommended for all such patients.[59] Repeat cystoscopy is necessary for women who experience recurrent bleeding because of the possibility of subsequent tumor development.[59]

OVARIAN CANCER

Twenty-one cases of ovarian cancer have been reported after radiation for cervical cancer.[20,35,37,40,58,59] Latency time until occurrence of ovarian cancer was greater than 5 years in the five cases reported by Fehr et al.[37] In eight other cases mean latency time was 13.8 years (range 7–31 years) (Table 13-1). Specific histology of the secondary ovarian tumors was not mentioned, nor was there any indication of unusual clinical characteristics or different response to therapy when compared to naturally occurring ovarian cancer. An increased risk for the development of ovarian cancer after cervical irradiation was not shown by Palmer et al. (O/E 1/1.7, relative risk 0.59), Fehr et al. (O/E 5/3.44, relative risk 1.5), or Czesnin et al. (O/E 8.7/18.1, relative risk 0.48).[20,37,40]

VAGINAL AND VULVAR CANCER

The association of vulvar or vaginal cancer simultaneous with or subsequent to the occurrence of cervical cancer is well-established.[95,96] However, after irradiation for cervical cancer the expected incidence of vulvar and vaginal cancer has been reported to be increased.[17] Cervical cancer patients treated only with surgery were reported to have a lower incidence of subsequent vulvar and vaginal cancers compared to cervical cancer patients who were irradiated.[97] Recently, a number of investigators have suggested that vulvar and vaginal cancers occuring after irradiation for cervical cancer are radiation-induced malignancies.[97-104]

Support for this contention comes from the observation that recurrences of cervical cancer usually develop within the first 2 to 3 years following completion of primary radiation therapy.[102,103] Less than 2 percent of recurrent cervical carcinoma will present after the tenth year following radiation treatment.[105,106] Therefore, it is likely that tumors occurring after 10 or more years are new primary malignancies, and may be related to prior radiation. This is further supported pathologically by the absence of recurrent cervical carcinoma in cases of subsequent vaginal cancer.[101] Murrad et al.[97] have determined that vaginal neoplasms which occurred 5 or more years after cervical irradiation had pathological features of primary vaginal cancer. They felt that such cases should be regarded as new primary malignancies which could possibly be induced by radiation.

Forty-one cases of vaginal cancer[20,101-104,107] and 11 cases of vulvar cancer[20,37,40,58,108] have been reported after irradiation for primary cervical cancer. The latency period was noted for 21 of the 41 cases of vaginal cancer and for six of the 11 cases of vulvar cancer. Mean latency time until occurrence of vaginal cancer was 14.1 years (range 6–26 years) (Table 13-1). Eighteen of these 21 cases had latency periods of 10 or more years. The latency periods reported prior to vulvar cancer were one and one-half years (two cases), greater than 5 years (two cases), 7 years and 14 years. Initial radiation therapy was in the standard range utilizing both internal and external radiation sources. Estimated absorbed vaginal radiation dose was reported by Edwards et al.,[107] and ranged from 5,300–9,700 rads.

The most common presenting symptoms of secondary vulvar or vaginal cancer were bleeding, pain, weight loss, thigh and leg edema, and an unusual vaginal discharge.[99,103] Geisler[103] reported that abnormal urograms were present in two-thirds of patients at time of diagnosis. One-half of these patients had partial ureteral obstruction and one-half had loss of function of one kidney. Treatment results with either surgery or radiation have been variable. Survival of less than 1 year with or without radiation has been reported by Geisler.[103] However, others have noted longer survival times after therapy with either surgery or radiation.[102,104]

Up to 41 percent of secondary tumors associated with cervical cancer are reported to occur after cervical irradiation.[96] Pride and Buchler[104] reported that 13.6 percent of all primary vaginal cancer occurred after cervical irradiation. The biologic behavior as well as survival for vaginal cancer is thought to be the same whether the tumor occurs naturally or after prior irradiation.[97] Since survival is improved by early diagnosis[109] close lifetime follow-up is necessary after cervical irradiation.[95,97,102,104] Geisler[103] has suggested periodic radiographic evaluation of the urinary tract for long term survivors. Whether this would be of additional benefit to careful, complete pelvic and cytologic examinations remains to be determined.

CERVICAL CANCER AND LEUKEMIA:

In contrast to earlier reports that showed a three-fold excess of leukemia in patients given low dose irradiation to the pelvis for benign gynecologic conditions,[1,110–112] an increased risk of leukemia has not been established with therapeutic doses of radiation in the treatment of gynecologic tumors. In fact, it would appear that in all studies reported to date (Table 13-2), there is no increased risk of leukemia after cervical irradiation.[59,113–117] However, one major criticism has been the short duration of follow-up time in many of these studies.[21]

In a review by Smith,[21] follow-up was considered to be incomplete in the initial report of Simon et al.[113] In Dickson's report, the median duration of follow-up was less than 10 years.[59] Zippin et al.[114] in their study of 497 patients had follow-up time ranging from 17–36 years and an increased incidence of leukemia was not observed. From an international study involving 31 institutions, both the early report[116] and the most recent 10-year update[117] covering more than 31,000 patients followed for more than 140,000 women years, failed to show an increase of leukemia. The observed and expected frequencies did not differ significantly among patients treated with external irradiation, internal implantation, or both.[117] However, follow-up was less than 10 years in 79 percent of these women, and it is possible that longer follow-up may show an increased incidence of leukemia.[117]

The observed lack of radiation induced leukemia after treatment of cervical cancer may involve a number of different factors. Analysis of port size and tissue dose may partially explain the absence of increased risk. Irradiation field size in cervical cancer patients is localized to the pelvis, whereas most associations of radiation with

Table 13-2. Risk for Leukemia After Radiation Therapy of Cervical Carcinoma

| Reference | Number of Patients | Leukemia Cases | | Relative Risk |
		Observed	Expected	
59	923	2	1.1	1.8
113	71,582	16	16	1.0
114	497	0	1	—
115	7,835	12	9.5	1.3
116	29,493	4	5.5	0.7
117	31,219	15	16.4	0.9

leukemia have been after total body exposure.[118–123] The anatomic distribution of dose may be important if large doses to small volumes of tissue cause cell sterilization rather than cell transformation. Myeloid cell death may occur within the localized port to such an extent that sublethal events are not manifested in this population. This can result in a decrease in leukemia incidence as seen in animal experiments[124] and after treatment of cervical cancer. As also observed in animal experiments, the level at which tumorigenicity increases, plateaus and decreases appears to be a function of the tissue irradiated.[125,126] Rodent myeloid leukemia increases and plateaus with doses less than 500 rads total, whereas kidney neoplasms do not begin to rise until doses are well over 500 rads and peak near 1500 rads.[125] Therefore, it is possible to have two tissues within a radiation port so that the dose given kills most of one tissue and is tumorigenic to the other tissue.

While cell sterilization may occur in pelvic bone marrow that is heavily exposed, it is difficult to explain why intermediate and presumably nonsterilizing doses of radiation to bone marrow outside the pelvic region were not leukemogenic.[117] If the length of the latent period for older persons is directly related to age at exposure, as suggested by studies of atomic bomb survivors,[121] then the older cervical cancer patients may not yet have been followed long enough for an increased risk of leukemia to become apparent. Also, women appear to be at lower risk of radiation induced leukemia and this sex difference in susceptibility may contribute somewhat to protection from leukemia.[6] Continued observation of treated patients should resolve these questions in the future.

SECONDARY TUMORS OCCURRING AFTER RADIATION FOR UTERINE AND OVARIAN CANCERS

A total of 26 cases of secondary tumors have been reported after therapy of uterine and ovarian cancers.[34,39,52,61,87,104,127–132] Primary treatment consisted of external radiation in all six cases of ovarian cancer with alkylating agents used in two cases. Both internal implantation and external radiation were initially used for 15 of 20 cases of uterine cancer, with external radiation administered to the remainder. Latency times until occurrence of secondary tumors was available in 24 of 26 cases. The largest group consisted of 13 colorectal cancers with a mean latency time of 15.2 years (range 5–30 years). Latency times for other specific secondary tumors were also similar to the latency times observed after radiation therapy of cervical cancer. These included soft tissue sarcomas (4.5,7,10 years), bone sarcomas (4,21,23 years), mixed mesodermal tumor of the uterus (1.5,7,11 years) and vaginal cancer (16,40 years). Survival was less than 1 year for two cases of mixed mesodermal tumor and one case of bone sarcoma. Because of the small number of cases in this series, meaningful estimates of risk were not obtainable. However, others have reported a significant increase in risk for solid tumors after irradiation for ovarian cancer.[15] These included uterine cancer (O/E 56/12.4, relative risk 4.5, 95 percent confidence interval 3.4–5.9), colon cancer (O/E 33/17.0, relative risk 1.9, 95 percent confidence interval 1.3–2.7), bladder cancer (O/E 9/3.2, relative risk 2.8, 95 percent confidence interval 1.3–5.3) and lymphoma (O/E 6/2.2, relative risk 2.7, 95 percent confidence interval 1.0–

5.9). As with women irradiated for primary cervical cancer, the recommendation for close, lifelong follow-up should also apply to women irradiated for primary uterine or ovarian cancers.

ACUTE LEUKEMIA AFTER THERAPY WITH ALKYLATING AGENTS ALONE OR IN COMBINATION WITH RADIATION FOR OVARIAN CANCER

Post therapeutic acute leukemia was first reported after alkylating agent therapy for ovarian cancer.[133] Since then, information has become available about 80 additional cases of acute leukemia occurring after administration of alkylators alone or combined with radiation for primary ovarian cancer.[134–166] Although acute leukemia is also reported to develop after only radiation therapy for ovarian cancer,[151,167] this is a rare occurrence, and probably does not contribute to an excess of acute leukemia as observed after alkylating agent therapy.[161] This section will review the characteristics of 81 cases of acute leukemia that developed after prior administration of alkylating agents.

Alkylating agents given to patients with advanced ovarian cancer have produced both improved survival and quality of life when compared to patients receiving either radiation or no therapy.[145,168,169] As previously mentioned, the carcinogenic properties of these drugs probably relates to their ability to bind to DNA and induce chromosomal abberations. Such abberations are seen in a much higher proportion of therapy related leukemias than in spontaneously developing leukemias.[141]

In leukemia occuring after therapy of ovarian cancer, the most frequently used alkylating agent was melphalan (Table 13-3). Einhorn et al.[162] have shown that melphalan induced several types of cytogenetic alterations in the cells of patients developing leukemia after treatment of ovarian cancer. One type of damage lead to sister chromatid exchange which corrected within several months after discontinuation of therapy. A second alteration was that of chromosomal rearrangement, which could persist for several years and probably arose from the faulty repair of melphalan induced DNA damage. Thirdly, the frequency of DNA cross-links was found to be increased. The authors felt that any of these types of genetic alterations could initiate leukemogenesis.[162]

Table 13-3. Primary Alkylating Agent Used for Ovarian Cancer Prior to the Development of 81 Cases of Acute Leukemia

Drug	Number of Cases	Percentage of All Cases
Melphalan	40	49
Chlorambucil	16	20
Treosulfan	11	14
Thiotepa	7	9
Cyclophosphamide	4	5
Uracil Mustard	3	3
TOTAL	81	100

Overall, Einhorn et al.[162] found that there was a statistically significant number of chromosome or chromatid abberations in the cells of previously treated patients compared to control cells (p<0.02). A similar finding of abnormal chromosomes in five of six previously treated patients compared to four of 21 non-drug exposed patients was made by Andersen et al.[160] Pedersen-Bjergaard et al.[159] have reported that in therapy related leukemia the cytogenetic defect was missing B or C group chromosomes, and in all banded cases there were deletions of chromosomes 5 and/or 7, a pattern clearly different from de novo acute leukemia. Each of their five cases analyzed had these types of chromosomal abnormalities after treosulfan therapy for ovarian cancer. Others have also noted abnormal karyotypes in patients who developed acute non-lymphocytic leukemia after alkylating agent therapy.[143,147,151]

The clinical picture of acute nonlymphocytic leukemia (ANLL) subsequent to therapy for another neoplastic disease appears to be different from that of patients with spontaneous ANLL. Foucar et al.[150] have suggested that therapy related acute leukemia be considered a specific clinicopathologic entity. This entity is characterized by chemotherapy and/or radiation therapy which is followed by a long interval before a brief preleukemic period. After this, there is evolution into a panmyelosis which is marked by increasing myeloblast counts, progressive morphologic abnormalities, major chromosomal abberations, poor response to anti-leukemia therapy and a short survival.[150] Preisler et al.[141] have also reported that at the time of diagnosis of therapy related leukemia, patients have lower leukocyte counts and a less cellular bone marrow which contains a lower proportion of leukemic cells.

For the 81 patients in this series, the mean age at the time of diagnosis of ANLL was 53-years-old (range 27–72 years old). Melphalan was the most common drug administered prior to the development of acute leukemia. This was followed by chlorambucil, treosulfan, thiotepa, cyclophosphamide, and uracil mustard (Table 13-3). Fourteen of the 81 patients received more than one aklylating agent and 46 patients had also received prior radiation therapy.

The suggestion that an increased risk of leukemia was related to a high total dose of drug was initially made by Einhorn.[148] Since then, Green et al.[161] have defined a high total dose category of greater than 700 mg for melphalan and a high total dose category of greater than 2,000 mg for chlorambucil. As shown in Table 13-4, leukemic risk appeared to be related to total dose of drug. Seventy-five percent of patients who received melphalan and 86 percent of the patients who received chlorambucil were in the high total dose categories. In their discussion of drug dose and leukemic risk, Greene et al.[161] noted that ANLL was not observed in treatment protocols in which a low total dose of melphalan was administered. For treosulfan therapy, Pedersen-Bjergarrd et al.[157] also found that the risk of ANLL appeared to be related to a high total dose of drug. In their experience, all eight patients who developed ANLL received greater than 100 grams of treosulfan.[157,159]

The mean latency time from the diagnosis of ovarian cancer until the development of ANLL was 53.0 months (range 16–118 months) for all patients. For patients treated with alkylating agents only, mean latency time was 57.4 months (range 16–96 months). After combined modality therapy, mean latency time was 48.9 months (range 16–18 months). Three of the four cases of ANLL that developed within 2 years after the diagnosis of ovarian cancer occurred in the combined modality group.

Table 13-4. Total Dose of Alkylating Agents for Ovarian Cancer Prior to the Development of Acute Leukemia

Drug	Number of Patients	Range of Total Dose (mg)
Thiotepa	4	150–840
Chlorambucil	1	1,000
Chlorambucil	6	2,000–7,740
Melphalan	5	310–680
Melphalan	15	710–3,120
Treosulfan	8	126–413 gm

Table 13-5. Morphologic Type of Leukemia Occurring After Therapy for Ovarian Cancer

Type of Leukemia	Number of Patients	Percentage
Myeloblastic	51	63
Myelomonocytic	16	20
Erythroleukemia	7	9
Undifferentiated	5	6
Monocytic	1	1
Plasma Cell	1	1
TOTAL	81	100

A preleukemic cytopenia consisting of unexplained anemia, leukopenia and/or thrombocytopenia was found in 83 percent of the cases. The duration of the preluekemic period ranged between 1 to 12 months prior to the diagnosis of acute leukemia. Acute myeloblastic leukemia was the most common morphological classification of the leukemias that developed after therapy of ovarian cancer (Table 13-5). The percentages of the morphologic types of leukemia occurring after ovarian cancer were similar to the percentages of the morphologic types of therapy related leukemias occurring after other tumors.[151] Mean survival after the diagnosis of leukemia was 3.6 months (range 0.5–18 months). Historically, there has been poor response to therapy and short survival of secondary leukemias occurring after ovarian cancer[148,151,157,161] and other primary tumors.[150,160,170–172] Preisler et al.[151] have suggested that the limited survival after therapy for secondary leukemia is due to the complications of prolonged bone marrow hypocellularity rather than leukemic drug resistance. Additionally, most patients with therapy related leukemia have been found to have chromosomal abnormalities, a feature which is prognostically poor for de novo ANLL.[173–175]

Using high dose cytarabine therapy, Preisler et al.[176] have recently reported a high response rate with eight of eleven complete remissions for secondary leukemia. They noted that six of seven patients who achieved a complete remission had abnormal chromosomes. With high dose cytarabine therapy it was suggested that chromosomal abnormalities may not continue to be a poor prognostic factor.[176] Therapeutic success with high dose cytarabine therapy of secondary leukemia has also been reported by Vaughn et al.[164] In four cases of ANLL occurring after therapy for ovarian cancer, there were two complete remissions.[164,165] In one of these cases, patient death was due to progressive ovarian cancer with leukemia in complete remission.[165]

At the time of diagnosis of acute leukemia, 71 percent of the patients were without clinical and/or pathological evidence of ovarian cancer. Since it is not possible to state at which point in treatment a cytotoxic drug becomes leukemogenic, it is important to determine when chemotherapy can be reasonably discontinued in patients without altering their prognosis. The second-look operation has provided the basis for determining response to prior therapy and need for additional treatment.[177-179] Smith and Rutledge reported a 5-year survival for 17 of 23 patients in whom chemotherapy was discontinued after a negative second look procedure.[180] A negative second look procedure has since become an indication to stop chemotherapy.[181] Because the occurrence of therapy related ANLL is rare with less than 1 year of therapy,[140] a second-look operation done after 10–18 months of treatment may aid in reducing the risk of secondary leukemia. Effective, new combinations of chemotherapy which include reduced amounts of alkylating agents may also lessen the risk of subsequent leukemia.

A cocarcinogenic effect between radiation and alkylating agents has been demonstrated in animal studies.[182,183] Although the majority of patients developing leukemia had combined modality therapy of ovarian cancer, their risk for leukemia has not been found to be significantly greater than after the administration of chemotherapy alone.[161] In studies of therapy related leukemia after Hodgkin's disease, there have been conflicting results as to whether an increased leukemogenic risk is due to combined modality therapy[184,185] or only chemotherapy.[186]

A number of facts suggest that the excess of ANLL occurring after treatment of ovarian cancer is primarily due to the administration of alkylating agents and not due to the natural history of ovarian cancer, selection bias, or chance. In an analysis of 4,324 women with ovarian cancer not treated with alkylating agents and recorded in the End Results Program, Reimer et al.[145] did not find an increased risk of leukemia. In the study of Pederson-Bjergaard et al.[157], half of the patients who developed leukemia had early stage ovarian cancer, also suggesting that alkylating agents and not the natural history of the disease were responsible for the occurrence of leukemia. Follow-up for women not exposed to alkylating agents has been longer and without an increased incidence of leukemia.[161] This further supports the etiologic role of alkylating agents for the development of leukemia.

Statistically, a number of studies have shown a marked increase in leukemogenic risk after use of alkylating agents. In their analysis of 5,455 women treated for ovarian cancer, overall, Reimer et al.[140] found ANLL to occur 21 times greater than expected (O/E 15/1.62, relative risk 9.95 percent, confidence interval 5.2–15.3). When treated for longer than 2 years after the diagnosis of ovarian cancer, the relative risk increased to 171, 95 percent confidence interval 88.5–299.5, when compared to historical controls. ANLL occurred in 0.3 percent of all patients treated in this study. For patients surviving 10 or more years, it was projected that 5 to 10 percent of these patients would develop ANLL. In their series of 553 patients treated with treosulfan, Pedersen-Bjergaard et al.[157] found an increased risk of leukemia (O/E 7/0.04, relative risk 175). They estimated that in the group of women surviving longer than 5 years,

7.6 ± 3.0 percent would develop leukemia. Similarly, Greene et al.[161] have reported increased risk of leukemia (O/E 12/0.18, relative risk 67, 95 percent confidence interval 34–116). They calculated that after 7 years from diagnosis, there would be a 9.6 ± 3.3 percent cumulative risk of leukemia in women treated with alkylating agents. The data from Einhorn et al.[162] have also suggested leukemogenic risk due to melphalan. They calculated that in patients who received greater than 300 mg of melphalan, the incidence of ANLL was 950 times higher than in the total female population. In patients who received 800 mg or more of melphalan, the calculated risk rose to 3600 times higher than the risk for the total female population.

In contrast, only the study of Kagan et al.[129] has suggested no significant increase in leukemogenic risk after therapy for ovarian cancer (O/E 1.0/0.12, relative risk 8.27, 95 percent confidence interval 0.18–39.5). However, their conclusion might be considered premature in lieu of the short duration of follow-up for most of their patients.

Despite the apparent risk of ANLL after chemotherapy for ovarian cancer, the overall survival curve for ovarian cancer may be only slightly affected.[157] In patients with ovarian cancer, the potential risk of ANLL should not be a deterrent to the administration of alkylating agents.[161] It is clear that the low possibility of a later leukemic death is preferable to an earlier death due to ovarian cancer. New treatment regimens that optimize primary therapy while minimizing potential late risks still need to be developed.[7]

ACUTE LEUKEMIA AFTER THERAPY FOR UTERINE CANCER

There are twenty cases of acute leukemia developing after therapy for uterine or fallopian tube cancer.[141,146,151,159,167,187–189] These cases have occurred after radiation, alkylating agents, and combined modality therapy. There is insufficient information to determine if excess ANLL has occurred after treatment of uterine cancer. It would appear, however, that the pattern of risk would be determined by the primary mode of therapy. For patients treated with radiation therapy, probably little excess leukemia would be expected as observed after radiation therapy of cervical and ovarian cancer. If alkylating agents were used, probably a slight increase in leukemic risk would exist. The clinical characteristics of cases of ANLL developing in this setting would probably be similar to cases of ANLL occurring after treatment of ovarian cancer. This has been observed in the cases reported by Morrison[186] and Reimer et al.[187] The recommendation that the potential risk of ANLL should not act as a deterrent to effective primary therapy should also apply to uterine cancer.

SUMMARY

The actual incidence of second tumors occurring after primary therapy for gynecological cancer is probably underreported. This problem is not addressed in several recent standard texts of radiation oncology or gynecologic oncology. Also lacking is a central location to which these cases can be reported.

It is of obvious importance to determine the iatrogenic risk of new malignancies so that new forms of therapy can be designed to lessen this complication. There appear to be certain subsets of patients whose clinical response to therapy may predict an increased risk of tumor. This is suggested in patients who develop colorectal cancer. Also, certain forms of therapy may make the later diagnosis of cancer more difficult, as has been noted for secondary uterine cancer. Only with more comprehensive reporting and analysis of these cases can such problems be addressed.

Finally, the long latency times that can separate treatment and secondary cancer should not be permitted to provide a false sense of security for either patient or treating physician. Adequate, periodic follow-up must be continued indefinitely for all patients previously treated for cancer.

REFERENCES

1. Hutchinson GB: Late neoplastic changes following medical irradiation. Radiol 105:645, 1972.
2. Chabner BA: Second neoplasm—A complication of cancer chemotherapy N Engl J Med 297:213, 1977.
3. Harris CC: A delayed complication of cancer therapy—cancer. J Natl Cancer Inst 63:275, 1979.
4. Shellabarger CJ: Radiation carcinogenesis: laboratory studies. Cancer 37:1090, 1976.
5. Mole RH: Late effects of radiation: Carcinogenesis. Br Med Bull 29:78, 1973.
6. Boice JD: Cancer following medical irradiation. Cancer 47:1081, 1981.
7. Messerschmidt GL, Hoover R, Young RC: Gynecologic cancer treatment: Risk factors for therapeutically induced neoplasia. Cancer 48:442, 1981.
8. Loveless A: Genetic and Allied Effects of Alkylating agents. London, Butterworths, 1966.
9. Farber E: Chemical carcinogenesis. N Engl J Med 305:1379, 1981.
10. Harris CC: The carcinogenicity of anticancer drugs: A hazard in man. Cancer 37:1014, 1976.
11. Miller EC, Miller JA: Mechanisms of chemical carcinogenesis. Cancer 47:1055, 1981.
12. Makuch R, Simon R: Recommendations for the analysis of the effect of treatment on the development of second malignancies. Cancer 44:250, 1979.
13. Schottenfeld D, Berg J: Incidence of multiple primary cancer. IV. Cancers of the female breast and genital organs. J Natl Cancer Inst 46:161, 1971.
14. Moertel CG: Multiple primary neoplasms-historical perspectives. Cancer 40:1786, 1977.
15. Reimer RR, Hoover R, Fraumeni JF Jr., et al: Second primary neoplasms following ovarian cancer. J Natl Cancer Inst 61:1195, 1978.
16. Newell CR, Krementz ET, Roberts TD. Excess occurrences of cancer of the oral cavity, lung, and bladder following cancer of the cervix. Cancer 36:2155, 1975.
17. Kapp DS, Fischer D, Grady KJ: Radiation induced tumors in patients subject to radiation therapy for pelvic neoplasms. Long Term Normal Tissue Effects of Cancer Treatment, April 13–15, 1981 Bethesda, Md (abs).
18. Schoenberg BS, Greenberg RA, Eisenberg H: Occurrence of certain multiple primary cancers in females. J Natl Cancer Inst 43:15, 1969.
19. Arneson AN, Schellhas HF: Multiple primary cancers in patients treated for carcinoma of the cervix. Am J Obstet Gynecol 106:1155, 1970.
20. Palmer JP, Spratt DW: Pelvic carcinoma following irradiation for benign gynecological disease. Am J Obst Gynecol 72:497, 1956.

21. Smith PG: Leukemia and other cancers following radiation treatment of pelvic disease. Cancer 39:1901, 1977.

22. Buchler D: Multiple primaries and gynecologic malignancies. Am J Obstet Gynecol 123:376, 1975.

23. Jacox, HW, Major G, Baker MR: Multiple heteromorphologic malignant tumors of the uterus. Radiology 32:51, 1939.

24. Fernandez-Colmeiro J: Le cancer primitif de l'uterus apres guerison par radiotherapie d'un antre cancer du même organe. Presse Med 57:565, 1949.

25. Zuspan FP: Development of endometrial carcinoma subsequent to irradiation for carcinoma of the cervix. Am J Obstet Gynecol 69:59, 1955.

26. Novak ER, Woodruff JD: Postirradiation malignancies of the pelvic organs. Am J Obstet Gynecol 77:667, 1957.

27. Page WG, Barnes L: Endometrial adenocarcinoma eleven years after pelvic irradiation for cervical epidermoid carcinoma. Am J Obstet Gynecol 75:175, 1958.

28. Krupp PJ, Sternberg WH, Clark WH, et al: Malignant mixed mullerian neoplasms (mixed mesodermal tumors). Am J Obstet Gynecol 81:959, 1961.

29. Mills DC: Endometrial cancer in patients previously irradiated for cervical cancer. Obstet Gynecol 22:280, 1963.

30. Edwards DL, Sterling LN, Keller RH, et al: Mixed heterologous mesenchymal sarcomas (mixed mesodermal sarcomas) of the uterus. Am J Obstet Gynecol 85:1002, 1963.

31. O'Connor KJ: Mixed mesodermal tumors of the body of the uterus following irradiation therapy for carcinoma of the cervix. J Obstet Gynecol Brit Commonwealth 71:281, 1964.

32. Norris HJ, Taylor HB: Postirradiation sarcomas of the uterus. Obstet Gynecol 11:102, 1981.

33. Thomas WO, Harris HH, Enden JA: Postirradiation malignant neoplasms of the uterine fundus. Am J Obstet Gynecol 104:209, 1969.

34. Chuang JT, VanVelden JJ, Graham JB: Carcinosarcoma and mixed mesodermal tumor of the uterine corpus. Obstet Gynecol 35:769, 1970.

35. Morton RF, Villasanta U: New cancers arising in 1563 patients with carcinoma of the cervix treated by irradiation. Am J Obstet Gynecol 115:462, 1973.

36. Kielbinska S, Tarlowska L, Fraczek O: Studies of mortality and health status in women cured of cancer of the cervix uteri. Cancer 32:245, 1973.

37. Fehr PE, Prem KA: Malignancy of the uterine corpus following irradiation therapy for squamous cell carcinoma of the cervix. Am J Obstet Gynecol 119:685, 1974.

38. Seydel GH: The risk of tumor induction in man following medical irradiation for malignant neoplasm. Cancer 35:1641, 1975.

39. Mindell ER, Shah NK, Webster JH: Postradiation sarcoma of bone and soft tissues. Orthop Clin N Am 8:821, 1977.

40. Czesnin K, Wronkowski Z: Second malignancies of the irradiated area in patients treated for uterine cervix cancer. Gynecol Oncol 6:309, 1978.

41. Varela-Duran J, Nochomovitz LE, Prem KA, et al: Postirradiation mixed mullerian tumors of the uterus. Cancer 45:1625, 1980.

42. Toongsuwan S, Suvonnakote T, Varthananusara C: Endometrial carcinoma following irradiation for cervical cancer: A case report. J Med Assoc Thailand 63:421, 1980.

43. Kwon TH, Prempree T, Tang CK, et al: Adenocarcinoma of the uterine corpus following irradiation for cervical carcinoma. Gynecol Oncol 11:102, 1981.

44. Corscaden JA, Fertig JW, Gusberg SB: Carcinoma subsequent to the radiotherapeutic menopause. Am J Obstet Gynecol 51:1, 1946.

45. Smith FR, Bowden L: Cancer of the corpus uteri following radiation therapy for benign uterine lesions. Am J Roentgenol 59:796, 1948.

46. Speert H, Peightal TC: Malignant tumors of the uterine fundus subsequent to irradiation for benign pelvic conditions. Am J Obstet Gynecol 57:261, 1949.

47. Hunter RM, Ladwich HV, Motly JF: The use of radium in the treatment of benign lesions of the uterus: A critical twenty year survey. Am J Obstet Gynecol 67:121, 1954.

48. Stander RW: Irradiation castration. A follow-up study of results in benign pelvic disease. Obstet Gynecol 10:223, 1957.

49. Afonso JF: Mixed mesodermal tumors of the uterus. West J Med 120:17, 1974.

50. Williamson ED, Christopherson WM: Malignant mixed mullerian tumors of the uterus. Cancer 29:585, 1972.

51. Rubin P, Ryplansky A, Dutton A: Incidence of pelvic malignancies following irradiation for benign gynecologic conditions. Am J Roentgenol 85:503, 1961.

52. Black, WC, Ackerman LV: Carcinoma of the large intestines as a late complication of pelvic radiotherapy. Clin Radiol 16:278, 1965.

53. Slaughter DP, Southwick HW: Mucosal carcinomas as a result of irradiation. Arch Surg 74:420, 1957.

54. Smith JC: Carcinoma of the rectum following irradiation of carcinoma of the cervix. Proc Roy Soc Med 5:701, 1962.

55. Quan SH: Factitial proctitis due to irradiation for cancer of the cervix uteri. Surg Obstet Gynecol 126:70, 1968.

56. Decosse JJ, Rhodes RJ, Wentz WB, et al: Late results of radium treatment of carcinoma of the cervix. Clin Radiol 23:528, 1972.

57. Localio A, Stone A, Friedman M: Surgical aspects of radiation enteritis. Surg Gynecol Obstet 6:1163, 1969.

58. MacMahon CE, Rowe JW: Rectal reaction following radiation therapy of cervical carcinoma. Ann Surg 173:264, 1971.

59. Dickson RJ: Late results of radium treatment of carcinoma of the cervix. Clin Radiol 23:528, 1972.

60. Bhagabati JN, Zaman N: Carcinoma of the sigmoid colon occurring after radiation therapy for carcinoma of the cervix. Ind J Med Sci 27:143, 1973.

61. Castro EB, Rosen PP, Quan SHQ: Carcinoma of large intestine in patients irradiated for carcinoma of cervix and uterus. Cancer 31:45, 1973.

62. Mortenson E, Nilsson T, Vesterhangae S: Treatment of intestinal injuries following irradiation. Dis Colon Rectum 17:638, 1974.

63. Qizilbash AH: Radiation-induced carcinoma of the rectum. Arch Pathol 98:118, 1974.

64. Greenwald R, Barkin JS, Hensley GT, et al: Cancer of the colon as a late sequella of pelvic irradiation. Am J Gastroenterol 69:196, 1978.

65. O'Connor TW, Rombeau JL, Levine HS, et al: Late development of colorectal cancer subsequent to pelvic irradiation. Dis Colon Rectum 22:123, 1979.

66. Kumar PP, Newland JR: Radiation oncogenesis. J Natl Med Assoc 72:687, 1980.

67. Martins A, Sternberg SS, Attiyeh FF: Radiation-induced carcinoma of the rectum. Dis Colon Rectum 23:572, 1980.

68. Shumsuddin AK, Elias GE: Malignant and premalignant changes after radiation therapy. Arch Pathol Lab Med 105:150, 1981.

69. Thar TL, Millin RR, Daly JW: Radiation treatment of carcinoma of the cervix. Semin Oncol 9:299, 1982.

70. Buie LA, Malmgren GE: Factitial proctitis. Trans Am Proctol Soc 29:80, 1930.

71. Wiernik G: Changes in the villous pattern of the human jejunum associated with heavy radiation damage. Gut 7:149, 1966.

72. Localio SA, Pachter HL, Gouge TH: The radiation-injured bowel. Surg Annual 11:181, 1979.

73. Cahan WG, Woodward HQ, Higinbothan NL, et al: Sarcoma arising in irradiated bone. Report of eleven cases. Cancer 1:3, 1948.

74. Arlen M, Higinbothan NL, Huvos AG, et al: Radiation-induced sarcoma of bone. Cancer 28:1087, 1971.
75. Weatherby RP, Dahlin DC, Ivins JC: Postradiation sarcoma of bone. Mayo Clin Proc 56:294, 1981.
76. Cade S: Radiation-induced cancer in man. Br J Radiol 30:393, 1957.
77. Bloch C: Postradiation osteogenic sarcoma: Report of a case and review of the literature. Am J Roentgenol 87:1157, 1962.
78. Phillips TI, Sheline GE: Bone sarcomas following radiation therapy. Radiol 81:992, 1963.
79. Brezina K: Ueber eine Beobachtung von osteonekrove und malignem Tumor nach gynekologischer Roentgenbestrahlung. Krebsartz, 20:265, 1965.
80. Steiner GC: Postradiation sarcoma of the bone. Cancer 18:603, 1975.
81. Castro L, Choi SH, Sheehan FR: Radiation-induced bone sarcomas. Am J Roentgenol 100:924, 1967.
82. Ianca I, Dobrscu G, Timofte D, et al: Sarcoma induced by radiotherapy. Oncol Radiol 8:443, 1970.
83. Fehr PE, Prem KA: Postirradiation sarcoma of the pelvic girdle following therapy for squamous cell carcinoma of the cervix. Am J Obstet Gynecol 116:192, 1973.
84. McSwain B, Whitehead W, Bennett L: Angiosarcoma: Report of three cases of postmastectomy lymphangiosarcoma and one of hemangiosarcoma. South Med J 66:102, 1973.
85. Rushforth GF: Osteosarcoma of the pelvic following radiotherapy for carcinoma of the cervix. Br J Radiol 47:149, 1974.
86. Babrock TL, Powell DH, Bothwell RS: Radiation-induced peritoneal mesothelioma. J Surg Oncol 8:369, 1976.
87. Kim JH, Chu FC, Woodard HQ, et al: Radiation-induced soft tissue and bone sarcoma. Radiol 129:501, 1978.
88. Tountas A, Fornaisien VL, Harwood AR, et al: Postirradiation sarcoma of bone. Cancer 43:182, 1979.
89. Chung CK, Struker JA, Cohen C, et al: Malignant mesechymoma developing 6 years after radical hysterectomy and postoperative radiotherapy for cervical carcinoma. Gynecol Oncol 12:367, 1981.
90. Pinkston JA, Sekine I: Postirradiation sarcoma (malignant fibrous histiocytoma) following cervical cancer. Cancer 49:434, 1982.
91. Dalinka MD, Ediken J, Kinkelstein JB: Complications of radiation therapy: adult bone. Semin Roentgenol 9:29, 1974.
92. McIntyre D, Pointon RCS: Vessical neoplasms occurring after radiation for treatment for carcinoma of the uterine cervix. J Roy Coll Surg Edin 16:141, 1971.
93. Duncan RE, Bennett DW, Evans AT, et al: Radiation-induced bladder tumors. J Urol 118:43, 1977.
94. Kennedy DR: Radiation-induced bladder cancer. Brit J Urol 53:74, 1981 (abst).
95. Kanbout AI, Klionsky B, Murphey AI: Carcinoma of the vagina following cervical cancer. Cancer 34:1838, 1974.
96. Buchler D: Multiple primaries and gynecologic malignancies. Am J Obstet Gynecol 123:376, 1975.
97. Murad TM, Durant JR, Maddox WA, et al: The pathologic behavior of primary vaginal carcinoma and its relationship to cervical cancer. Cancer 35:787, 1975.
98. Lee RA, Symmonds RE: Recurrent carcinoma in situ of the vagina in patients previously treated for in situ carcinoma of the cervix. Obstet Gynecol 48:61, 1976.
99. Latour JPA, Fraser WD: The problem of late local recurrence of carcinoma of the cervix. Can J Surg 4:5, 1961.

100. Geelhoed GW, Henson DE, Taylor PT, et al: Carcinoma in situ of the vagina following treatment for carcinoma of the cervix: A distinctive clinical entity. Am J Obstet Gynecol 124:510, 1976.

101. Koss LG, Melamed MR, Daniel WW: In situ epidermoid carcinoma of the cervix and vagina following radiotherapy for cervical cancer. Cancer 14:353, 1961.

102. Hynes JF: Cancer of cervix uteri, late local recurrence or late radiation cancer. Del Med J 35:1, 1963.

103. Geisler HE: Carcinoma of the cervix or vagina 10 or more years after therapy: recurrence or new primary? J Ind State Med Assoc 67:711, 1974.

104. Pride GL, Buchler DA: Carcinoma of the vagina 10 or more years following irradiation therapy. Am J Obstet Gynecol 127:513, 1977.

105. Graham JB, Sotto LSJ, Paloncek FP: Persistent and recurrent cancer of the cervix, in carcinoma of the cervix. Philadelphia, W.B. Saunders Company, 1962, pp. 447–449.

106. Van Herik M, Decker DG, Lee RA: Late recurrence in carcinoma of the cervix. Am J Obstet Gynecol 108:1183, 1970.

107. Edwards MC: Carcinoma of the vagina following treatment of carcinoma of the cervix with radiation therapy. J Ark Med Soc 64:46, 1967.

108. Woodruff DJ, Hildebrandt EE: Carcinoma in situ of the vulva. Obstet Gynecol 12:414, 1958.

109. Perez CA, Arneson AN, Galakatus A, et al: Malignant tumors of the vagina. Cancer 31:36, 1973.

110. Alderson MR, Jackson JM: Longterm follow-up of patients with menorrhagia treated by irradiation. Brit J Radiol 44:295, 1971.

111. Doll R, Smith PG: The long-term effects of x-irradiation in patients treated for metropathia haemorrhagica. Brit J Radiol 41:362, 1968.

112. Smith PG, Doll R: Late effects of x-irradiation in patients treated for metropathia haemorrhagica. Brit J Radiol 49:224, 1976.

113. Simon N, Brucer M, Hayes R: Radiation and leukemia in carcinoma of the cervix. Radiol 74:905, 1960.

114. Zippin C, Bailar JC, Kohn HI, et al: Radiation therapy for cervical cancer: late effects on life span and leukemia incidence. Cancer 28:937, 1971.

115. Wagoner JK: Leukemia and other malignancies following radiation therapy for gynecological disease. Unpublished Doctoral Thesis, Harvard School of Public Health, Boston, 1970.

116. Hutchison GB: Leukemia in patients with cancer of the cervix uteri treated with radiation: a report covering the first 5 years of an international study. J Natl Cancer Inst 40:951, 1968.

117. Boice JD, Hutchison GB: Leukemia in women following radiotherapy for cervical cancer. Ten year followup of an international study. J Natl Cancer Inst 65:115, 1980.

118. March HC: Leukemia in radiologists. Radiol 43:275, 1944.

119. March HC: Leukemia in radiologists in a 20 year period. Am J Med Sci 225:202, 1950.

120. Folley JH, Borges W, Yamawaki T: Incidence of leukemia in survivors of the atomic bomb in Hiroshima and Nagasaki, Japan. Am J Med 13:311, 1952.

121. Ichimani M, Ishimora T, Belsky JL: Incidence of leukemia in atomic bomb survivors belonging to a fixed cohort in Hiroshima and Nagasaki 1950–71. Radiation dose, years after exposure, age at exposure, and type of leukemia. Japan Radiat Res (Tokyo), 19:262, 1978.

122. Court-Brown WSM, Doll R: Mortality from cancer and other causes after radiotherapy for ankylosing spondylitis. Brit Med J 2:1327, 1965.

123. Lyn JL, Klauble MR, Gardner JW, et al: Childhood leukemia associated with fallout from nuclear testing. N Engl J Med 300:397, 1979.

124. Major IR, Mole RH: Myeloid leukemia in x-ray irradiated CBA mice. Nature 272:455, 1978.

125. A report of the United Nations Scientific Committee on the effects of atomic radiation; ionizing radiation: Levels and effects Vol II: Effects 379, 1972.

126. United Nations Scientific Committee on the effects of atomic radiation. Sources and effects of ionizing radiation. Publ E771x1, New York, United Nations, 1977.

127. Chekharina EA, Aseer LV, Christova NM: Rhabdomyoblastoma of the anterior abdominal wall developing after irradiation. Vopr Onkol 13:100, 1967.

128. Gudgeon DH: Mixed mesodermal tumor of the uterus occurring after radiotherapy. Proc Roy Soc Med 61:1281, 1968.

129. Kagan AR, Ryoo MC, Tawa K, et al: Secondary neoplasms in treated ovarian cancer. Gynecol Oncol 13:356, 1982.

130. Sadore AM, Block M, Rossof AH, et al: Radiation carcinogenesis in man: New primary neoplasms in fields of prior therapeutic radiation. Cancer 48:1139, 1981.

131. Park HH, Komorowski R: Hemangiosarcoma of the abdominal wall following irradiation therapy of endometrial carcinoma. Am J Clin Pathol 66:810, 1976.

132. Inada S, Vanai S, Yamasaki R, et al: A light and electron microscopic study of a case of radiation-induced malignant giant cell tumor of the soft tissue. J Dermatol 6:47, 1979.

133. Sypkens Smith CG, Meyler L: Acute myeloid leukemia after treatment with cytostatic agents. Lancet 2:670, 1970.

134. Allen WSA: Acute myeloid leukaemia after treatment with cytostatic agents. Lancet 2:775, 1970.

135. Kaslow RA, Wisch N, Glass JL: Acute leukemia following cytotoxic chemotherapy. JAMA 219:75, 1972.

136. Greenspan EM, Tung BG: Acute myeloblastic leukemia after cure of ovarian cancer. JAMA 235:418, 1974.

137. Hague T, Luther C, Faguet G, et al: Chemotherapy-associated acute myelogenous leukemia and ovarian carcinoma. Am J Med Sci 272:225, 1976.

138. Sortel G, Jafan K, Lash AF, et al: Acute leukemia in advanced ovarian carcinoma after treatment with alkylating agents. Obstet Gynecol 47 (suppl):675, 1976.

139. Khandekar JD, Kurtides ES, Stalzer RC: Acute erythroleukemia complicating prolonged chemotherapy for ovarian cancer. Arch Int Med 137:355, 1977.

140. Reimer RR, Hoover R, Fraumeni JF, et al: Acute leukemia after alkylating agent therapy of ovarian cancer. N Engl J Med 297:177, 1977.

141. Preisler HD, Lyman GH: Acute myelogenous leukemia subsequent to therapy for a different neoplasm: Clinical features and response to therapy. Am J Hematol 3:209, 1977.

142. Blythe JC: Acute leukemia after melphalan treatment for ovarian carcinoma. J Med Assoc Ala 56:42, 1977.

143. Buskard NA, Boyes DA, Grossman L: Plasma cell leukemia following treatment with radiotherapy and melphalan. Can Med Assoc J 117:788, 1977.

144. Masterson BJ, Snyder TE: Second primary malignancies in patients with ovarian carcinoma treated with radiation and chemotherapy. J Kan Med Soc 78:283, 1977.

145. Young RC, Chabner BA, Hubbard SP, et al: Advanced ovarian adenocarcinoma. A prospective clinical trial of melphalan (L-PAM) versus combination chemotherapy. N Engl J Med 299:1261, 1978.

146. Morrison J, Yon JL: Acute leukemia following chlorambucil therapy of advanced ovarian and fallopian tube carcinoma. Gynecol Oncol 6:115, 1978.

147. Kapadia SB, Krause JR: Ovarian carcinoma terminating in acute nonlymphocytic leukemia following alkylating agent therapy. Cancer 41:1676, 1978.
148. Einhorn N: Acute leukemia after chemotherapy (Melphalan). Cancer 41:444, 1978.
149. Shetty MR, Freel R: Therapy-linked leukemia: A case report. Gynecol Oncol 7:264, 1979.
150. Foucar K, McKenna RW, Bloomfield CB, et al: Therapy-related leukemia. Cancer 43:1285, 1979.
151. Zarrabi MH, Rosner F: Acute myeloblastic leukemia following treatment for nonhematologic cancer: Report of 19 cases and review of the literature. Am J Hematol 7:357, 1976.
152. Klaassen DJ, Boyes DA, Gerulath A, et al: Preliminary report of a clinical trial of the treatment of patients with advanced stage III and IV ovarian cancer with melphalan, 5-fluorouracil, and methotrexate in combination and sequentially: A study of the clinical trials group of the National Cancer Institute of Canada. Cancer Treat Rep 63:289, 1979.
153. Ortonne JP, Thirolet J, Coiffet CJ: Pyoderma gangrenosum, cystadeno-carcinome ovarien traites par melphalan et leucemie aigue myeloblastique. Ann Dermatol Venereol (Paris) 106:251, 1979.
154. Bezwoda WR, Hofman K, Bothwell TH, et al: Bone marrow damage due to melphalan and other cytostatic agents. S Afr Med J 58:479, 1980.
155. Haas JS, Mansfield CM, Hartman GV, et al: Results of radiation therapy in the treatment of epithelial carcinoma of the ovary. Cancer 46:1950, 1980.
156. Potish R, Adcock L, Brooker D, et al: Sequential surgery, radiation therapy and alkeran in the management of epithelial carcinoma of the ovary. Cancer 45:2754, 1980.
157. Pedersen-Bjergaard J, Nissen NI, Sorenson HM, et al: Acute nonlymphocytic leukemia in patients with ovarian carcinoma following long term treatment with treosulfan (Dihydroxybusulfan). Cancer 45:19, 1980.
158. Kapadia SB, Krause JR, Ellis LD, et al: Induced acute non-lymphocytic leukemia following long term chemotherapy. Cancer 45:1315, 1980.
159. Pedersen-Bjergaad J, Philip P, Mortensen BT, et al: Acute nonlymphocytic leukemia, preleukemia and acute myeloproliferative syndrome secondary to treatment of other malignant diseases. Clinical and cytogenetic characteristics and results of in vitro culture of bone marrow and HLA typing. Blood 57:712, 1981.
160. Anderson RL, Bagby GC, Richert BK, et al: Therapy-related preleukemic syndrome. Cancer 47:1867, 1981.
161. Greene MH, Boice JD, Greer BE, et al: Acute nonlymphocytic leukemia after therapy with alkylating agents for ovarian cancer. N Engl J Med 307:1416, 1982.
162. Einhorn N, Eklund G, Franzen S, et al: Late side effects of chemotherapy in ovarian cancer. Cancer 49:2234, 1981.
163. Einhorn N: Personal communication, 1982.
164. Gerad H, Wiernik PH: Unpublished data.
165. Vaughan WP, Karp JE, Burke PJ: Effective chemotherapy of acute myelocytic leukemia occurring after alkylating agent therapy or radiation therapy for prior malignancy. J Clin Oncol 1983 (in press).
166. Vaughan WP: personal communication, 1983.
167. Faber M. Borum K: Leukemia and a malignant tumor in the same patient. Br J Haematol 8:313, 1962.
168. Smith JP, Rutledge FN, Delclos L: Postoperative treatment of early cancer of the ovary: a random trial between postoperative irradiation and chemotherapy. Natl Cancer Inst Monogr 42:149, 1975.
169. DeVita VT Jr, Wasserman TH, Young RC: Perspectives on research in gynecologic oncology: treatment protocols. Cancer 38:509, 1976.

170. Cadman EC, Capizzi RL, Bertino JR: Acute nonlymphocytic leukemia. Cancer 40:1280, 1977.

171. Rosner F, Grunwald H: Multiple myeloma terminating in acute leukemia. Am J Med 57:927, 1974.

172. Rosner F, Grunwald H: Hodgkin's disease and acute leukemia. Am J Med 58:339, 1975.

173. Trujillo JM, Cork A, Hart J, et al: Clinical implications of aneuploid cytogenetic profiles in adult acute leukemia. Cancer 33:824, 1974.

174. Sakurai M, Sandberg AA: Chromosomes and causation of human cancer and leukemia. XI. Correlation of karyotypes with clinical features of acute myeloblastic leukemia. Cancer 37:285, 1976.

175. Golomb HM, Vardiman JW, Rowley JD, et al: Correlation of clinical findings with quinacrine-banded chromosomes in 90 adults with acute nonlymphocytic leukemia. N Eng J Med 299:613, 1978.

176. Preisler HD, Early AP, Raza A, et al: Therapy of secondary acute nonlymphocytic leukemia with cytarabine. N Engl J Med 308:21, 1983.

177. Wallach RC, Kabakow B, Jerez E, et al: The importance of second-look surgical procedures in the staging and treatment of ovarian carcinoma. Semin Oncol 2:243, 1975.

178. Smith JP, Delgrado G, Rutledge F: Second-look operation in ovarian carcinoma. Cancer 38:1438, 1976.

179. Piver MS, Shashikant BL, Barlow JJ, et al: Second-look laparoscopy prior to proposed second-look laparotomy. Obstet Gynecol 55:571, 1980.

180. Smith JP, Rutledge FN: Chemotherapy in advanced ovarian cancer. Natl Cancer Inst Mnogr 42:105, 1975.

181. Katz ME, Schwartz PE, Kapp DS, et al: Epithelial carcinoma of the ovary: current strategies. Ann Int Med 95:98, 1981.

182. Shellabarger CJ: Effect of 3-methylcholanthrene and radiation, given singly or combined, on rat mammary carcinogenesis. J Natl Cancer Inst 38:73, 1967.

183. Vogel HH Jr, Zaldivar R: Cocarcinogenesis: the interaction of chemical and physical agents. Radiat Res 47:644, 1971.

184. Borum K: Increasing frequency of acute myeloid leukemia complicating Hodgkin's disease: a review. Cancer 46:1247, 1980.

185. Coleman CN, Williams CJ, Flint A, et al: Hematologic neoplasia in patients treated for Hodgkin's disease. N Eng J Med 297:1249, 1977.

186. Pedersen-Bjergaard J, Larsen SO: Incidence of acute nonlymphocytic leukemia, preleukemia, and acute myeloproliferative syndrome up to 10 years after treatment of Hodgkin's disease. N Eng J Med 307:965, 1982.

187. Wagner K: Roentgen and leukaemie. Krebsarzt 8:330, 1953.

188. Mayeda K, Yamamoto S, Miyata H, et al: A study on the incidence of leukemia developing after therapeutic irradiation of cancer of breast and uterus. Nippon Acta Radiol 28:1122, 1968.

189. Reimer RR, Groppe CW: Acute nonlymphocytic leukemia. Ann Int Med 90:989, 1979 (letter).

190. Smith JP, Rutledge FN: Chemotherapy in advanced ovarian cancer. Natl Cancer Inst Monogr 42:105, 1975.

Index

Page numbers followed by f represent figures; page numbers followed by t represent tables

Actinomycin D
  in gestational trophoblastic disease, 257f, 257-258
  in ovarian cancer, 161
Acute nonlymphocytic leukemia
  morphologic type, 289t, 289
  after ovarian cancer therapy, 287-291
  after uterine cancer therapy, 291
Adenomatous hyperplasia, of the uterus, and estrogen intake, 205
Adjuvant adriamycin, trial in high-risk early endometrial carcinoma, 239, 240f
Adjuvant chemotherapy, and cervical carcinoma,
  111-112
Adnexal spread, endometrial carcinoma and, 223,
  223t
Adriamycin
  adjuvant, trials in, 239, 240f
  endometrial carcinoma and, 235, 236t, 237t
  in ovarian cancer, 161
Adriamycin-based combination chemotherapy, 103t,
  103-104
Adriamycin-Cytoxan, in treatment of ovarian cancer, 147
Adriamycin-methotrexate combination chemotherapy, 104t, 104
After loading technique, in radiotherapy, 73
Alkylating agents
  in treatment of ovarian cancer, 157-160
    development of acute leukemia and, 287-291
    response rates for, 157-159, 158t, 159t
    suboptimal, 145-146, 146t
  secondary cancer following use of, 276
American Cancer Society, cervical cytology guide-
  lines of, 49
Angiography, for gynecologic neoplasms, 22-23
Antibodies
  for herpes simplex virus type-2, prevalence rates
    of, 38-39
  for infectious agents in cervical intraepithelial
    neoplasia, 42-43
Antiestrogen, in ovarian cancer treatment, 163, 188
Antigen, in ovarian cancer, 125-126
  carcinoembryonic, 123
  tissue polypeptide, 124
Antimetabolites, in treatment of ovarian cancer, 160

Arteriography, and hepatic metastases, 22
198 Au, in treatment of ovarian cancer, 141-142

Barium studies, metastasis and, 5
B1-glycoprotein (SP1), hCG and, 269
Bilateral salpingo-oophorectomy, 57
Biopsy
  in metastatic cervical cancer, 24f, 25f, 25
  radiation therapy for cervical cancer and, 85
  in second look operation in ovarian cancer, 134-
    135
Births, number related to endometrial carcinoma,
  204-205
Bleomycin-mitomycin combination chemotherapy,
  for cervical cancer, 98t, 98-100
Blood pressure, endometrial cancer and, 209
Bone sarcoma, postirradiation, 281-283
Brachytherapy, for cervical cancer, 69-70
Brain metastases
  in choriocarcinoma, 15, 16f
  in trophoblastic disease, 261-262, 261f
Bulky endocervical carcinomas, management con-
  troversies and, 81-82

Carcinoembryonic antigen, and therapeutic response in ovarian cancer, 123
Cervical carcinoma, 11, 12f
  bulky endocervical carcinomas and, 81-82
  chemotherapy for, see Chemotherapy; Systemic
    chemotherapy
  and circumcision, 37
  CT scan of, 16, 17f
  descriptive epidemiology of, 34-36
  evolution of treatment for, 69-71
  factors influencing prognosis of, 69t
  FIGO classification of, 52-53, 52t
  genesis of, 43-44
  and herpes simplex virus type-2, 37-42
  histology and pathogenesis of, 33-34
  and infectious agents, 42-43
  metastastic, percutaneous lymph node biopsy of,
    24f, 25f, 25
  microinvasive, see Microinvasive cervical cancer
  para-aortic irradiation and, see Para-aortic irra-
    diation

301

Cervical carcinoma *(continued)*
  patterns of infiltration in, 68-69
  radical hysterectomy for, 54-56
  radiotherapeutics for, *see* Radiotherapy
  recurrent, 58-60
  risk factors in, 36-37
    and secondary tumors, 277-278
    latency times for, 279t
    staging laparotomy for, 53-54
    surgery vs. radiation for, 80-81
Cervical cone biopsy, 51-52
  confirming diagnosis by colposcopy, 50, 50t
Cervical cytology
  abnormal findings evaluation in, 51f
  diagnostic procedures in, 50-52
  false negative rate in, 47-48
  ovarian cancer and, 122
  sampling techniques in, 48
  screening frequency in, 49-50
Cervical intraepithelial neoplasia, 33-34
  cervical cone biopsy and, 51-52
  and herpes simplex virus type-2, 37-42
  and other infectious agents, 42-43
Cervix
  carcinoma of, *see* Cervical carcinoma
  involvement in endometrial carcinoma, 223-224,
    223t
  irradiation of, *see* Irradiation, cervical
CHAMOCA regimen, in high risk gestational tro-
    phoblastic disease, 263, 263t, 264t, 264, 265t
Chemo-immunotherapy, in treatment of suboptimal
    ovarian cancer, 149-150
Chemotherapy
  for cervical carcinoma, 94
    adjuvant, 111-112
    combined with radiotherapy, 110-111
    future directions in, 112-113
    regional, 107-109
    systemic, *see* Systemic chemotherapy
    transcatheter intraarterial, 28f, 28
  combination, *see* Combination chemotherapy
  for endometrial carcinoma, 235-238
  hydatidiform mole and, 254
  infusional, and radiation, 87-88
  in metastatic gestational trophoblastic disease,
    259f, 259-260, 263-266
  for ovarian cancer, 143, 145
    in advanced cases, 155-156, 157t
    effect of residual disease on response to, 178t
    high dose, 185-186
    intraperitoneal, *see* Intraperitoneal chemother-
      apy
    prognostic factors in, 166-169
    and second look operation, 133, 134
  secondary cancer following, 276
  sequential, 264-265, 265t
Chest radiography, for pulmonary mestastasis, 4f,
    5
Chlamydia trachomatis, dysplasia and, 42, 43
Chlorambucil, endometrial carcinoma and, 237t
Choriocarcinoma
  angiography of, 23f

metastatic
  in the brain, 15, 16f, 261, 261f
  in the liver, 262f, 262
  pulmonary, 4f, 5
Cigarette smoking, as factor in endometrial cancer,
    210
Circumcision, cervical carcinoma and, 37
Cis-diammine dichloroplatimun (CDDP)
  percutaneous nephrostomy and, 26
  transcatheter management and, 26, 28
Cisplatin
  in cervical cancer, 96-97, 97t
  in combination chemotherapy, 100-103, 165t, 165-
    166
  in ovarian cancer, 162, 165t, 165-166
Cis-platinum
  endometrial carcinoma and, 236t, 236-237
  in gestational trophoblastic disease, 265-266
  high dosage in ovarian cancer, 185t, 185-186
Colorectal cancer, following pelvic irradiation, 279-
    281
Colposcopy, 50-51, 50t
Combination chemotherapy
  for endometrial carcinoma, 237-238, 237t, 238t
  in ovarian cancer, 163, 164t, 165t
    with cisplatin, 165t, 165-166
    without cisplatin, 164t, 164-165
  in suboptimal ovarian cancer, 146-149, 149t
Combined radiotherapy-chemotherapy
  for cervical cancer, 110-111
  for early endometrial carcinoma, 229
  in ovarian cancer, 190t, 190
Computed tomography, for gynecologic neo-
    plasms, 11, 13-17, 18f, 19f
Computerized axial tomography, in ovarian cancer,
    127
Curettage, hydatidiform mole and, 253-254
Cyclophosphamide, endometrial carcinoma and, 237,
    238t
Cyst, ovarian, 6f, 11, 14f
Cystadenocarcinoma, of the ovary
  bilateral, 11, 13f
  psammomatous calcification of, 2f
  with solid nodules, 7f
Cystadenoma, in pelvis, 6f
Cytarabine therapy, for secondary leukemia, 289-
    290
Cytologic tumor grade, in ovarian cancer, 166f, 166-
    167
  vs. survival, 167, 168f, 169
Cytology
  cervical, *see* Cervical cytology
  for ovarian cancer, 122-123
Cytomegalovirus, dysplasia and, 42, 43
Cytoxan-Adriamycin-cisplatin, survival vs. clinical
    response in ovarian cancer, 156, 157t

Diabetes mellitus, as risk factor in endometrial can-
    cer, 209
Dianhydrogalactitol, in ovarian cancer, 162
Diethylstilbesterol, in ovarian cancer, 163

Dilatation, hydatidiform mole and, 253-254
Directed biopsy, in colposcopic evaluation, 51
Disseminated disease, in advanced or recurrent endometrial carcinoma, 232-239
Dose requirements, in radiation therapy, 75
Dose-response relationship, in cervical carcinoma, 72
Dose-response relationship, in cervical carcinoma, 72
Dosimetry, of intracavitary irradiation, 73-74
  in the Manchester system, 74
  of the M.D. Anderson system, 74-75
Double alkylator therapy, for ovarian cancer, 157-158

Early invasive carcinoma, radiotherapeutic management of, 76-78
4'-epi-doxorubicin, in ovarian cancer, 162
Epipodophyllotoxins, in ovarian cancer, 161
Endocervical curettage, in abnormal cervical cytology evaluation, 51f, 51
Endometrial carcinoma, 10f, 10
  clinical characteristics of, 216, 216t
  diagnosis of, 219-220
  future directions in, 210
    for advanced or recurrent disease, 240
    for high-risk early disease, 239, 240f
  incidence of
    age and, 202, 203f
    nationality and, 201, 202t
    race and, 202t, 202-203, 203f
    and time, 200, 200t, 201t, 201
  management of
    in advanced or recurrent disease stage, 230-239
    in early disease stage, 226-230
  pathology of, 216-217, 217t, 218t
  pretreatment evaluation of
    pathologic factors in, 221-225
    patient evaluation and, 225-226, 226t
    prognostic factors in, 220-221, 220t
  recurrence of, 219, 228t
  risk factors in
    hormonal, 203-209, *see also* Estrogen; Menopausal estrogen; Progestogen
    non-hormonal, 209-210
  spread patterns of, 218-219, 218t, 219t
Endometrium, carcinoma of, *see* Endometrial carcinoma
Enzymes, in ovarian tumors, 125
Estrogen, in endometrial carcinoma
  postmenopausal use, 201
  as risk factor
    endogenous, 203-204
    exogenous, 205-208, *see also* Menopausal estrogen
Exenteration, pelvic, recurrent ovarian cancer and, 132-133
External beam therapy, 71-72
  combined with intracavitary irradiation, 75
External radiation therapy, for cervical cancer, 70-71

Extrauterine spread, endometrial carcinoma and, 223-224
Extravascular infiltration, of actinomycin D, 257f, 258

Factitial proctitis, 280
Fibrosis, postirradiation, in cervical carcinoma, 21f, 21
Field size, in radiation therapy, 75-76
FIGO, *see* International Federation of Gynecologists
Fletcher-Suit's Tandem, in intracavitary irradiation, 72-73, 73f
5-fluorouracil
  endometrial carcinoma and, 237, 237t, 238t
  ovarian cancer and, 160
Fractionation, 88

Gall bladder disease, endometrial cancer and, 209-210
Genetics, as factor in endometrial cancer, 210
Germ cell malignancies, of the ovary, 169-170
Gestational trophoblastic disease, 249-250
  intensive treatment multiple agent, 264, 265t
  metastatic
    high risk, 260-266
    low risk, 258-260
    moderate risk, 260
  non-metastatic, 256-258
Glucose tolerance, abnormal, as risk factor in endometrial cancer, 209
Gonadotropin, *see* Human chorionic gonadotropin
Gynecologic Oncology Group
  and chemotherapy
    combination study in ovarian cancer, 147, 148
    new agents tested, 96t, 97
  and microinvasive cervical cancer, 56
  protocol 34 schema, 239, 240f
  and single agent cisplastin trials, 96-97, 97t
  and treatment of borderline ovarian cancer, 140

HCG, *see* Human chorionic gonadotropin
Heavy particle radiation, 87
Hematometra, 10f, 10-11
Hepatic artery embolization, for metastatic choriocarcinoma, 27f
Herpes simplex virus
  type-2
    experimental studies on, 37-38
    role in cervical cancer, 43-44
    seroepidemiologic studies on, 38-40
    virologic studies on, 40-41
  types of, 37
Hexamethylmelamine
  endometrial carcinoma and, 235-236, 236t
  in ovarian cancer, 161
Histocompatibility specificities (HLA), 256
Histologic grade, in endometrial carcinoma, 217, 217t, 218t, 221, 221t, 222t, 224t
  and receptor status correlations, 234t, 235
HLH, *see* Human luteinizing hormone

Hormone therapy
for disseminated endometrial carcinoma, 233-235
for ovarian cancer, 162-163, 187-188
see also Estrogen; Progestogen; Individual hormone names
Human chorionic gonadotropin (HCG)
in gestational trophoblastic disease
measurement of, 266-269
metastatic, 258, 260, 264-265, 266
non-metastic, 256
and HLH, 267
in hydatidiform mole, 250
following molar evacuation, 255, 256
Human luteinizing hormone (HLH)
and HCG, 267
radioimmunoassay for, 267
Human tumor stem cell assay, and in vitro drug sensitivity testing, 191-192
Hybridization techniques, and herpes simplex virus type-2 DNA sequences, 41
Hydatidiform mole, 11, 12f
diagnosis of, 250, 251f, 252f, 253
post-molar follow-up practices in, 255-256
treatment of, 253-255
Hydroxyurea, and radiation therapy, 110, 110t
Hypoxic cell sensitizers, 87
Hysterectomy
hydatidiform mole and, 254
postradiation therapy, 57-58
radical, see Radical hysterectomy
standard, for invasive disease, 56-57
Hysterography, for gynecologic neoplasms, 23
Hysterotomy, hydatidiform mole and, 254

Immunofluorescence techniques, and herpes simplex virus type-2 antigens, 41
Immunotherapy, for ovarian cancer, 186-187
Infiltration, pattern characteristics in cervical carcinoma, 68-69
Infusional chemotherapy, and radiation, 87-88
International Federation of Gynecologists
classification of cervical carcinoma, 52-53, 52t
clinical staging system for endometrial carcinoma, 218t, 219t
Intra-arterial therapy, in chemotherapy for cervical carcinoma, 107-108, 108t
Intracavitary irradiation
after loading techniques in, 73
combined with external beam therapy, 75
dosimetry of, 73-75
in management of early invasive carcinoma of the cervix, 76-77
combined with parametrial external irradiation, 77, 77f
plus whole pelvic irradiation, 77-78
typical system in, 72-73, 73f
Intraperitoneal chemotherapy, for ovarian cancer
past and present techniques compared, 180
phase I and II trials in, 181-185
Tenchkoff catheter in, 180-181, 181t

Intraperitoneal human ovarian antitumor serum, 189-190
In vitro drug sensitivity testing, in ovarian cancer, 190-192
Irradiation
bone and soft tissue sarcoma following, 281-283
cervical
leukemia following, 285-286, 285t
ovarian cancer following, 283-284
secondary cancer following, 275-276, 276-277, 279t
urological cancer following, 283
uterine cancer following, 278
vaginal and vulvar cancer following, 284-285
intracavitary, see Intracavitary irradiation
para-aortic, see Para-aortic irradiation
pelvic
colorectal cancer following, 279-281
plus intracavitary irradiation, 77-78

Kavorkian cervical biopsy, in second look operation, 135

Lactic dehydrogenase, in ovarian cancer, 123
Laparoscopy, in ovarian cancer, 126-127
Laparotomy
as complication in radiation therapy for cervical cancer, 85
second look, in ovarian cancer, 150-151
staging of, 53-54
Leiomyoma, of uterine corpus, 22
Leukemia
acute, see Acute nonlymphocytic leukemia
following cervical irradiation, 285-286, 285t
Liver metastases
from ovarian neoplasm, 11
in trophoblastic disease, 262f, 262
Locoregional disease, in advanced or recurrent endometrial carcinoma, 231-232, 232t
Lymphadenectomy
cervical cancer and, 53-54
as complication in radiation therapy for, 85
postradiation therapy and, 57-58
standard hysterectomy and, 56
Lymphangiography, for gynecologic neoplasms, 17-22
Lymphatic network, in cervical carcinoma, 68
Lymph nodes
involvement in endometrial carcinoma, 222t, 223, 224t
metastases from cervical carcinoma, 16-17, 19f
percutaneous biopsy of, 24f, 25f, 25
see also Lymphatic network

m-AMSA, in ovarian cancer, 162
Manchester system
dosimetry in, 74
in radium brachytherapy, 70
M.D. Anderson system, dosimetry in, 74-75
Medroxyprogesterone, endometrial carcinoma and, 237, 237t, 238t

Megavoltage irradiation, 71
Melphalen
  endometrial carcinoma and, 237, 237t, 238t
  in ovarian cancer, development of acute leuke-
    mia and, 287-288, 287t, 289t
  prior to second look laparotomy, 159t, 159-160
Menopausal estrogen, and risk of endometrial can-
    cer, 205, 206t
  and periodic interruption of use, 207-208
  time factors associated with, 205, 207
  type and dose of, 207
6-Mercaptopurine, in ovarian cancer, 162
Metastasis
  to brain, *see* Brain metastases
  to liver, *see* Liver metastases
  mesenteric, 8f
  nodal
    from cervical carcinoma, 16, 19f
    from ovarian carcinoma, 18, 20f
  omental, CT of, 11, 14f
  patterns in ovarian cancer, 179
  pulmonary, 4f, 5
  submucosal and serosal, from ovarian carci-
    noma, 3f
Methotrexate, in ovarian cancer, 160
Methrotrexate/Citrovorum protocol, in gestational
    trophoblastic disease, 257t, 258
Microinvasive cervical cancer, 56
  radiotherapeutic management for, 76
  standard hysterectomy for, 56-57
Mitomycin-Vincristine (Oncovin)-Bleomycin regi-
    men, for cervical cancer, 99-100, 99t
  with cisplatin, 100-101, 101t
Molar pregnancy, hydatidiform mole and, 250, 252f,
    253
Monoclonal antibody
  hCG and, 269
  in immunotherapy, 187
Mullerian inhibiting substance, in immunotherapy,
    187
Multimodality treatment, of advanced ovarian can-
    cer, 188-190
Mycoplasma pneumoniae, and dysplasia, 42
Myometrial invasion, endometrial carcinoma and,
    221-222, 222t, 224t

National Cancer Institute, and ovarian cancer stud-
    ies
  and combination chemotherapy, 147-148
  trials of intraperitoneal chemotherapy, 181-185
Neutrons, 87
Nitrosoureas, and ovarian cancer, 160
Nuclear magnetic resonance, in ovarian cancer, 127

Omental cake, 8f
Omental metastasis, CT of, 11, 14f
Oral contraceptives, endometrial cancer and, 208,
    208t, 209
Osteosarcoma, 282
Ovarian cancer
  acute leukemia following therapy for, 287-291

antigens associated with, *see* Antigens
borderline or low potential malignancy, 140-141
chemotherapy for, *see* Alkylating agents; Chem-
    otherapy; Combination chemotherapy; Indi-
    vidual drug names
clinical manifestations of, 120-121
cytology and, 122
diagnosis of, 121-122
enzymes associated with, 125
etiology of, 178-179
following cervical irradiation, 283-284
hormone therapy for, 187-188
immunotherapy for, 186-187
incidence of, 119-120
investigative techniques in, 126-127
multimodality treatment for, 188-189
patterns of metastases in, 179
potential role for investigational therapies for,
    192t, 193-194
recurrent, radical surgery for, 131-133
with resectable disease, therapy for, 141-144
secondary tumors after radiation for, 286-287
and second look operation, 133-135
small residual disease and, 144-145
staging of, 127-128
suboptimal, therapy for, 145-150
surgical management of, 128-131
true, options for, 141
tumor markers in, 123-124
Ovarian germ cell malignancies, 169-170
Ovarian function, radical hysterectomy and, 55-56
Ovary
  angiography of, 22
  carcinoma of, *see* Ovarian cancer
  computed tomography of, 11, 13f, 14f
  conventional radiography of, 2f, 3f, 4-5
  lymphangiography of, 17-18, 20f
  and transcatheter management, 26
  ultrasonography of, 6f, 7f, 7, 8f, 9

P-32, in treatment of ovarian cancer, 142-143, 144-
    145
Papillomavirus, dysplasia and, 43
Pap smear, ovarian cancer and, 122
  see also Cervical cytology
Para-aortic irradiation, in invasive cervical carci-
    noma, 82-83
  prophylatic, 84
  therapeutic, 83-84
Parametrial external irradiation, and intracavitary
    irradiation, in treatment of cervical cancer,
    77, 77f
Paris technique, in radium brachytherapy, 70
Pelvic examination, and ovarian cancer, 122
Pelvic exenteration
  recurrent ovarian cancer and, 132-133
  survival and operative mortality rates in, 58-60,
    59t
Pelvis
  and calcification within uterine fibroid, 3f, 5
  irradiation of, 77-78

Pelvis *(continued)*
    sagittal sonogram through, 6f
    and sarcoma of the uterus, 2f
    transverse sonogram of, 6f
Penile cancer, cervical carcinoma and, 37
Percutaneous biopsy, for gynecologic neoplasms,
    24f, 24-25, 25f
Percutaneous nephrostomy, for gynecologic malig-
    nancy, 26
Peritoneal cytology, endometrial carcinoma and,
    222t, 223
Pfannenstiel incision, in management of ovarian
    cancer, 129
Piperazinedione, endometrial carcinoma and, 236t,
    237
Piperazinidine, in ovarian cancer, 162
Pneumography, for gynecologic neoplasms, 24
Point A concept, in Manchester system, 74
Polycystic ovary syndrome, and risk of endometrial
    carcinoma, 204
Postradiation therapy hysterectomy, 57-58
Prednimustine, in ovarian cancer treatment, 163
Pregnancy, molar, hydatidiform mole and, 250,
    252f, 253
Premenopausal women, endometrial carcinoma in,
    204
Proctocolitis, 280
Progestational agents, in treatment of endometrial
    carcinoma, 233-235
Progesterone, in ovarian cancer therapy, 162-163,
    187-188
Progestin, in treatment of endometrial carcinoma,
    233, 233t
    and receptor status correlation, 234t, 235
Progestogen, lack of, endometrial cancer and
    endogenous, 204-205
    exogenous, 208-209
Punch biopsy, 51, 52

Radiation
    exposure to, as risk factor in endometrial cancer,
    210
    fractionation of, 88
    heavy particle, 87
    infusional chemotherapy and, 87-88
Radiation therapy, *see* Radiotherapy
Radical hysterectomy
    for cervical carcinoma, 54-56
    as complication in radiation therapy, 85
Radical surgery, in recurrent ovarian cancer, 131-
    133
Radiography, conventional, for gynecologic neo-
    plasms, 4-6
Radioimmunoassay
    for hCG, 267-268
    for hLH, 267
Radioisotopes, in treatment of ovarian cancer with
    resectable disease, 141-143, 144-145
Radioreceptorassay, for hCG, 268
Radiosensitizers, in cervical cancer

Radiotherapeutics, *see* Radiotherapy
Radiotherapy
    alkylating agents and, 290
    for cervical cancer, 69-71
        combined with chemotherapy, 110-111
        complications in, 84-86
        management of, 76-78, 79t, 79-80
        vs. radical hysterectomy, 55-56
    concepts of, 71-76
    dose requirements in, 75
    for early endometrial carcinoma, 229, 230t
    and field size, 75-76
    future modalities for, 86-88
    hysterectomy following, 57-58
    management of, 77-80
        controversies in, 80-84
    for ovarian cancer, 143-144
    see also Intracavitary irradiation; Irradiation
Radium brachytherapy, development of, 69-70
Radium implants, radical hysterectomy and, 56
Recurrent cervical carcinoma, surgical management
    of, 58-60
Regan alkaline phosphatase isoenzyme, in ovarian
    cancer, 125
Residual tumor mass, vs. survival in ovarian can-
    cer, 167, 167f, 168f, 169
Retroperitoneal nodes, CT of, 11, 13f

Salpingo-oophorectomy, bilateral, 57
Sarcoma, bone and soft tissue, postirradiation, 281-
    283
Scalene node biopsy, surgical staging and, 54
Second look laparotomy, in ovarian cancer, 150-151
    alkylating agents and, 159-160, 159t
Second look operation
    acute leukemia and, 290
    in ovarian cancer, 133-135
Serum alpha fetoprotein, and therapeutic respone in
    ovarian cancer, 124
Sexual activity, and onset of cervical carcinoma, 36-
    37
Society of Gynecologic Oncologists (SGO), mi-
    croinvasive cervical cancer and, 56
Soft tissue sarcoma, postirradiation, 281-283
Southwest Oncology Group
    and mitomycin-vincristine-bleomycin trials, 99-
    100, 99t
    and multidrug cisplatin combination vs. single
    agent cisplatin trials, 101, 102t
Spirogermanium, in ovarian cancer, 162
Standard hysterectomy, for invasive disease, 56-57
Stockholm technique, in radium brachytherapy, 69-
    70
Supervoltage radiation therapy, 71
Swann-Ganz catheter, in management of ovarian
    cancer, 129
Systemic chemotherapy, for cervical carcinoma
    combination regimens in, 97-104
    randomized trials in, 105t, 105, 106t, 106-107
    single agents in, 95-97

Tamoxifen
in endometrial carcinoma therapy, 234, 235t
in ovarian cancer therapy, 163, 188
Tenchkoff catheter, in intraperitoneal chemotherapy for ovarian cancer, 180-181
complications of, 181t, 181
Teratoma, ovarian, 8f
Therapeutic ratio, 71
and external beam therapy, 71
Tissue polypeptide antigen, in ovarian cancer, 124
Transcatheter intraarterial chemotherapy, for cervical cancer, 28f, 28
Transcatheter management, for gynecologic malignancy, 26-28
Trichomonas vaginalis, and dysplasia, 42, 43
Trophoblastic disease, *see* Gestational trophoblastic disease
Trophoblastic neoplasms, of uterine corpus, 22, 23f
and transcatheter management, 26, 27f
Tumor excision, in ovarian cancer, 131
Tumor markers, in ovarian cancer, 123-124

Ultrasonography
in detection of ovarian cancer, 126
for gynecologic neoplasms, 7-15
Urological cancer, following irradiation for cervical cancer, 283
Uterine cancer
acute leukemia following therapy for, 291
secondary to cervical cancer, 277-278
secondary tumors after radiation for, 286-287
Uterine cervix
computed tomography of, 16-17, 17f, 18f, 19f
conventional radiography of, 5-6
lymphangiography of, 19f, 19-22, 21f

and transcatheter management, 26, 28f, 28
ultrasonography of, 11, 12f
Uterine corpus
angiography of, 22-23, 23f
computed tomography of, 15f, 15, 16f
conventional radiography of, 3f, 5
lymphangiography of, 18-19
and transcatheter management, 26, 27f
ultrasonography of, 9f, 9-11, 10f, 12f
Uterine fibroid, 9f
calcification within, 3f, 5
computed tomography of, 15f, 15

Vaginal cancer, following irradiation for cervical cancer, 284-285
Vascular invasion, endometrial carcinoma and, 223
Veneral disease, cervical carcinoma as, 36
Venography, ovarian, 22
Vesico-vaginal fistula, CT of, 16, 18f
Vinblastine, in ovarian cancer, 161
Vincas, in treatment of ovarian cancer, 161
Vincristine, in ovarian cancer, 161
Vindesine, in gestational trophoblastic disease, 266
Viral antigens, in herpes simplex virus type-2 infection, 40-41
Viral proteins, in herpes simplex virus type-2 infection, 40-41
VP-16
for drug-resistant choriocarcinoma, 264
endometrial carcinoma and, 236t, 237
Vulvar cancer, following cervical irradiation, 284-285

Walton Report, cytological screening and, 49

Yoshi 864, and ovarian cancer, 160